Respectful TREATMENT

Practical Handbook of Patient Care

Second Edition

Respectful TREATMENT

A Practical Handbook of Patient Care
Second Edition

Martin R. Lipp, M.D.

Associate Clinical Professor
Department of Psychiatry
University of California, San Francisco
San Francisco

Elsevier
New York • Amsterdam • Oxford

Elsevier Science Publishing Co., Inc.
52 Vanderbilt Avenue, New York, New York 10017

Sole distributors outside the United States and Canada:
Elsevier Science Publishers B.V.
P.O. Box 211, 1000 AE Amsterdam, The Netherlands

© 1986 by Elsevier Science Publishing Co., Inc.

This book has been registered with the Copyright Clearance Center, Inc. For further information please contact the Copyright Clearance Center, Inc., Salem Massachusetts.

Library of Congress Cataloging in Publication Data

Lipp, Martin R., 1940-
    Respectful treatment—a practical handbook of patient care.
    Rev. ed. of: Respectful treatment—the human side of medical care. c1977.
    Includes bibliographies and index.
    1. Medicine and psychology. 2. Physician and patient. 3. Humanistic psychology. I. Lipp, Martin R., 1940- Respectful treat—the human side of medical care. II. Title. [DNLM: 1. Mental Disorders. 2. Physician-Patient Relations. 3. Psychiatry. WM 100 L765r]
    R726.5.L56   1986   610.69′6   85-27422
    ISBN 0-444-01001-7

Current printing (Last digit):
10 9 8 7 6 5 4 3 2 1

Manufactured in the United States of America

to the memory of my grandparents, who taught me about respect; and of my parents, with whom I learned so much about illness

Contents

Preface

Never disregard a book because the author of it is a foolish fellow.
—Lord Melbourne

. . . I remain a black in a white world. . . . I never cared about acceptance as much as I cared about respect.
—Jackie Robinson

When the original edition of *Respectful Treatment* was published, it had the advantage of being one of a kind: the only contemporary handbook for the generalist that applied practical psychiatry to the general hospital setting. Since then, many other books have focused on the same territory, inevitably some good and some less so, but all of them (to my knowledge) written by psychiatrists wanting to help nonpsychiatric physicians with behavioral problems of medical practice.

In the interval, I have undergone my own evolution, and the new edition of *Respectful Treatment* reflects the changes of its author. Where earlier I was an academic, I am now a physician in the community. Instead of inpatients, I work with outpatients. Where formerly I worked as a consultation-liaison psychiatrist, I have for the past ten years worked exclusively as an emergency room physician and ambulatory care doctor, treating patients with myocardial infarctions, broken bones, bladder infections, and runny noses. I've had my emotional ups and downs, too, experiencing divorce, a couple of malpractice suits, and the predictable mid-life crisis.

Somewhat humbled by life's events, I now wish I knew as much about doctor-patient interaction as I thought I knew when I wrote the first edition. Further, my views on what is euphemistically known as "humanistic medicine" have also changed; whether for the better or not, I'll let you be the judge.

Over the past three-quarters of a century at the very least, there have been well-intentioned, spirited, solidly funded attempts to "humanize" medical care. The Phipps Pavilion and the first university department of psychiatry at Johns Hopkins were established in the expectation that psychological insights would be incorporated into medical practice and the doctor-patient relationship would change for the better. A tabulation of the time, money, anguish, and rhetoric devoted to similar efforts would fill the equivalent of several metropolitan phone books.

And yet, has it made a difference? I would be surprised if you could get more than a few percent of practitioners or patients to say that the emotional climate of the doctor-patient relationship is better now than at *any* time in the past. And how much, really, does it matter?

Take, on the one hand, a humanistically oriented physician, well intended and reasonably well trained, but often better at the interpersonal aspects of patient care than at the highly technical superscientific parts of the job (a suitable description of me at various stages of my medical career). On the other hand, take a physician more impressed with laboratory values and technical procedures and the latest research reports about *Bacillus fragilus,* someone who tends toward the arrogant and is insensitive and aloof in the bargain. Can you say that one or the other will obtain detectably superior results with the overwhelming majority of patients?

I gradually concluded that except for a few fuzzy percent, all the researchers in Rockville, Maryland, would be hard pressed to demonstrate any significant difference.

Despite *all* the rhetoric to the contrary, you can be an effective doc with a minimum of sensitivity, warmth, tenderness, and compassion. Where some doctors might seduce their patients into taking their meds, you can badger and bully yours, and the patients will or won't get well in the same proportion. You can put in an endotracheal tube or chest tube with empathy, or you can put it in with brusque disdain, and it won't make any difference to their PaO_2. The patients may attribute their improvement to your tender mercies or they may say angrily they got well despite them, but their clinical course may be otherwise identical.

So why bother writing a handbook on the psychological aspects of medical practice when much of the content may fairly be regarded as inconsequential in the clinical evolution of your patients' disease?

Ah, there's the nub of it: as a physician, you're often concerned not only with the patient's objective improvement, you're concerned about how the patient feels about that improvement and the relationship you share. You are concerned about colleagues and nurses and technicians and clerical staff, and whether they think you are a decent human being, as well as a competent pill pusher.

We're talking about more than mere image problems here. One gets tired of hearing from hospital and clinic administrators that one has botched another interaction with a patient. It spoils the working day to have patients or staff always angry or upset. And, on the positive side, there's a reassuring sense of mastery to be had when one can not only read an EKG, one can also read a patient in a potentially unpleasant situation and can operate on those readings to prevent potential disaster, not only in cardiac arrhythmias, but also in doctor-patient interaction.

The task of this handbook is to help you answer several questions: (1) In a given patient with a given medical disorder, how can I sort out the relative contributions of functional and organic components? (2) To the degree that a given disorder has a functional etiology, what can and should I do myself, and when should I call in a consultant? (3) When a patient of mine becomes a management problem, how do I figure out what to do about it?

In addition, I will discuss the changing nature of the doctor-patient relationship and the implications of these changes in clinical practice and in our own lives, a heady task indeed.

The information presented here mostly represents conventional wisdom accepted and promulgated by consultation psychiatrists all over the country. I have profited from the ideas of many such, and have referred the reader to many excellent sources in the bibliography at the end of each chapter. However, some ideas presented here are clearly my own. This is particularly true with my suggestions regarding psychiatric diagnosis, the alcoholic and psychotic patients, antidepressants, and psychotherapy. Where my views differ significantly from the conventional ones, I have clearly labeled them as being unconventional.

Several additional cautions are appropriate. Although I deal with numerous topics under separate headings, few can be dealt with clinically in such isolation. Treatment must be based on adequate evaluation, and the physician who consistently implements treatment while slighting evaluation may be satisfying his or her own need to treat rather than the patient's need to be treated.

Although the intent of this handbook is to make problem-solving suggestions available to those responsible for patient care, there is no substitute for listening to the patient. The wily consultant in every field knows that the quickest, easiest, surest route to clinical problem solving lies in giving the patient an opportunity to tell you what is going on within. Wherever possible, I have tried to be concise and pragmatic;

however, much of the person-oriented approach to patients relies not so much on data and tasks as on philosophy and understanding. I therefore sometimes have provided more detailed comments to clarify philosophic perspectives.

Though most of us strive to approach the patient as a human being rather than as an object, our actions don't always match our intent. The reasons are many. In part, we don't know how to do it. We have enough difficulty relating to family, friends, and colleagues as humanely as we would like, let alone patients. We cannot count on our mentors to teach us the mystical art because many don't know it themselves, having trained and thrived in academic programs with other priorities. But all of us—practitioners, teachers, students, hospital staff, patients—still have individual needs for respect, understanding, and consideration. If we can't help one another, all our lives are going to be a lot more aggravating; and none of us needs more aggravation than we have already.

This handbook offers factual information to bolster strength in dealing with such difficult clinical challenges, and perspective to help you bear the frustration and personal suffering when ideal solutions seem elusive. The only solution often will be to develop equanimity in facing the insoluble. *You* are your most important resource. To preserve yourself, to foster your own growth while serving the patient, to assist you in finding satisfaction in respectful patient care—that is the task to which this volume is dedicated.

A further word about respect: like Jackie Robinson, who felt alien in a predominantly white world, many of our patients feel alien in the medical environment we take for granted. They don't know the language; they don't fully comprehend the culture; they feel awkward, ignorant, powerless, and defensive—even separate from whether they are sick or well. All in all, it's not a setting designed to bring out the best in them. And frankly, most modern medical institutions—multi-doctor group practices, large clinics, and hospitals—are not ideally designed to bring out the best in us either. The time pressure, the disease-oriented focus, often the rotation system of traineeship, the sheer numbers of people involved with the patient, and the complexity of their interactions mitigate against it. The truth is that dealing with a suffering or hopeless or disfigured patient as one human being to another subjects health-care personnel to personal stress which, for many, is simply not worth the cost. Most of the problems discussed here cannot be solved in the way we would prefer. Many problems are products of our social and health-care systems themselves. They are difficulties that will linger or recur as long as we are involved with clinical medicine. Yet treating the patient with respect, and being ac-

corded respect in return, can make the process not only more endur-
able but even enjoyable.

The word *respect* can be defined variously, but definitions always
seem to me to be unsatisfactory. Each of us knows whether he or she is
being treated respectfully. I always address adult patients as "Sir" or
"Ma'am," a sometimes awkward remnant of my upbringing, but respect goes beyond mere words. Respect is an expression of understanding of other people, a recognition of their significance, an affirmation that what they say and do and think and experience matters to you
and that you care about what happens to them and how they feel about
it.

Your style of showing respect may differ from mine, but I write in
the hope that my experiences, practices, and opinions will be useful to
you, if only to stimulate you to develop and refine your own clinical
practices.

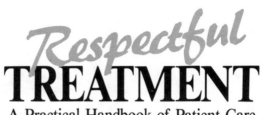

TREATMENT

A Practical Handbook of Patient Care

Second Edition

1

Problem Patients

Coincident self-interest is the mother of all alliances.
—Adapted from Henry Kissinger

If you're not part of the solution, you're part of the problem.
—Eldridge Cleaver

To be put off by the difficult or provocative or uncooperative patient is to fail to understand the nature of helplessness and the diversity of potentially adaptive responses to such feelings.
—Meyer Ben Feival

One of the areas in which traditional psychoanalytic teaching is weakest, I think, is in interpreting misbehavior in the doctor-patient relationship. The deficiency is a natural consequence of the psychoanalytic focus on psychopathology in the individual. We all can learn something by concentrating on individual misbehavior and trying to understand it in terms of the psychodynamic evaluation of a character structure, but we lose something, too: a broader understanding of the interactional and contextual source of problems. Besides, such retrospective explanations have little predictive value; virtually anyone is likely to become (or be perceived as) a problem patient if the conditions promote such behavior or perceptions. That is especially true for physicians and other knowledgeable health professionals. When *you,* for example, get sick and are hospitalized, how cooperative and charming are you likely to be when you are cared for by an assortment of inexperienced medical students, rushed house officers who haven't slept in 24 hours, and nurses who are overworked and underpaid? No fair guessing. You simply have to experience it before you can answer accurately.

Although certain behavioral patterns inevitably stress the doctor-patient relationship, such stress does not mean that either the patient or the doctor has a character disorder; both may do well in other situations. For example, take a chauvinistic, highly competent, proudly self-sufficient, physically active middle-aged man. Put him at absolute bed rest and have him cared for by hovering female relatives, female nurses, and female physicians, and a conflict is likely. It isn't useful to talk about the patient's "counter dependence related to early weaning and oedipal fears" or to characterize the female professionals as "acting out sublimated maternal nurturing fantasies" or "subjugating the male patient through castrating, controlling behavior." Few individuals appreciate being thought about in such terms. The fact is that the patient and care givers are mismatched, and his health care would proceed more amicably if he were looked after by a matter-of-fact and respectful male physician, with many clinical gray hairs, who emphasizes activity as tolerated and self-care whenever possible.

There is a tendency in medicine to think of "difficult" patients as crazy; their behavior, superficially, seems inexplicable on any other basis. There is also a tendency to use blame as a weapon of subjugation. The latter is rarely successful, and an accusatory approach adds stress to the relationship and increases the original problem.

The following situation is an example. You are a house officer and you have just presented a case to your attending. The patient is an intelligent but very edgy man in his fifties who complains of malaise and vague abdominal symptoms that don't fit neatly into any package. Initial studies reveal nothing abnormal except for some borderline liver-function tests and a barely palpable liver. After a vigorous discussion and considerable disagreement among the treatment team, the attending suggests that you should do a liver biopsy next. You go in to get the patient's consent, with the premonition that he may be hard to convince. Given that you first establish rapport with the patient and put the thoughts into your own words, which of the following statements are you likely to make?

1. "The next step in your evaluation is a liver biopsy."
2. "The wisest course now is to perform a liver biopsy."
3. "We need to biopsy your liver in order to maintain the standard of care we think is appropriate."
4. "If I were in your shoes, I would want to have a liver biopsy."
5. "The staff was divided, but the attending's judgment was that you should have a liver biopsy."
6. "We struggled with this decision, and now you may want to struggle with your own thoughts and feelings before acting on our advice."

Obviously there is no one right answer. Certainly many clinicians would lean toward the first two alternatives either as openers or as rejoinders if the patient questioned another approach. Alternatives 1 and 2 present the advice in a way that appears to be objective and tends to reduce patient noncompliance to the level of irrationality. The advantage of "objective" approaches is also a disadvantage because these alternatives ignore the fact that the decision is also based on the value systems of those most intimately involved, patient and doctors.

Alternatives 3 and 4 recognize that human beings are involved on at least one side of the negotiation and therefore facilitate a greater range of responses. Treatment of the patient's protopathic problem is no longer presented in a monolithic fashion, but rather as a function of the needs and values of the persons involved in the transaction. The advantages of this approach are again the same as the disadvantages: the patient can more easily question whether his or her needs are the same as the doctors', or say that he or she perceives the needs differently than does the doctor, or even ask for another opinion. The doctor who takes these middle approaches or their equivalents must be prepared to deal with such questions.

Alternative 5 recognizes the realities of the decision-making process. By divulging that the staff does not agree, Alternative 5 validates the patient's right to question. The attending's authority can be given great weight, or not, depending upon how the conversation proceeds.

Alternative 6 is the most open and honest, because it reflects both what happened, and what you expect the patient to do, namely struggle with the decision. Nonetheless, this approach is used rarely because of the qualities that also make it appealing. Many consider such openness and honesty unprofessional, antitherapeutic, and undermining of the patient's trust in the health-care giver. However, in many cases, openness and admission of subjective values may be useful.

With the preceding information as background, we now can discuss the whys and wherefores of who becomes a problem patient, and in what circumstances.

A problem patient is any patient who interferes with your work as you see it. Not every reader will view each type as a problem for himself or herself. Ask yourself these questions: (1) What are my expectations of myself in this situation? (2) To whom do I feel primary obligation? (Consultant? Family? Patient? Everyone?) (3) What are my expectations of the patient? (To shut up? To be compliant? To be appreciative?) (4) What are my perceptions of the ideal doctor-patient relationship? Where do I get my goodies? What kinds of behavior do I personally find most upsetting? (5) What are the patient's expectations of me, what sort of psychic rewards is he or she looking for, and what sorts of behavior does he or she find particularly exasperating in a physician?

If you view disease as one response of the organism to multiple stresses, the medical complaints represent *your* point of entry into a multiproblem system. In that sense, many patients probably are not functioning ideally even aside from the issue of illness. It's a wonder, then, that so many patients cooperate rather than pose problems for us who care for them.

Usually a patient *becomes* a problem when he or she *has* a problem to communicate to others.

It is most useful to learn to view problem behaviors as potentially multicausal. That is, problems may be related to the patient's personality style, disease process, or the hospital or clinic milieu. We always will want to attempt to measure medical components of behavior (i.e., those that are an expression of underlying disease or perhaps of drug side effects), and we will want to make allowances for the patient's baseline character, if we know the patient well enough to estimate realistically what that baseline might be. However, most problems have an interpersonal component, which makes the problem ours as well as the patient's. In this context, the most useful approach is, "How can we work this out together?"

What is a problem for you will depend on your perceptiveness, values, tolerance, and skill in understanding behavior as a symptom. Your tolerance may vary due to how much sleep you had the night before, and other demands being made on you currently. However, certain patterns emerge for most of us.

Your tolerance for diverse behavior in patients will depend on your tolerance for diversity in general. If character differences interest you, you may find the "types" discussed here to be among your more fascinating patients. All problem patients, after all, represent personalities we encounter in everyday life as neighbors and acquaintances, transplanted to a patient-care setting. To attempt to modify basic character structure in a patient is akin to trying to remold a cousin or friend—possible, but improbable. It makes more sense to accept people as they are.

It's worth emphasizing that certain characteristics in physicians tend to bring out certain characteristics in patients. Rigidity in a physician tends to elicit rigidity in a patient, anger tends to elicit anger, and aloofness in the face of the needy patient may result in greater expressions of dependency on the patient's part.

The most important question to ask when a patient's behavior seems to be troublesome is, "Whose problem is this?" If the problem is heavily influenced by the patient's personality and your response to it, then the suggestions offered in this chapter will be particularly useful.

If a problem with a hospitalized patient is also a consequence of limited tolerance for normal illness behavior on the part of the nursing staff, it's appropriate to ask why. Maybe somebody just needs a vacation. Maybe you need additional personnel assigned to the hospital ward (good luck on this one!). Maybe you have to limit elective admissions for a few days. Maybe you have to eliminate a few administrative or teaching conferences which soak up too much staff time. The problem patient is seldom a problem only for us physicians. The hospital has an informal reward-and-punishment system in which staff lowest on the education and status totem pole play the most important role.* When nurses' aides and orderlies take a dislike to a patient, it requires extraordinary self-restraint on their part to do their customary conscientious job with such minor but important considerations as how long the patient is left on the bedpan, whether the coffee is brought cold or warm or the telephone and ice water are kept within reach, and dozens of other similar activities of daily hospital life.

Consider that the "problem" may be *your* problem—which is not to put you down, but rather to recognize your humanity. Each physician—indeed, each person—has individuals of certain types who arouse strong internal reactions. I may be easily irritated by passive-dependent patients, whereas you or your colleague may be turned off by the argumentative or denying patient.

I don't mean to imply (as some of the literature unfortunately does) that problems the physician perceives in the patient always are rooted in the physician, that the preselection in medical schools creates a stereotypic physician who can't tolerate patients who are other than stoical, respectful, obedient, rational, and reliable. People with these characteristics are easy for *anyone* to deal with, not simply physicians. If in doubt, ask a lawyer or hair stylist or mechanic what attributes make the ideal client and what make the reverse; you will find that many share your prejudices.

While every physician can deal with the occasional denying or complaining patient, many savvy physicians keep this ability a secret. They know that if they get a reputation for being adroit (among their col-

---

*Because so much patient care depends upon the nursing staff, we should understand that the nursing profession is going through turmoil. Widespread dissatisfaction in nursing stems from the fact that a nurse can progress in salary and status only by moving away from patient care. For instance, one report revealed that staff R.N.s spend only 40% of their time devoted to patient care, head nurses, 15%, and supervisors, 7%. Nurses are poorly paid compared to many other professionals with similar levels of training. Hospital nursing is hard, back-breaking work; and many nurses feel that the rewards and recognition are not commensurate with the extraordinary demands placed on them. Morale is low among the nursing staff of many complex medical centers. An average, annual staff turnover rate of 70% may climb to 200% in some major metropolitan hospitals. (This is in contrast to an annual turnover rate of 20% among public school teachers.) Many new titles among the nursing staff (nurse clinician, nurse practitioner) represent attempts by the nursing profession to develop career paths within clinical nursing which will result in greater rewards and recognition. The relative acceptability and status of these labels is not yet certain, and itself represents a source of contention for many in nursing.

leagues) and nice (among their patients), they quickly will accumulate a huge patient load, which includes a lot of folk that no one else wants to see. A great way to build up a private practice, it may be less adaptive to a salaried physician in a busy clinic practice. The young doctor usually aspires to be popular; the older physician knows better.

However, assuming that you want to do your best most of the time, there are a few precepts to keep in mind.

1. Patients who suffer greatly generally need more, and usually end up appreciating more. If you can resolve differences with potentially difficult patients, many of them will become your most ardent supporters. They know they wouldn't receive the same respectful treatment from just anyone.

2. Approach the patient in the most empathetic manner possible. Despite the degree to which either my patient or I are nerds or fools, we will do best focusing on other aspects of our respective personalities.

3. Merely because a patient requests (or the behavior implies) a certain type of response does not mean you have to comply, any more than the patient automatically has to comply with yours. Principles of conflict resolution require that both parties to a dispute begin to feel that their interests are being paid appropriate respect and attention.

4. Know your own level of tolerance. To the degree that you control your schedule, see that the patients you perceive as problems remain a manageable number. Mark their charts in some way, or keep a roster for the scheduler's reference. Space them out, or bunch them up—whatever works best for you.

5. Do not respond at a gut level when a patient's behavior upsets you. Monitor what is going on inside yourself, and reflect upon it. In reading this chapter, you are already doing some of what needs to be done. You are thinking about your own behavior and how to improve it.

6. Discuss problem patients with colleagues, especially those who know you well, are psychologically savvy, and whom you like and trust. They can often zero in on potential solutions that escape you when you are emotionally overwrought. You probably already ask for assistance with a puzzling EKG or murky diagnostic challenge. Try not to be more reticent with problems in the doctor-patient relationship.

7. And finally, while this chapter emphasizes the "normality" of the problem patient, and sees the source of such problems as interactive (involving both doctor and patient) rather than intrapsychic, occasionally such problems are due to psychosis in the patient. In the event of frank delusions or hallucinations, refer to the measures described in the chapter on Psychiatric Emergencies, and call in a psychiatric consultant.

The Angry Patient

Anyone can become angry—that is easy, but to be angry with the right person, to the right degree, at the right time, for the right purpose, and in the right way—that is not easy.

—Aristotle

I done wrassled with an alligator; I done tussled with a whale. . . ./Only last week I murdered a rock; Injured a stone, hospitalized a brick/I'm so mean I make medicine sick.

—Muhammad Ali

Anger is related to, but not necessarily identical with, irritation, hostility, verbal abusiveness, belligerence, and lack of cooperation. Anger is a normal part of the illness experience for many individuals, and it is crucial that physicians not get defensive in the face of such anger. Because the patient is angry does not necessarily mean that he or she is angry at *you;* even if the anger is directed at you, it does not necessarily mean that you are a direct stimulus of that anger.

The amount of hostility you perceive in a patient will vary directly with the proportion of anger directed at you personally. That is, a patient who is displeased with a nurse or consultant will not seem to you to be a hostile person. The patient who aims displeasure directly at you is much more likely to be labeled "hostile" by *you.*

If you are a person who expresses anger directly and encourages patients to do the same, your patients are more likely to express their anger directly at you and less likely to bitch and moan about you to others. Conversely, if you are uncomfortable with anger and convey this by your manner, the patients are more likely to subdue their anger in your presence and talk about it with their families and their lawyers.

Long-term hospitalized patients are sometimes sufficiently bored so that picking on staff represents a diversion, one that emphasizes what independence they have, compensates for feelings of being impaired, and brings them up to the level of equals in their own minds. Sometimes this takes the form of abusive humor shared with other patients. Usually this is a good sign that the patient has gotten beyond the needy, dependent stage.

However, the doctor also can foster anger in a patient by being distant, defensive, blaming, or impolite. Lack of humility on our parts is occasionally seen by patients as an indication for taking us down a peg or two, especially if they feel they have been humiliated by their illness and the process of seeking care.

It is usually most useful to see anger as a symptom and an indication to seek out the cause. Angry patients seldom express their anger merely for the purposes of punishing the people around them. Anger is heavily situation dependent. If there is absolutely no discernible reason for the anger, look for pathophysiologic sources.

Whether anger is kept inside or let out in the form of verbal expression or physical aggression depends upon the intensity of feelings, situational constraints, expected outcome of exhibiting anger, and an individual's customary personality style.

It's useful to remind ourselves that anger has many positive functions. For many people, anger is both scary and satisfying at the same time. Many individuals treasure their anger, and allow themselves to express their rage as a gift they give themselves but rarely. Anger is a vitalizing emotion, endowing an individual with a sense of potency, a feeling of being in charge. As emotions go, it is high in communication value. You tend to pay more attention to a man who says he is angry than to one who says he is a bit miffed. Anger can be intimidating and make the individual expressing it feel more secure. Like the porcupine's spines, it tends to keep people at a distance. Anger has considerable instrumental value; it has the power to instigate action, whether constructive or not. Finally, anger provides a way for externalizing conflict. Depression frequently results from anger turned inward; depression turned outward in the form of anger tends to put the responsibility for change on factors external to the individual.

It's important to note that all these functions of anger are as relevant for the physician as they are for the patient. Therefore, the temptation to meet the patient's anger with anger of your own is sometimes considerable.

Anger kept inside can be a major barrier to amicable relations between doctor and patient. Conversely, ventilated anger, handled with appropriate responses by the parties involved, can provide the basis for a good relationship.

Anger in patients usually results in one of three responses from medical staff—anger right back, "There, there, now," or avoidance. Each sometimes works, and I'll have more to say about ideal responses shortly. Some internal reactions are to feel threatened or guilty.

Take the following example. You have been caring for a 44-year-old man, hospitalized with pancreatitis for several days. He has a sales job in a local brewery, and he's not happy about being away from work and about being away from his sons, for whom he obviously cares a good deal. From time to time, he's been in considerable discomfort, and he has been unhappy with many aspects of his treatment—initially, his nasogastric tube and the intravenous fluids, and now a bland and admittedly unappetizing diet. Nonetheless, he is clearly improving. However, on rounds today, the patient explodes, seemingly inexplicably, holding you accountable for the hospital's many deficiencies, some of which he itemizes: the lab technician botched his venipuncture, the patient down the hall was screaming and kept him awake all night, the nurse tried to give him somebody else's medication, which fortunately he was "too smart" to let happen, and the pain medication has been inadequate to control the discomfort. Which of the following responses would you choose?

1. "Don't be angry; there's no reason to be so upset."
2. "Those things could have happened to anyone. Don't take it so personally. In any event, I'm not responsible."
3. "What was the name of the lab technician? What was the name of the nurse? Give me some more details."
4. "Nobody talks to me that way. I simply won't tolerate that behavior. Don't you ever talk to me that way again."
5. "Gee, I'm awfully sorry those things happened; we have to tighten up ship around here. I'll try to see those things don't happen again."
6. "Perhaps you'd rather have another physician. If you like, I'll withdraw from the case and turn your care over to another doctor."
7. "Look, this kind of talk isn't getting us anywhere; why don't we just concentrate on your pancreatitis and try to get you out of here as soon as we can?"
8. "You don't know how hard I've been trying; it's not easy to be a doctor at this hospital. I wish you would appreciate what I'm trying to do for you."

Like other examples cited in this book, there is obviously not one simple, correct answer. The kind of response that you choose depends upon your own style, but it is useful to attempt to understand what led to choosing the response. Did you choose to preach? To argue? To interrogate? To punish? To apologize? To withdraw? To sidestep? To defend?

There are some good general rules for responding to anger in patients. Like all rules, they must be adjusted to fit the situation, but I urge you to review these considerations in your own mind before responding by shooting from the hip.

1. Allow the patient to ventilate, and treat his or her reaction with respect. Grant his or her perspective and the naturalness of the feelings. Try to be glad that the feelings were expressed rather than kept inside. Say, "If that's what your experience was, I can certainly understand why you're so upset." Or, "I'm glad you're calling the shots just the way you see them." Try to remember the positive functions that expression of anger can serve. "I'm glad you're telling me these things. It's people like you who help to keep us on our toes."

2. Avoid becoming defensive. Try not to argue or preach or take the patient's anger as a personal attack against yourself. Never take sides with the patient against another member of the staff as a means of

directing anger away from yourself. Say, "I understand your concerns. I am concerned too. I would certainly welcome any suggestions that you may have."

3. Retain control of the situation consistent with the amount of responsibility you carry, but recognize that patients carry ultimate responsibility for themselves and need to retain some control too. Say, "I'm glad you recognized the error in medications, and I'm glad to see you involved in the details of your own care." Work out whatever compromises seem suitable. Say, "You and I will have to come to some understanding about your pain medication, but I'm afraid my influence with the clinical pathology lab is limited. I hope you spoke to the laboratory technician directly."

4. When the patient is angry, maintain a thoroughly professional and respectful stance. Unless you are extremely skillful, do not respond with humor—the patient may think that you aren't taking the matter seriously. Avoid informality; if the patient is at all suspicious, he or she may see warmth as a ploy rather than an expression of your good intentions.

5. Be careful to keep the patient informed on details relevant to his or her circumstances. Say, "Yes, you aren't the only person who is concerned about the noise down the hall. However, that patient is quite ill, and sedating him is not as easy as it sounds. That person's doctor has to balance sedation with side effects, and I'm afraid it's a difficult task. I'm sorry that you and others were disturbed. We all hope that things will be better tonight."

6. If an angry situation erupts and gets out of hand, try not to leave it at that. Don't let one unpleasant interaction interfere with your usual standards concerning thoroughness and continuity of care. For instance, if the conflict occurs in your office, give yourself and the patient a chance to cool off. That evening or the following day, call the patient and express what you probably feel. "I'm sorry that situation ran away with us. I'd like very much to work things out between the two of us and, at the very least, to see that your health-care needs are well served. Shall we try again?" Most people will respond to such an overture; and, even with those who don't, it's reassuring to know that you have tried your best.

The Dependent, Passive Patient

Nothing is ours, Lucilius, save only our time. And yet we let the first comer deprive us of our sole and fleeting fortune.
—Seneca

The chronophage is generally a man who has very little to do himself, and not knowing what to make of the time on his hands, decided to fill it up by devouring yours. The audacity of the animal passes all belief.
—André Maurois

Intermittent dependency is a fact of life for most of us. Everyone finds a shoulder to lean on a useful resource from time to time. Sometimes that shoulder can be appropriately provided by one's physician, both because illness results in increased dependency for most of us, and because the illness situation is the most important culturally sanctioned circumstance in which an adult can say to another, "Help me."

An extraordinary percentage of patients seen in any primary care practice come to their physicians for reasons related to temporary dependency, to sense that somebody cares, to be told it's okay to take a few days off, to be reassured that their temporary neediness is not a basic character flaw. The overwhelming majority of these, though presenting with supposedly physical complaints, will feel successfully treated with nothing but symptomatic care and a few minutes of respectful attention from their physician.

There's a moral in there somewhere.

Health professionals are often called "care givers" with the implication that patients come to health professionals to be taken care of. Doctors mostly enjoy taking care of people—certainly up to a point—and we generally get along best with patients who are willing to accept an appropriate amount of "caretaking" from us. However, we differ widely, both physicians and patients, in how we define an appropriate amount. The patient who gets labeled "overly dependent" is one who is seen as expecting others to do all the work in order to change from a state of illness into a state of health, and is unwilling to do however little or however much can be done in order to assist that process. Furthermore, such individuals are usually perceived as gobbling up vast quantities of the physician's precious time for reasons that make no apparent sense to anyone but themselves.

"Excess" dependency occurs most often in individuals with some bona fide medical disorder, and particularly in older patients who are under coexistent psychological or social stress. This latter group tends to bring out all the feelings in a physician that one has concerning potential dependency by one's own parents. Consequently, responses often are quite personal.

With a patient whom we gradually come to see as overly dependent, our interactions usually follow a certain pattern. First, the patient makes needs known, implicitly or explicitly. We then do what we can to satisfy the patient's requests. When our response fails to satisfy the patient, usually we try again. And again. And again. How long all this

continues depends upon our frustration tolerance versus patience ratio
for the people involved. Ultimately, the frustration is likely to result in
anger or withdrawal. Neither response seems to help things much,
either for the patient or for the soulful satisfaction that the doctor gets
from his or her work.

Internally, most physicians feel annoyed with themselves and with
the patients, but have difficulty articulating the reasons for that annoy-
ance. There is often a sense of helplessness and guilt. The patient
seems to defeat every effort to help, and the doctor is torn between
vain, repeated efforts and a desire to avoid the patient entirely. Patients who are particularly irritating are those who add a note of urgency to their requests, perhaps with tears, and those who up the ante
by presenting themselves as being giving and caring persons. The hospitalized patient says, "I took out Mr. Snort's bedpan for you," making it clear that while he or she appears generous, repayment in full is
expected. The outpatient brings you a box of cookies or says, I've told
everyone how grateful I am for your help.

Usually, physicians have most difficulty with this kind of patient
when the physician is feeling overworked and underrewarded. If you
are not being adequately nurtured at any given time, someone else's
cry of need may arouse anger and aggression on your part rather than
compassion. If you have never been adequately nurtured, your tolerance for needy patients will be zero.

Dependency has many meanings, both to doctor and to patient. It
represents an expression of general neediness, a means of maintaining
human contact, and a way of controlling a relationship. Being given
something, a gesture or an emotion or an object, often represents love,
caring, or affection. Illness, to many individuals, means not only being
taken care of but also represents a stress which may tend to exaggerate
any neediness in the person's character structure. Illness is sometimes
the only situation in which any given person feels he or she can show
dependency needs, and so those that have been stored up for months
come out with a vengeance.

Physicians are customarily individuals who do not allow many of
their dependency needs to show on the surface. Indeed, many of us are
not consciously aware of having any dependency needs at all. However, those needs are there in all of us, and many of us are a bit
frightened by them. It is because of this that dependency in patients
may be particularly rankling. We resent most in others what we won't
permit in or perceive as a threat to, ourselves.

Only by accepting your own dependent needs will you come to
accept the dependent needs of others without making a moral judgment
as to their appropriateness.

One way of dealing with a dependent person who is perceived as a time-gobbling leech is to use unmitigated brutality: point out all the patient's deficiencies in the nastiest possible fashion. This has the appeal of immediate effectiveness with all but the most masochistic of individuals, but, alas, it also cheapens you in the process. Physicians who resort to such crude responses are, if viewed in an empathic manner, usually fearful that if they show the slightest kindness to the dependent patient, they will be consumed by an insatiable appetite for nurturance.

Fortunately, there are other approaches. The first step in adequate treatment of the dependent patient involves the development of tolerance for dependency and some feelings of comfort in its presence. If you manage to perceive dependency as something other than a personal threat, you will do much better in your relationship with the patient.

Try approaching the issue of dependency as a paradox. "It must be awfully difficult for an ordinarily self-sufficient person like you to be so dependent on others for so many basics of daily living." This helps patients understand that you are not trying to define them totally by their dependent needs, and that you understand that they are complex persons. A comment like this brings the issue out into the open, and does so in a way that almost no one will ever object to.

Next, try to see the dependency as a symptom. Ask, "Why does the patient prefer to be helpless rather than independent?" without making the question an indictment. What is it that the patient really wants? Satisfaction of generalized neediness? Maintaining human contact? Exerting some control over the relationship with you? Try to satisfy some of the patient's needs for special attention. Give the patient the feeling that you care. In other words, be willing to gratify the patient's dependent needs for at least a little while. Say, "You just relax and let me take care of you." In general, allow the patient a period of time in which you ask relatively little, but give a little extra of yourself. Most such patients respond extremely well to small gestures on our part: a pat on the hand, fluffing up the bedridden patient's pillow before you leave.

If you are jealous of your time, as of course most of us are, learn to give something other than time. One reason doctors write so many prescriptions is that physician and patient may perceive handing the patient the paper as a gift, one that takes little time. Rather than stuffing the patient with powerful chemicals, however, the same principle can be adapted to other uses: using the prescription to write instructions ("Don't forget to take orange juice with your blood pressure pills"), requests ("Bring in an exercise log on your next visit"), and phone numbers (self-help groups for diabetics or whatever). An inspired "gift" is helping dependent patients to feel needed. Say, "I have another patient who is having the same problem that you overcame last year. Could I ask her to give you a call?''

Probably you will feel more comfortable giving your time to such patients if you are confident that the gift is finite. You won't want to lure many patients out of their shells if you are afraid you can never get them back in long enough to draw your appointment to a close. In other words, you must learn to feel comfortable setting limits before the patient's needs outdistance your resources.

However, it is important not to appear impatient, rejecting, or punishing when doing so. Explain what you are doing and why. Offer concessions. Say, "I'm not going to be able to spend as much time with you today as I would like to, but here's what I'm going to try to do."

Avoid getting caught up in the details of the patient's dependent requests. Instead, focus on the emotional needs which sprouted the specific requests, but try not to rub the patient's nose in it while you're doing so. Say, "I think you're just feeling lousy today and you're going to need some special care and attention." However, say that *only* if you can do so empathically.

The Complaining, Demanding Patient

Arrogant, pompous, obnoxious, vain, cruel, persecuting, distasteful, verbose, a show-off. I have been called all of these. Of course, I am.
—Howard Cosell

The kinship between the angry patient and the complainer is obvious, but there are also important differences that make it worthwhile to separate the two.

The patient with a complaint does not represent a unique entity. Every ordinary person can find plenty to complain about in life, more so during illness, and particularly while in the benevolent clutches of a physician or complex medical center. However, only a minority of patients actually do complain to the doctor or staff, and a much smaller group do so with any regularity.

Complaints are best seen as a process, a means of communication. Complaints are vehicles for expressing dissatisfaction or discomfort. It's important to emphasize that complaints in and of themselves do not necessarily require a response in the form of any specific action. While complaints may focus upon matters of personal discomfort, medical treatment, or the hospital or clinic environs, it is useful to ask, Why has this patient chosen to express a complaint rather than remaining passive and quiet like most patients?

Complaints occur most frequently among several groups of patients. The first are those individuals who genuinely have something upsetting to complain about. We never should neglect this possibility, even though other factors may also be playing a part. Second, complaints tend to be most prominent among particular groups, certain long-term and chronic patients in particular. The usual pattern is that the patient becomes progressively more disenchanted with health-care, at the same time that he or she becomes increasingly more knowledgeable about the varieties of ways in which his or her own care might be managed. The ratio between the amount of experience the patient has had with his or her condition and the amount of experience the physician has had with the same condition, tends to increase exponentially in all but the most expert and specialized of physicians. The patient begins to feel that there is little the physician can provide that the patient can't, except mobilization of medical services. The patient comes to resent the physician as an obstacle rather than as a facilitator of medical care. The patient *knows* he or she needs a catheter irrigated, yet the nurse refuses to comply unless so ordered by the physician. We physicians, in turn, do not like to be told what to do, especially by patients. The potential for resentment and friction is obvious. The medical environment becomes a major focus in chronic patients' lives, and, like most of us, they seek to put their stamps on it.

Some locations in a medical facility seem to be magnets for complaints, particularly those that process a high volume of patients in relatively impersonal contacts in which the patient's view of his or her needs may differ radically from that of staff. Screening nurses are often special targets for complaints, as are drop-in clinics in general, and as are emergency rooms where sick but not critical patients may be shunted to the sidelines.

Often complaints stem from brusqueness, impersonal behavior, and insensitivity on the part of ward staff. Frequently, however, the patients don't complain about these qualities or even about these individuals directly, but rather about seemingly trivial matters only marginally related to specific staff. It sometimes takes a tenacious mind to ferret out the Byzantine evolution of such complaints.

One patient-type whose complaints are frequent is the compulsive individual who copes with stress by mastering detail. This individual tends to be logical and self-disciplined, orderly, precise, punctual, and cost-conscious. Requiring knowledge and data in order to cope best, this patient seeks them by asking questions and may be quite obstinate when such information is not forthcoming. This patient can become very upset at lapses in routine. The more stressful the circumstances, the more compulsive he or she becomes, and complaints usually develop proportionately. Such attention to detail can be an asset when patient and doctor are working together but an obstacle when the two are not working toward the same goal.

Sometimes complaints have strong cultural components. Suffering with a certain amount of dramatic flair is highly esteemed in some ethnic groups—indeed, it is an expected sign of situation-appropriate behavior—and it is only when your patient begins to brood silently that you need to become worried that he or she may be overwhelmed by circumstances. Another culturally sanctioned behavior sometimes perceived by physicians as criticism has to do with the self-consciously masculine patient who uses aggression as one route to establish bonding. For example, the patient may say "Doc, you have the worst handwriting on the face of this earth" in the same way he might say to his favorite basketball buddy, "You can't dribble worth diddley" as a prelude to saying "Let me buy you a beer."

A truism about complaints is that no one likes them. No one likes to be complained about, and no one likes to be seen as a complainer. Both parties tend to feel guilty. However, as long as you don't feel responsible for the patient's suffering, you won't get defensive, and possibilities for coexistence are enhanced.

Patterns of responses to a series of complaints tend to follow a predictable sequence. The first complaint results in a response; the complaint repeated results in a diminished response; the complaint made yet again results in no response; repeated again, the complaint results in an aversive response.

Like other problem behaviors discussed in this chapter, complaints are most usefully seen as symptomatic behavior. That is, complaints are a way for the patient to express feelings of dysphoria, though the precise nature of that discomfort may stem from fear, anxiety, loneliness, generalized neediness, insecurity, and the like. Many people find it difficult to articulate what they really want or feel, and complaints become an indirect means for self-expression. These feelings are invariably exacerbated by illness, but they may predate the illness as well.

The first task for the physician is to develop his or her own frustration tolerance, in part for self, and in part as a prelude to helping the patient develop frustration tolerance. It helps to keep your sense of humor and to see as adaptive the patient's capacity for suffering noisily. Only after you have sorted out what reactions complaints stir up in you—regardless of the consequences to the patient—can you hope to approach their solution in a comfortable manner.

It's no fun, as a person who wishes to help, to be subjected to complaints. The most useful way to see the unhelpable or help-rejecting complainer is to see the patient as someone who seeks, but cannot perceive or accept, the help that we are able to give. The challenge is to empathize without shoving your own particular variety of help down the patient's throat.

At all costs, avoid prolonged bickering over trivia. Stay away from arguments about the medical profession in general or the merits of your hospital, clinic, or office relative to others the patient might have chosen. Refrain from joining in on criticism of previous physicians. Be empathetic. (Say, "If that's how you experienced it, it certainly must have been unpleasant!") But remember (without necessarily saying so) that there is always more than one perspective to any difference of opinion.

Let the patient know that whereas you care how he or she feels and appreciate the need to ventilate, your job is to remember and focus on the health problems that brought the patient to your office: "I don't want to interrupt, but why don't you finish the story while I'm doing your sigmoidoscopic examination?"

Any time you label a person a "complainer," ask, "What is this person trying to tell me?" Look for the message behind the complaints.

As with other problem patients, fasten onto the paradox: "It must be frustrating for you to feel such dissatisfaction and be unable to alter our behavior to suit your needs." With some patients, you can also acknowledge your own frustration: "I would really like to be of more help to you, but I have my own limitations. It's frustrating for me not to be able to do things to your satisfaction."

More than any other patient, the chronic complainer needs a primary physician who is willing to see the patient at regular intervals over time. The patient should never be hospitalized for diagnostic studies unless compelling reasons exist, and the chief challenge is to prevent iatrogenic illness or injury.

For patients whose complaints reflect a compulsive need for control, do what you can to see that they have full access to all data relevant to their conditions. Understand that they need control over anxiety, not over the technical aspects of care per se, though some participation in the latter may help. Avoid getting bogged down in minutiae with these patients, but recognize that they especially value the scientific and technological aspects of care. Give them respect for their desire to know, for their attempts to understand, and for their high standards. Give them responsible tasks which will occupy their attention, such as keeping their own intake and output records, charting their own "out-of-bed" time, and responsibility for changing their own dressings if they wish.

As medical care gets more complicated and its organization more laden with bureaucracy, the patient has a much wider choice of places to lodge complaints: patient-assistance offices, chiefs of services, hospital directors, medical societies, licensing boards, and the like. Whenever your patient complains to you personally, be grateful. Working out complaints between the two of you allows for the utmost growth for each of you and also for the relationship you share. Try to let your manner show all of your patients that if they have any complaints you want to hear them. If a patient lodges a formal complaint with an administrative office, think about calling the patient up directly to express your regret that any difficulties occurred.

Always remember to ask for suggestions from colleagues; and, if the breach with the patient is beyond repair, arrange for the orderly transfer of care to another physician.

The Denying Patient

Refuse to be ill. Never tell people you are ill; never own it to yourself. Illness is one of those things which a man should resist on principle at the outset.
—Bulwer-Lytton

When viewed from the patient's perspective, denial makes a lot of sense. Frankly, if I had to choose either conscious or unconscious suffering, I think I often would choose the latter. Lack of awareness just might be a blessing. Denial, in fact, is a matter of day-to-day existence: few of us can face the full implications of the human vulnerability of our leaders, the fact of carcinogens in our food and water, or the ever-present danger of nuclear accidents.

Physicians are most concerned with denial as a response to the fact of illness. However, we must see denial in a broader social context than that. Denial has many cultural determinants. Older people tend to do it more than younger people. The people who deny the most are, understandably, the people with the most to deny: persons with multiple problems. The more stresses a person has at a particular time, the less able he or she is likely to be to face the full implications of all of them.

When a patient uses denial, we must recognize that that patient has been so shaken by the awareness or the suspicion of illness and its potential seriousness that he or she has not been able fully to deal with it. The fact that the patient is seeing us at all represents an important achievement. We must not punish him or her for it by demanding that fate be confronted, as we imagine we might handle such circumstances.

By virtue of coming to us, the patient is saying "I know at least some of what's happening, but I want to see myself, and I want you to see me, as healthy, intact, and able." There are multiple levels of denial, both as to degree, and as to the conscious acceptance of fact, significance, and affect:

Delusion. "This isn't me. I'm not here. This isn't happening."

Minimization. "This is happening; I am here; but this isn't serious."

Repression. "I know I am sick, but I keep forgetting the details."

Blunted Affect. "I know I am sick; I know what is happening; but I have no feelings about it."

Suppression. "I know what is happening; but as long as I try not to think about it, I don't feel so bad."

Despite the fact that denial is often adaptive for the person using it, physicians often find denial irritating because they see it as an obstacle to good treatment—"How can I help him if he doesn't accept what's wrong with him?" The physician responds emotionally with frustration, anger, and bewilderment—It's so obvious—how can she be denying it when it's right in front of her eyes? Many physicians feel obliged to confront the patient with the patent falsehood of the patient's position *vis–à–vis* illness. This customarily leads to greater anxiety for the patient, with consequent increased denial, increasingly strident confrontations by the physician (and sometimes family), with the patient finally either decompensating or eloping from treatment.

Denial can create problems for the physician when the patient chooses to focus on one aspect of a condition without acknowledging other perhaps even more important aspects. For example, the terminal cancer patient may appear unwilling to accept the prognosis, but nonetheless keeps asking the physician, "Why am I losing all this weight?" Physicians often find such questions extremely frustrating. In fact, it is this frustration which offers a guide to approaching the patient effectively. In some respects, the physician's frustration reflects the frustration the patient also feels at a lack of control over destiny. An appropriate response for the physician therefore is, "It must be awfully frustrating for you to want to get well so badly and nonetheless to be losing weight." A response of this general nature identifies the patient's paradox and places the physician in an empathetic and nonadversary situation.

Another approach is to focus on your own emotional response without pitting yourself against the patient. As the man with severe emphysema sits in your office for the hundredth time—dyspneic, coughing, with a cigarette pack peeking out of his shirt pocket—one potential approach is to say, "It upsets me to see what you are doing to yourself, but I will continue to do my best for you, even if you can't cut down your smoking." Try to remain firm, gentle in your reasonableness, the ally of your patient always.

The physician's task is to respect the patient's way of coping with stress and to see tactics like denial as a part of a broadly normal sequence of reactions to the fact of illness. Denial usually follows a predictable pattern; with time and decreased anxiety on the patient's part, the denial will lessen. Therefore, denial is best approached indirectly. Anything you can do to lessen the patient's anxiety is likely to be helpful. Focusing on the denial per se or the facts being denied usually will lead only to more anxiety and therefore more denial.

The Overly Affectionate Patient

There is only one kind of love, but there are 1,000 imitations.
—La Rochefoucauld

The doctor-patient relationship has enormous potential for intimacy. That intimacy represents a powerful tool for the enhancement of patient care, but this potential for good is also matched by a potential for problems. It is with patients with whom you have the greatest intimacy that you are likely to have your most dramatic successes and your greatest troubles. The dividing line between "a useful amount of intimacy" and "too much intimacy" is often difficult to draw and subject to considerable individual and circumstantial variation.

The terms used to describe the overly affectionate patient vary somewhat: adoring, worshipping, respecting, admiring, seductive. The patient appears to want more from the relationship than simply interacting on the basis of illness and its treatment. In style, patients like this come across as flirtatious, teasing, inviting, or pressuring. They tend to be highly personal in manner, forthcoming, seeming to demand a similar response from their physician. They often have a self-dramatizing or even charming character. They may ask physicians and other medical personnel very personal questions. While some of these approaches may seem frankly sexual in nature, they may in an older patient take on maternal or paternal characteristics.

In return, the medical personnel tend to label such patients with predictable tags. If the patient is a premenopausal woman, she is likely to be called "hysterical." An older woman may be labeled a "Jewish mother" or an "Italian mother," depending upon the patient's ethnicity or that of the staff. A man may be labeled a "Romeo" or "God's gift to women." In general, these patients tend to be colorful and lively, and those who can do so effectively often exhibit considerable sexual strutting.

It's important for us as physicians to recognize the adaptive value for a patient, especially in an impersonal hospital, to be able to reach someone else on a personal level. Flirting with the nurses, for example, usually *does* result in the patient gaining for himself a clear identity in the hospital milieu, and having staff recognize him as an individual separate from all the other patients on the ward. If a patient approaches you as a potential friend or lover, that's a patient whose name you will not forget. The patient will have succeeded in raising himself or herself above the level of being just "another gastrectomy in Room 432." The patient who comes across seductively, sexually or not, often feels as though you won't pay special attention to him or her unless you get special attention in return. The patient's behavior therefore should be seen as an attempt by that patient to win you as an ally.

Seductive or "overly personal" behavior occurs most often in persons who feel the need for special attention or recognition. It also tends to occur in patients who have found such a behavior style effective in the past; for example, persons who are or have been physically attractive or who are warm and vital by nature.

Some physicians never seem to have any problems with "overly personal" patients. There is an obvious message here; certain kinds of physicians tend to elicit certain kinds of behaviors in their patients. Some doctors foster very personal kinds of interactions between doctor and patient. Thus, there are seductive physicians as well as seductive patients.

The problem is really a double one: the seductive patient and the seducible doctor, or the seductive doctor and the seducible patient. The available information certainly suggests that, when sexual liaisons develop between physician and patient, such intensely personal involvement with patients occurs at times of personal neediness for the physician—e.g., when he or she is feeling particularly depressed or lonely. At such times, it is often not clear who is the seducer and who is the seduced.

I want to emphasize that sexual arousal and involvement with patients, while perhaps the most dramatic form of intimate interaction between doctor and patient, is nonetheless only one aspect of the broader area of emotional and personal intimacy with patients. However, it is also usually the most difficult to talk about with colleagues or friends, let alone with the patient. Imagine the following example. You are in the process of examining a young man with a chronic orthopedic problem such as a medial meniscus injury. The patient is a handsome, likeable, professional athlete. During the course of your complete physical examination, you do a rectal exam and check the patient for inguinal hernias. In the course of this process, the patient develops what is without any doubt a solidly turgid erection.

How do you respond, both internally and externally? If you are a woman, do you automatically assume that the patient has a heterosexual interest in you? If you are a male, do you assume that the patient has a homosexual interest in you? Do you assume it is simply a reflex response to your manual examination? Do you treat the matter with humor and make a joke about the patient's erection? Do you pretend it didn't happen? (We call that denial in patients!) Do you become very businesslike? Will you say something to "put the patient in his place"?

Will you want to avoid the patient? There are obviously a variety of ways to respond, and a good deal of room for individual variation and style.

Nonetheless, there are a few useful guidelines. Behavior has meaning, both to the patient and to yourself, and you ignore that meaning at your mutual peril. Regardless of the factors that predisposed the patient to this particular display, he is likely to have some feelings about it after the fact, just as you do. Sidestepping the issue entirely will seldom enhance your relationship, and is most likely to be a reflection of your anxiety in dealing with such matters. There is a major irony here in that the more troubled you are by such patients and such behavior, the more likely you are to try to handle such problems alone, and the more uncomfortable you will feel in asking another professional for assistance.

For the sake of the present discussion, I will ignore any potential reflex components in the above example, and instead concentrate on the meaning of very personal and/or intimate behavior to the parties involved. Most commonly, intimate or seductive behavior indicates a need on the patient's part to be noticed, and a desire for a personal relationship as opposed to an impersonal one. This seductive behavior can easily be interpreted as bravado by anyone observing it. If you take this bravado at face value, you may well miss the anxiety that prompts it. It may well represent a cover for feelings of helplessness on the part of the patient. Occasionally the patient's seductive behavior is designed to make authority figures appear more accessible and humble, particularly in the face of an illness which makes the patient feel defective and unattractive. Often, it is this fear of decreased personal attractiveness, sexual and otherwise, that prompts seductive behavior. The latter is therefore most usefully seen as a bid for approval.

Physicians, in turn, usually struggle not only with the tactics of responding to the patient's behavior, fearful of being rejecting, hurting, or appearing stuffy, for instance, but also with the emotional impact on their own psyches. How would I act if I were in the patient's shoes? How do I feel about my own personal and sexual attractiveness? How needy am I feeling for approval and admiration from my patients? Am I in fact feeling seducible? And does that possibility frighten me?

It's important to recognize that personal and intimate relations between physician and patient are not all necessarily evil or destructive. Most physicians feel particular closeness with some of their patients, and it is perhaps an inhuman physician whose heart is never tugged by a patient at all. However, intimacy is also an identifiable hazard for the physician. It represents a situation in which the patient's needs become blurred with your own, and you run the risk of not being able to sort out what you are doing for the patient and what you are doing for yourself.

That's dangerous for most of us, because maintaining the primacy of the patient's needs is an extremely important ethic in medicine. Physicians run the risk of losing their own self-respect when they cease behaving in a way that says to the patient, "You can trust me. I will not confuse your needs with my own."

There are several guidelines for physicians in such situations. First, you should see seductive behavior as symptomatic behavior; the patient is asking you for a positive response, and the range of potential positive responses is broad. Withholding a positive response usually results in more stereotypic behavior on the patient's part. Potential positive responses include: "You appear to be doing quite well," "You seem to have made quite a hit with the nursing staff," and "You may have a bum knee but there's nothing wrong with the rest of you."

Second, in general, acknowledge the patient's overtures without feeling that you have to respond to them exactly as you are being asked to respond. Ignoring the overtures entirely is rarely the preferred method, unless you are too anxious to deal with them in any other way. It's not so much what you say, as letting your manner and tone say, "You are a unique and decent person; I see you as an individual; I will give you the best care I can."

Third, you must learn to set limits for seductive behavior that are comfortable for yourself, but not punitive towards the patient. The limits most appropriate for you may differ from those that are best for your colleagues. However you assess your limits of comfort, avoid going beyond them. Don't set yourself up for any resentment or guilt. Say, "I really appreciate your invitation for dinner, but I find it very difficult to take good professional care of patients with whom I am socially and personally involved. Since that takes such a high priority with me, I simply must decline."

Keep the patient's needs separate from your own. Be especially wary of intimate involvement with patients when you are yourself feeling needy. Know your own vulnerabilities, and treat them with respect. You practice medicine for a long time, but you may know any given patient relatively briefly. Don't get involved in relationships that will jeopardize your professional self-respect or effectiveness over the years to come.

Acknowledge that anyone sick or hospitalized for a long time is likely to feel sexual neediness and some need for enhancement of self-esteem. This is natural enough, and hopefully will not merit any disapproval from you. Give symbolic attention, reassurance, and approval whenever you can, but do not become enmeshed with the patient.

Finally, discussing positive feelings openly with a patient can be very helpful, but it requires a lot of skill and soul-deep self-assurance. Discussing mutual attraction and still maintaining a professional relationship is extremely tricky; unless you are experienced in this matter, request a consultation with someone with greater experience. Do not try it alone. Whenever possible, get the input and perspective of someone you know and trust.

The Chronic Schizophrenic

When you look directly at an insane man, all you see is a reflection of your own knowledge that he is insane, which is not to see him at all. To see him you must see what he saw.

—Robert Pirsig

It has long been established that physicians who are not psychiatrists have little enthusiasm for taking care of chronic schizophrenics. Actually, when you look at practices of most psychiatrists—made up largely of depressed and neurotic patients—you may conclude that even psychiatrists are not very keen on seeing chronic schizophrenics.

However, with the closing of many state hospitals and the concomitant emphasis on keeping chronic psychiatric patients in the community, ambulatory schizophrenic patients are likely to be part of every physician's case load.

Why is it that physicians are so wary of caring for such people? There's no need for us to feel defensive about it; our reluctance to become involved with this group is widely shared by the population at large. Some of it must stem from the stigma long attached to the mentally ill, a stigma that persists despite centuries of efforts designed to convince us that the "mentally ill" are similar to everyone else.

While anyone can experience depression or panic in their lives, and almost everyone can become psychotic under sufficiently catastrophic social and/or biochemical conditions, chronic schizophrenia is indeed a condition apart from the norm. Regardless of our "scientific" nomenclature, the general public considers such folk "crazy" and therefore to be regarded with some apprehension and even repugnance. We physicians too are products of our culture and therefore share some of these emotional perspectives. So, too, are the schizophrenics themselves, and their self-perceptions are heavily tainted by the dominant cultural attitude. You won't find many with much self-esteem.

Clinically, problems in caring for these people derive from (1) the basic nature of the disease; (2) medical staff's feelings of awkwardness; and (3) the patients' cachectic self-esteem.

Chronic schizophrenics commonly are alienated "loners;" consequently, relating to others, including health-care personnel, is not something they can do comfortably or skillfully. Their affect often seems blunted; they are not people with whom you can easily share a belly laugh or a tender moment. Their thinking—to the extent you can assess it—seems tortuous and confused or leaden, paralyzed by indecision. How can you have a collaborative relationship with a person when you can't even share a rational discussion and when your confidence in the patient's compliance is essentially nonexistent?

Most chronic schizophrenics in the community who come to the office of nonpsychiatric practitioners are mental hospital "graduates" who seek you out for one of two reasons: (1) they have a medical problem which needs attention, or (2) they need help with managing antipsychotic medications and no psychiatrist is readily available.

Surprisingly, managing medical problems can be remarkably straightforward. If the patient is functioning well enough to be out of the psychiatric hospital, he or she can usually attend to the necessities of health-care. The key is to maintain a manner which is, in a word, professional. Be formal without being cold, welcoming but without false warmth or awkward heartiness, respectful and honest but without being judgmental. Understand that while you are concerned about the patient's reliability, the patient simultaneously has the same questions about you. Be especially trustworthy. Don't make promises you can't keep and don't pretend to be anything but what you are: a physician who can be trusted to do a competent job in a straightforward manner, who expects a reasonable attempt at responsible patient behavior in return.

The principal challenge in juggling psychotropic medications in ambulatory schizophrenics is overcoming disbelief of the dosage levels involved. While most physicians have experience prescribing chlorpromazine at the 25- to 50-mg level (or the equivalent with other antipsychotic medications), many become uncomfortable when the dosage reaches levels 10 or 20 times greater, as often will be the case in patients recently discharged from large and probably understaffed psychiatric hospitals. It's a widely accepted axiom in psychiatry that the people who tolerate large doses of major tranquilizers best are those who need it most.

Nonetheless, most nonpsychiatrists in such positions usually consider lowering dosage levels an important priority. It is reasonable to aim for the lowest dose consistent with accomplishing desired goals, especially after the patient has reached a stable living situation in the community, but in order to do the task well, you have to have a clear idea of what it is you are trying to do.

Write down one or more "target symptoms" which you hope to spare the patient by prescribing medications. Typical examples are auditory hallucinations ("Tell me if the voices come back"), compulsive repetitive acts ("I want to know if you start washing your hands more than once an hour again"), or paranoid behavior. Usually, target symptoms can be identified by reviewing the patient's history prior to the last psychiatric hospitalization, or by talking with reliable persons who have assumed something of a caretaker role in the patient's life (these include relatives, members of the same church, directors of board-and-care homes, et cetera). Obviously, it is helpful if you can monitor the patient's progress, not only by what the patient says, but also via your own observation of the patient's hygiene and appearance, the reliability with which appointments are kept, and so on, and with the observations of others. Patients like this are often treated best by multiple brief appointments, every few weeks or every month.

Once you are convinced that the patient has achieved relative stability, you can begin the task of lowering dosage levels. Proceed slowly and methodically. Lower the dosage 10% to 15% every month or so. One technique is to offer the patient "drug holidays" in which meds are skipped; for example, every Sunday. Remember, almost all drugs in this category have an extremely long half-life at the tissue level and, if you lower the dosage now, you won't see target symptoms—assuming they will appear—for several days or even weeks. If target symptoms do reappear, resume previous dosage levels (you may also need to give a few additional doses until tissue levels are once again adequate).

If you need to hospitalize your patient for medical problems, remember that you may have to raise dosage levels temporarily to help cover the additional stress that hospitalization often entails. Be sure to instruct nursing staff about target symptoms, and be wary of side effects and drug interactions (discussed elsewhere in this book) if the patient's medical condition is complicated or requires many medications.

Bibliography

Alper PR: Surefire steps to soothe the savage patient. *Medical Economics* (March 18) 1985; pp 131–136

An Abstract for Action, Report of National Commission for the Study of Nursing and Nursing Education (JP Lysaught, Director). New York, McGraw-Hill, 1970

Anstett R: The difficult patient and the physician-patient relationship. *J Fam Pract* 11:281–286, 1980

Baughan DM, Révicki D, Nieman LZ: Management of problem patients with multiple chronic diseases. *J Fam Pract* 17:233–239, 1983

Bird B: *Talking with Patients.* Philadelphia, Lippincott, 1955

Dahlberg CC: Sexual contact between patient and therapist, in *Medical Aspects of Human Sexuality.* July 1971, pp 34–56

Davis JM: The mystery and the magic—a defense of "difficult" patients. *Postgrad Med* 74:265–266, 1983

Duldt BW: Anger—an occupational hazard for nurses. *Nurs Outlook* September 1981, pp 510–518

Geyman JP: Malpractice liability risk and the physician-patient relationship. *J Fam Pract* 20:231–232, 1985

Groves JE: Taking care of the hateful patient. *N Engl J Med* 298:883–887, 1978

Hutchinson HH: Why patients are angry. *J Med Assn State Alabama* May 1983, pp 14–21

Kahana RJ, Bibring, GL: Personality types in medical management, in Zinberg NE (ed): *Psychiatry and Medical Practice in a General Hospital*. New York, International Universities Press, 1964

Klein D, et al.: Patient characteristics that elicit negative responses from family physicians. *J Fam Pract* 14:881–888, 1982

Lipp M, Weingarten R: Hazards in the practice of medicine. *Am Fam Physician* 12:92–96, 1975

Martin AR: Exploring patient beliefs. *Arch Intern Med* 143:1773–1775, 1983

Nesheim R: Caring for patients who are not easy to like. *Postgrad Med* 72:255–266, 1982

Ramesar S, McCall M: Coping with the negative therapeutic response in psychosocial problems in family medicine. *Can J Psychiatry* 28:259–262, 1983

Ross CE, Mirowsky J, Duff RS: Physician status characteristics and client satisfaction in two types of medical practice. *J Health Soc Behav* 23:317–329, 1982

Siegler M: The physician-patient accommodation. *Arch Intern Med* 142:1899–1902, 1982

Southgate LJ, Bass MJ: Determination of worries and expectations of family practice patients. *J Fam Pract* 16:339–344, 1983

Steinweg KK: The disgruntled patient—how family practice residing programs handle requests for a physician change. *J Fam Pract* 11:257–260, 1980

Thomas KB: Seeing the schizophrenic. *Emerg Med* March 15 1980:25–32

———: Temporarily dependent patient in general practice. *Brit Med J* 1:625–626, 1974

Whitenack DD, McGaghie WC: Towards an empirical description of problem patients. *Family Med* 16:13–16, 1984

2

Tough Places to Work

To write prescriptions is easy, but to come to an understanding with people is hard.

—Franz Kafka

To ward off disease or recover health, men as a rule find it easier to depend on healers than to attempt the more difficult task of living wisely.

—Rene Dubos

Myths envelope our lives. The images we present to ourselves and to others are reflections of reality, but the reverse is true as well: reality is a consequence of what we perceive it to be.

In medicine, a large part of our self-perceptions is heavily influenced by the labels attached to what we do. Different specialties (dermatology, cardiac surgery, psychiatry) have different connotations for every one of us; and, similarly, the varying locations in which physicians practice their craft tend to carry emotionally laden meanings as well. Each has its own challenges and satisfactions.

The places discussed in this chapter have been chosen because their realities clash with our expectations, and because physicians, especially novices, can find them gruesome places to work in.

Ambulatory Care Clinics

From these principles Ford established the final proposition of the theory of industrial manufacture—not only that the parts of the finished product be interchangeable, but that the men who build the product be themselves interchangeable parts.

—E. L. Doctorow

The tough thing about outpatient clinics is that they are supposed to be so easy. In medical school, most clinical teaching focuses on the seriously ill, hospitalized patient, presumably with the tacit assumption that outpatient medicine is the simple stuff, something even the dumbest student in the class can master.

While family medicine departments sometimes shift the focus to outpatients, they often do this so unrealistically that the young physician is unprepared to become an effective member of a high-volume outpatient medical practice. In teaching students the laudable principles of comprehensive, family-centered, highly personal medical care, the dominant and growing reality of health-care in this country is selectively ignored; i.e., that physicians are increasingly working as employed dispensers of health-care for large organizations who cater to huge volumes of patients in an endeavor that policy makers view largely as a cost-containment mechanism.

The naive doctor and naive patient try to think of themselves as leading characters in a Marcus Welby drama, but institutional practices usually enforce different standards of behavior, largely derived from production-line design: get the patient in quickly, get him or her out quickly, don't waste supplies or time, don't make any major mistakes, and don't make too much noise.

In the days of third-party-supported, fee-for-service practice, the norm was to encourage the patient to want the best, to do everything possible for the patient, spare no expense, take whatever time is necessary, and charge the patient and his or her insurance companies accordingly. Obviously, such a system favored errors of commission over errors of omission. However, during the next decade, the economic basis of medical care will undergo dramatic change, and so will our styles of practice. The norm increasingly will be that the compensation for treating patients will be negotiated up front (through prepaid health plans, preferred-provider organizations, diagnostically related groups, or various entitlement programs), and the net income of the physician (or the organization employing the physician) will be the negotiated compensation minus the cost of providing care to the patient. In a deft stroke of the pen, the policy shift now favors errors of omission (omitted time, tests, procedures) rather than errors of commission, a dramatic change in practice style for most of us, and one which will require difficult adjustments for both doctor and patient. The trick increasingly is to change patients' attitudes from utilizing services "because they have already been paid for," to utilizing services "only when they are necessary." Simultaneously physicians must learn to temper the notion of "maximum therapeutic effort for everyone" and instead, learn to give good care efficiently, walk a tightrope, and balance both quality and cost.

The emphasis on cost-containment favors centralized planning and administration, and the economics of scale, which means that individually crafted medical care is going the same direction as the individually crafted suit of clothes. In terms of physicians, it means that if you are not now working for a large corporation or institution, you probably will be if you continue to practice for very many years.

Such organizations have numerous virtues, freeing the physician from many of the hassles inherent in running a private office—especially in these days of unending reports, forms, administrative procedures, practice marketing, and subtleties of personnel management, litigation, and the like—but they also pattern professional life in a manner that differs considerably from the starry-eyed expectations of most medical students.

Consider, for example, a primary care physician fresh out of a residency. In addition to being a competent M.D., she is also a nice person and widely perceived to be such. She spends time with patients, listens well, is compassionate, answers phone messages conscientiously, doesn't gripe when asked to see patients for absent colleagues, is generous in providing formal and informal consultations to physicians in other specialties, and is willing to "take on" patients whom other docs regard as a nuisance or unattractive. Here is a doctor heading for burnout if ever there was one.

Rapidly, she will accumulate a huge case load of ordinary patients, with a disproportionate share of "difficult" patients. Because her patients have to pay nothing (or only a token fee) to see her, they will tend to seek appointments often. Because she gives her time freely, she will always be running late, staying longer hours than her colleagues, and probably coming in when she is not on call. She will feel overloaded, pressured, and not in control of her practice, and it will begin to bother her that—in contrast to colleagues in a fee-for-service practice—there seem to be no immediate rewards for working harder and seeing more patients than the doc in the next office. Soon she will feel obliged to cut corners to handle the volume, and these at-first-small, compromises in her standards will bother her more than they would a less conscientious colleague. She will try to trim her practice of patients, but will find this far more difficult than it was accumulating them. If she is like many, she will then try the time-honored procedure of "turfing" (farming out patients to consultants—low back pains to orthopedists, migraines to neurologists, prostatitis to urology), but usually will find that the patients are turfed right back to their "primary doctor." It is at this point, when she feels helpless in the face of volume overload and sees nothing that will significantly alter the pattern of practice for years in the future, that she may start erecting emotional barriers for protection against patients and reconstructing personal standards of practice which seem more practical in the face of evolving perceptions of clinical realities.

We can also generalize a bit about the patients who come to see our young doctor. They all will have paid for treatment in advance—either through some prepayment program or an entitlement system—and will *feel entitled* to all benefits that are a part of their health-care program. Often the contractual relationship is between the program and the patient. While the patient wants a physician who is both competent and "nice," the identity of the individual physician is secondary. It is service that they expect, and the doctor is merely the agent for providing it.

To work in such a setting, most physicians need to develop a core set of skills that are somewhat different from (though not entirely unrelated to) those necessary in a typical fee-for-service setting. Of course, you need knowledge, technical ability and decisiveness, but also endurance, adaptability, a sense of humor, a basic liking for people, and a knack for both tolerating and understanding verbal abuse from patients and your administrators. The following specific skills are highly recommended:

1. *Rapid Bonding.* You need to be able to form a working relationship quickly. Learning how the patient wishes to be addressed and introducing yourself by name is helpful. Good eye contact is crucial. Establishing an emotional connection helps (e.g., "You have a great sunshine smile," or "You look like you're in pain") as does any common interest ("I see from your shoes that you're a jogger, too"). Find out what works for you and use it.

2. *Time Management.* Know how much time you can spend with a patient and use it effectively. Be sociable in manner but don't socialize extravagantly. Get into the reason for the patient visit promptly ("Describe what is wrong"), and retain control of the patient interview always, even while giving the patient time to contribute ("Is there anything that I might have missed or that you would like to add?"). Especially important are developing an ability to interrupt the patient without being rude, or without foreclosing important information, and comfortably drawing the patient's visit to a timely conclusion. The amount of time you have available (whether 10 minutes or 45) is less consequential than your ability to structure that time for the combined benefit of you and your patient.

3. *Assessing for Compliance.* Patients are no better listeners than their doctors; neither can remember much of what transpired between them 24 hours later. Likewise, doctors are no better at following orders than patients. (Do you fill out all paper work as you are instructed to do?) What is important is making sure that you and the patient are working toward the same goals and that the two of you agree about what is most important. After giving instructions, say, "Now tell me

what you are going to be doing for this condition until the next visit.''
Ask, "Do you see any major problems in follow-through here?''

4. *Planning for System Screw-Ups.* The rule is: The system will
screw up. Lab results will be lost. The patient's appointment for cardiac catheterization will get postponed interminably. Whenever you
solve one problem, another will rise to take its place. You need to be
the patient's advocate, but you can't take all the responsibility on
yourself. Enlist the patient's assistance: "If we screw up and you don't
hear from us, please call to jog my memory." Have some system for
maintaining continuity where it is needed, despite system failures (3" ×
5" cards, an urgent attention file, a periodic review ledger, et cetera).
Recognize that system failures are inevitable everywhere, not unique
to your particular setting. Don't feel a failure or that you work in a
lousy place when bad things happen. Just do the best you can.

Just as the system will screw up, so, too, will you and your colleagues. If you haven't yet made any errors that have resulted in death
or significant morbidity to one of your patients, you haven't been in
practice very long. As a human being you are limited by finite patience,
knowledge, skill, energy, understanding, and sensitivity, and these limitations will be much more obvious in a high-volume outpatient practice than they would be in a low-turnover academic research ward.
You need to be accepting and forgiving with yourself, and with patients
as well. Do the best you can, but recognize that your best will not reach
a uniformly glowing standard every hour of every day.

5. *Balancing the Workload.* You must constantly be making
choices. If I spend more time with this patient, I'll have less time with
others. If I open my heart with this unfortunate patient, will I have the
emotional reserves to carry me through the day? I want to do my share
of the work, but I don't want people taking advantage of me. I was
trained to be thorough, but I obviously can't be equally thorough with
everyone. I was told I must cure disease and relieve suffering,
but usually the best I can do is alleviate symptoms and chip away at
suffering. Priorities and realistic goals must be set and respected,
and you must know and maintain what is a reasonable workload for
you.

6. *Toughness and Sensitivity.* You meet a lot of angry people in
outpatient clinics, people who are angry at their illness, the life circumstances which made them vulnerable to that illness, and of course the
health-care system itself. You have to be strong enough to take a lot of
guff, but not so tough that you lose the human sensitivity that makes
the role of physician (and you) so special. Try not to interpret normal
illness behavior as "guff." Be grateful when patients ask questions or
voice a criticism. Say, "Thank you for bringing that to my attention."
Avoid becoming defensive and avoid adversary stances.

7. *Finding Soulful Satisfactions.* No matter what kind of medicine you practice, whether outpatient pediatrics or neurosurgery, after a while most of it gets to be routine. You can see only so many sore throats (or subdural bleeds for that matter) before they lose their excitement. Ironically, the problems you have been most thoroughly trained to deal with (the cardiac arrests, lumbar punctures, drug interactions) will probably be less taxing than the foibles of the doctor-patient relationship—complaints about you by patients, squeezing newly troubled patients into an already busy schedule, dealing with the emotional consequences of being the defendant in a malpractice suit, and so on. Eventually, most of us get less joy from coming up with esoteric diagnoses (usually, the tougher the diagnosis, the more grief in store for the patient), and instead get more satisfaction from comfortable mastery of routine tasks and from human interaction with patients and co-workers. If you are lucky, you will learn to take time with patients, not so much for their sake as for your own: helping them to feel better not merely because of your technical skills, but because of who you are as a person.

Major Surgical Wards

Hospitals are not safe for children or other living things.
—Adapted from an antiwar slogan

The locations discussed in the next few sections have several things in common. Individuals not accustomed to them usually admit to finding them very stressful, staff members tend to take pride in saying the places aren't stressful "once you get used to them," and each location tends to be extraordinarily busy, with staff dashing in one direction or another, attending to thousands of details, leaving little time for relaxed introspective discussion.

Most patients enter each of these locations with the hope that highly specialized technology will result in cure or significant remission. In each case the patient, far more than the average person admitted to the hospital, willingly submits to extraordinarily difficult and uncomfortable treatment procedures.

Every doctor loves the idea of the dramatic cure and relishes being a hero to patient and coworkers. Major surgical wards in particular attract physicians whose responsibilities give them a godlike quality, and both they and their patients often get trapped in a set of expectations that are doomed to failure. Each location requires that the doctor regularly discuss with the patient the possibility of death, yet the response of many patients, especially initially, is one degree or another of denial.

The doctor also is tempted to use considerable denial concerning the patient's prognosis; high expectations sustain the morale of such places, and high morale is essential to high performance. Nursing stations of such wards commonly have signs posted with slogans such as, "The difficult we accomplish immediately—the impossible takes a bit longer." This optimism, despite the regular if not daily contact with human suffering and deterioration, adds an air of unreality to the place, though no one likes to be confronted with such incongruity.

All major surgical wards are high-risk/high-gain places. Daily contact with agony recedes from conscious awareness in favor of the chance to achieve dramatic cures. Placid types seldom feel at home here. Aggressive outbursts occur more frequently here than any other place in the hospital. Irritation, anger, biting or sardonic humor—all are regular parts of social interaction, though most often directed at outsiders: "I told that hippopotamus in the lab to get those results STAT. Why the hell are they keeping us waiting?"

Since technical competence is so highly prized, confessions of inadequacy are customarily taboo. It's very difficult to say to a colleague: "I just feel inept in talking to the family about the prognosis, and I sure would appreciate your help." Instead, the temptation is to bluff it through or avoid the task completely, or order some subordinate to do it because "I haven't got the time."

However, I believe that confronting each of the issues discussed results in progressively less discomfort in future confrontations, and increasingly frequent personal satisfaction as a consequence of being a human as well as a technical resource to patients and families. Once you overcome fear of being overwhelmed by the human needs, your level of satisfaction in such interactions can reach astounding proportions.

Seeing death and suffering all around can, if you are fortunate, help you become more reflective about your own existence, but the process will require accepting personal mortality without being weighted down by its inevitability, and confronting the gap between ideal and realistic solutions without feeling inadequate.

Never underestimate the value of discussing matters of mutual concern openly with colleagues—not only technical matters such as the management of a tricky metabolic acidosis but the more complex problem of managing that acidosis in a sullen, slowly dying patient with an omnipresent, supersolicitous family—when you find the task flat-out depressing.

In addition to having all the problems of patients in general, surgical patients undergo an experience in which they totally relinquish control of their destiny to a surgical team, most members of which they do not know and perhaps have not even met. During this time when patients are completely unconscious, their bodies are invaded by strangers. Most patients approach surgery with high hopes; it is only these hopes that let them undergo the experience—patients dread not only the relinquishment of control, but also the hazard, the prospect of discomfort, and the expense.

Actually, most surgery is well tolerated emotionally by patients. That's not the issue. Whether psychological complications occur in 0.01% or 10%, you will still want to do what you can with all your patients to make the experience of surgery as minimally traumatic as possible. What is at issue is how you can do so with the least personal cost to yourself. Your chances of achieving this are best if you (1) incorporate a therapeutic patient-centered manner into your own personal style so it won't take too much out of you, (2) identify high-risk patients, (3) mobilize other hospital resources when the patient needs them, and (4) have some skills in reserve to bring to bear when necessary.

Individuals consent to operations with varying degrees of awareness. Externally, most patients appear reasonably composed and committed to the idea of a surgical procedure. Internally, however, there is often turmoil and fear, which raise the patients' levels of concern regarding many aspects of their lives, not only the surgical procedure. Because the prospect of operation in and of itself can be so anxiety producing, most patients are eager to believe in the surgeon's power to cure, and they find it reassuring to see the surgeon as someone who is special and omnipotent. The fear of mutilation, pain, and death is balanced somewhat by imbuing the surgeon with superhuman powers. Scratch the surface of such idolatry, and you will often find a very anxious patient.

Just as we can make some general statements about what the surgical experience is like for most patients, there are some broadly relevant descriptions of what it is like to be a surgeon. As with any such generalization, all the details are unlikely to be applicable to any given specific situation or person. However, if you are a surgeon, the odds are that you conform to a certain pattern. Your professional life is based upon a commitment to long hours and hard work. You are used to regular and intense pressure, and you take emergencies as a matter of course. You make your rounds to see your patients early in the morning, and you're often in the operating room until late. You are never totally free of your professional responsibilities; being a surgeon is almost as basic a fact to your existence as being a human being. You expect and are used to a training program which is hierarchically structured, often with a pyramid system in which each succeeding level of training becomes more and more exclusive. Competitiveness is a way of life, and you are used to an authoritarian milieu—when you tell someone who works with you, Do it! you expect that it will be done. You tend to be stoic by nature, and you are impatient with dependence. You prefer concrete to fuzzy concepts, and, consequently, murky emotions and interpersonal conflicts may be distasteful to you. Many of your patients' fears may seem irrational and ridiculous, and rather than being patient, it is easier to respond stereotypically; in (1) denial ("There's nothing wrong with him—tell him just to tough it out"), (2) withdrawal ("I haven't got time for that sort of stuff—maybe I'll just skip her on rounds today"), (3) compartmentalization ("The patient is obviously nuts—we'd better call in a shrink"), and (4) narcotization ("Give him demerol, thorazine, seconal, anything—we've got to get that man to shut up—I can't stand it any longer!").

Because of the nature of the surgical experience for most patients, and the nature of surgical work for many surgeons, major surgical wards tend to follow a fairly predictable pattern. Most dramatic to an outsider is the fact that the surgeon is hardly ever on the ward, and is therefore inaccessible both to patients and ward staff most of the time. When on the ward, the surgeon's contacts with the patients are likely to be brief, with time to deal only with certain kinds of essentials: wounds, intake and output, lungs, bowels, and infection. The surgeon is simply not available enough to really take responsibility for the patient's comprehensive care, and it is often difficult for the surgeon to find time to be able to discuss psychological issues with potential resource people. The human aspects of care come principally from the nurses and, occasionally, a social worker assigned to the ward; these individuals, however, seldom have real decision-making power and often end up feeling caught in the middle and needful of support themselves. Nonetheless, they have a unique potential contribution to the patient of human sensitivity and compassion, and they tend to take to their roles more enthusiastically when their value is recognized by the surgeon. When they do their job well, the surgeon is relieved of considerable responsibility for necessary aspects of patient care. Their ability to tolerate fear, weakness, and indecision on the patient's part will make the hospital milieu seem more supportive and accepting and consequently less frightening to the patient.

The special psychological tasks concerning surgical patients can be grouped in three categories: (1) preoperative assessment, (2) preoperative preparation, and (3) postoperative treatment and problems.

PREOPERATIVE ASSESSMENT

The function of preoperative assessment is to evaluate the patient's ability to cope with the psychological and physiologic demands of the operative procedure, and to identify the patient who is especially at risk for psychological problems. You will want to pay particular attention to factors that predispose to confusion, postoperative or otherwise. Your next task is to identify the patient's current anxiety level. Every patient should be expected to have some preoperative anxiety, however well he or she manages to cope with it. If there is absolutely no anxiety present, the postoperative period will probably come as a dramatic shock to the patient and be very frightening indeed. Any patient who has seen another suffering through the postoperative period has a realistic basis for fears. A useful means for assessing possible escalation of anxiety is to ask the patient how he or she has fared with previous operations. Was the procedure tolerated well physically and emotionally? If the patient has not had previous surgical experience, ask about the experiences of friends and family. Did the operations result in relief from suffering, or were they themselves a source of extended suffering? Ask in particular whether the patient or any acquaintance has had previous knowledge of or experience with the kind of procedure anticipated for the patient. Ask patients what their anticipation is concerning the outcome of surgery. If they defer to your greater technical expertise, say, "I'm not asking you to decide your prognosis yourself; I simply find it useful to know whether my patients are approaching an operation optimistically or pessimistically." Watch the patient's manner of responding. Don't necessarily take a verbal answer at face value. Does the patient look worried? Anyone with prominent anxiety will profit from special preoperative psychological support.

Allow the patient time to ask questions. Remember that questioning serves many functions in addition to that of simply gathering information. It is a means for patients to check on your knowledge, to reassure themselves that they are being cared for by someone who is competent and able. For many individuals, questioning represents a style of coping with anxiety; they will feel better when they have a few facts to help organize their thinking, even though you may not think that the facts are related directly to the patient's condition or the procedure he or she is about to undergo.

It's useful to ask yourself some questions, too, as you talk with the patients. You will want to assess the patient's ability to cope with the routine problems of the procedure. Is he or she someone who is likely to follow instructions to breathe deeply? To cough? To adhere to a dietary regimen? To ambulate as instructed? If the patient is undergoing a particularly difficult procedure, or the patient's physical condition puts him or her at risk for certain physical complications, does this patient have the psychological reserve to meet such extra stresses? How has he or she dealt with such stresses in the past? Are family and friends supportive?

Assess your own psychological state as well as the patient's. If you are performing an operation which you know well, and you are feeling confident and emotionally comfortable, the patient will be reassured by your calm and assured manner. If you are feeling anxious, either about the operation or your private life, the patient may sense your anxiety and find your presence not nearly so reassuring. It is also useful to assess your own motivation for performing the operative procedure. Are you comfortable with the indications for the operation, and the choice of the procedure as opposed to others? Are you operating solely out of conviction, or partly at the behest of the patient and/or colleagues? An operation is not psychotherapy; therefore, you need to know when you are operating partly for psychological reasons, either yours, your colleagues', or the patient's.

There are no psychological contraindications to surgical procedure. Even the grossly psychotic patient can undergo emergency surgery and often do quite well, particularly with appropriate human and chemotherapeutic support. However, any nonemergency operation should proceed only after you have carefully weighed the indications for the operation with potential risk factors. Patients who are at risk include the following:

1. The psychotic or paranoid patient. Any patient who is hallucinating or is grossly delusional will almost inevitably present management problems. Elective operations on such individuals should proceed with great care.

2. Patients with a previous history of decompensation under stress. Patients who haven't handled stress well in the past may not handle it well in the present. Find out if there were special circumstances that made the patient's previous experiences more difficult, and whether the patient has additional resources now which will help him or her to survive the impact of the contemplated operation.

3. Patients who are remarkably ambivalent about giving consent. If you or the patient's family almost has to twist the patient's arm in order to get the consent form signed, the whole procedure may be more trouble than it's worth. Anyone who is that ambivalent is going to have difficulty marshaling the psychological resources to cope with the stress of operation. Any procedure of any magnitude should be postponed until the patient can say with some conviction, "This is what I want for myself."

4. Patients who don't expect to survive or improve. Like the patient who is ambivalent about consent, those who sign freely but don't expect to benefit by a procedure, should seldom be operated upon. Most are quite depressed, and may be choosing an operation as a form of ritualized suicide. Such patients, if they survive the operation at all, often simply wilt away in the postoperative period.

5. The patient with unrealistic expectations, or one who is seeking surgery for "the wrong reasons." Persons who have unrealistic expectations of what surgery is likely to accomplish are setting themselves up to be disappointed. In addition, they are setting up the surgeon to be a failure, in that the patient perceives the surgeon to be promising to deliver something which is impossible. Being an unwitting accomplice in such endeavors not only will lead to disappointment for both of you, but also to inevitable iatrogenic complications and malpractice suits.

6. Patients with deteriorating relationships with the hospital staff. In order for patients to survive operative experiences satisfactorily, they must be able to work effectively with the hospital staff whose job it is to help them. When such relationships are marked by stress and anger before operation, the prospect is for continued stress and aggravation after operation. Whenever possible, operations should be postponed in such circumstances, or the patient should be on a different ward, or should have a different surgeon. In the absence of one of these alternatives, you proceed at your own risk.

7. The patient with multiple previous surgeries. Any elective procedure on such a patient should advance with care, particularly with reference to the patient's expectations concerning outcome. Thoughtfully assess the patient's psyche as well as the cardiopulmonary function. Are both you and the patient working toward the same goal? How realistic is it?

8. Patients with very high or nonexistent anxiety. As discussed before, these patients are high risk for psychological problems in the postoperative period.

9. Patients facing enormously invasive or mutilating operations. If you want to achieve not only a technical success, but a human success, assess the patient's psyche as carefully as bodily function. Make sure that he or she understands the consequences of the procedure being undertaken, and that he or she has the emotional and social support necessary to achieve a reasonably successful outcome, given what the physical limitations will be.

PREOPERATIVE PREPARATION

Getting the patient into an ideal frame of mind to face a major surgical procedure takes time, for the hospital staff and also for the patient, to assimilate what needs to be known and to develop a reasonable emotional perspective. Ideally, there are many individuals involved: the surgeon, the family doctor, the anesthesiologist, and people from the nursing staff of the recovery room and the intensive care unit to which the patient will be sent. Each one attempts to let the patient know what can be expected as a natural course of the prospective procedure and in the way of support from the staff involved. The patient has a chance to do some anticipatory coping so that what can be seen, heard, felt, and tasted later will not be frightening. The idea of involving so many individuals in this preparatory process helps to promote continuity of care during the course of the patient's operation and recovery, but there is also a danger of contradictory information from the various professionals involved. Each must speak only about areas of personal expertise, and the physician must encourage the patient to ask questions if divergent information has been received from the various professionals involved.

It's important to let matters come up naturally. First, broadly outline what the patient can expect. Then, sketch in the details, to the degree that the patient wishes or that you feel is necessary if you anticipate problems. Remember that you can never reassure the patient completely; these are fears based on reality.

Preparation falls into two categories; technical and emotional. Technical information includes most of the data that must be conveyed under the rule of informed consent. Again, the amount of detail depends upon the patient's level of interest and sophistication. Remember that many of the patient's questions may represent an attempt to gain some control of the situation and cope with anxiety rather than a desire for information per se. You will, of course, tell the patient about the general nature of the procedure, its likely duration, the length of the hospital stay, and the amount of time required for recuperation outside of the hospital. You will talk about the range of expected results, including the possibility or probability of scars and disfigurement. You may wish to use drawings and statistics to add clarity to your presentation, but watch for the emotional impact of these devices on the patient, as well as their effect upon his or her understanding.

You will want to be sensitive to what effect "being out of commission for a while" will have on the patient's life in general. While the patient may be under anesthesia for only a few hours, he or she may be obtunded or potentially delirious for a matter of many days. If, for example, the end of the month is only five days away, the patient may believe that he or she will be able to write the rent check and take care of bills after the operation. In fact, the patient might be better advised to take care of these details before operation or formally allocate such responsibility to someone else.

It's important to recognize, and to convey to the patient, that "some things we regard as routine will not be routine to you, things like tubes, drains, pain, helplessness, and passivity." Let patients know that you understand they are facing an emotional as well as a physical ordeal, and they will not be demeaned in your mind by acknowledging this to you.

The evening before surgery is a difficult time for most patients. Most feel totally alone. Unless given appropriate sedation, the patient may struggle with insomnia and nightmares. If you can, stop by to see the patient, however briefly, just to let him or her know that you care.

POSTOPERATIVE TREATMENT AND PROBLEMS

The principal human problems of the postoperative period—delirium, depression, dependency, the patient who refuses to get well, and pain—are dealt with elsewhere in this book.

In addition to the specific suggestions given under each of those headings in other chapters, your overall goal will be to restore the patient to psychological and physiologic equilibrium. You will want to help fortify natural coping styles, give the patient opportunities for control and mastery, and avoid coming into conflict over the details of treatment. You will seek to have the patient see you as an ally, not an adversary. In particular, you will want to be alert for signs of confusion, particularly in elderly patients, and provide whatever prophylactic or other treatment is necessary.

Special-Care Units

There are many varieties of special-care units: respiratory care units (RCU), cardiac care units (CCU), medical intensive care units (MICU), surgical intensive care units (SICU), burn units, neurosurgical units, et cetera. Whatever their designation, they are centers of technologic sophistication. Human and emotional needs usually take a back seat to technologic requirements—some would say that emotional and philosophic issues are even selectively ignored. Outsiders who wander in have their senses besieged by the sounds of mechanical life and the odors of disease, putrifaction, and even death.

Typically, special-care units are constructed as one large room, with everyone visible from the nursing station and often in sight of one another. If a patient is conscious, he easily can see others who aren't. There are seldom windows, pictures, flowers, or outsiders. Ungrounded, plug-in appliances such as TVs or radios often are forbidden. Usually family can come into the unit only when they are escorted, and often must be gowned, gloved, and masked. In many respects, the unit personnel may seem more like guards than helpers, and, for the patient, any contact with staff is seen as resulting in pain more often than not.

Virtually everyone is confined to bed and totally dependent upon staff for the bare essentials of daily life. One can't even defecate without assistance because the procedure requires a bedpan. All of this involves an exposure and neediness that most adults, certainly when healthy, would regard as humiliating. The more severe the illness or injury, the more immobilized the patient is likely to be, tied to the hospital bed by urinary catheters, intravenous tubing to one or both arms, centrovenous pressure lines, chest tubes, nasogastric tubes, monitoring devices, bed rails, and—perhaps for good measure—physical restraints.

It's difficult to describe the experience of being a patient in such a unit. Almost all are obtunded, because of the nature of their medical condition and because they are heavily medicated. So much is subjective and difficult to articulate, let alone to quantify. The inconveniences, noise, routinization of daily experience, exposure—all tend to become a blur in the patient's mind. Many blessedly have amnesia for much of their experience in such units. However, some things stand out with extraordinary clarity.

For example, the experience of dyspnea, so common in many such units, is extraordinarily vivid to the patient, and often difficult for the doctor or nurses to comprehend. Dyspnea is a totally subjective feeling, not definable in terms of blood gases or ventilatory capacities. It's a feeling of air hunger, of being smothered, of life drifting away always tantalizingly just out of reach. The major problem is terror, and a vicious cycle often develops: fear of dyspnea produces panic; the patient then struggles harder, resulting in increased breath hunger, which results in yet more panic. There is a tendency to avoid all activity, and the dyspneic patient will cling to a respirator like a toddler clutching a security blanket. It is often extremely difficult for staff to be patient with such behavior.

The doctor's role in such units often involves great responsibility, but also great authority. The emotional stresses are considerable, and increased by fatigue. Physicians in such roles often find it difficult to relate to the patient as a human being; in many ways the patient seems more a biologic preparation. Many physicians emotionally distance themselves from their patients, and consequently come across as aloof and uninvolved to those few patients who are alert.

The physician who is located full-time on a special unit is more like a scientist than like a "good old doc," and primary care physicians tend to feel out of place in such units. The enormous investment of time and energy and attention to detail is balanced by the chance for incredible achievements. When these exciting gains occur, the physicians radiate good humor and have the emotional energy to be extremely giving to their patients. When these gains don't occur, or, even more difficult, when there are a series of difficult losses, the physician is likely to feel irritable, personally responsible, sometimes even worthless and incompetent. The tendency is to give heroic amounts of energy and seek heroic achievements, which others less involved in the patients' care may regard as vain attempts to wrestle the patient away from the inevitable prognosis.

Because the patients are so sick in the special units and because the physician is so often absent, the hour-by-hour patient care falls heavily upon the nursing staff. Depending upon the specific hospital and personalities involved, special-unit nurses tend to perform roles that are legally medical in nature.

Even more than other nurses in a busy medical-surgical hospital, the intensive care unit nurse is someone who must take hard work and considerable responsibility in the stride of daily activities. The work is intense and emotionally demanding. Many patients are incontinent, unable to speak, and physically mutilated. Day-to-day activities often have a real blood-and-guts flavor to them. There is constant input on the nurses, and constant demands on their productivity and effectiveness. In addition to usual nursing skills, they must also be mechanics and technicians. It sometimes takes great commitment and personal character not to replace the nurse–patient relationship with a nurse–machine relationship, which often seems emotionally much safer. At least the monitors don't die, and faulty ones are easily replaced by ones identical in appearance and function. When a physician is not present on the unit, the nurse must often make split-second diagnostic and therapeutic decisions. A good intensive care unit (ICU) nurse is far better at reading electrocardiograms than most noninternist physicians.

Though such generalizations are not universally applicable, intensive care unit nurses have a reputation for being action oriented, bright, quick, restless, impatient—in short, they are great sprinters, but not so good at patiently enduring the long haul. The same qualities which give them great emotional strength at working with the acutely ill tend also to make them intolerant of patients with weak spirit, and intensive care unit nurses are often at their least effective with long-stay patients or patients with chronic problems.

Even more than in other parts of the hospital, the head nurse on a special unit is not only an administrator, but a highly trained professional who is likely to see students and interns on short rotations through the unit as intruders, and more trouble than they are worth. There is a tendency for nurses to "burn out" on such units and want to move on to something else. The turnover rate in personnel is generally high.

The principal human problems that occur on special units vary a bit, depending upon the type of unit involved (see Table 2.1). Specific problems are discussed in other sections of this book; for example,

Table 2.1 Human Problems Associated with Special Units

Burn Unit	Pain, disfigurement, chronicity
SICU:	Delirium, absent authority figures, a compulsion to act, denial in staff as well as patients
CCU:	Anxiety, the trauma of cardiac arrests, (Patients generally not as obtunded as on other units)
RCU:	Anxiety, dependency, chronicity, air hunger
MICU:	Numerous consultants and diffusion of responsibility, intellectualization, concentration on "scientific data" to the exclusion of the patient

"intensive care unit syndrome," or ICU psychosis, is discussed under Delirium. Though associated with intensive care units, this phenomenon may be a consequence of the kinds of patients sent to intensive care units, their ages, and the severity of their illnesses.

Dialysis Units

A hospital unit devoted to renal dialysis in patients with chronic kidney disease has many similarities to the special units just discussed, and I will avoid repetitious statements here. However, there are some significant differences, mostly related to the extended stretch of months and years that patients spend on such units and the extraordinary commitment they must make to dialysis as a way of life. A chronic renal patient shares many features with any patient with any chronic illness.

However, almost unique to the dialysis patient is the experience of being continuously dependent upon a machine, together with an extended "staff family" to sustain daily life. The dialysis machine and the old iron lung are both somehow symbolic of the triumph of machines over man: each is a huge man-made monster designed to replace or augment natural organ function. It is easy to underestimate the psychological cost of continued, necessary reliance upon such technologic achievements. The patient's relationship with the machine becomes the most important single relationship in his or her life. Old relationships are at least partially replaced, and the daily life of the patient is dramatically disrupted by spending, e.g., eight hours a day, three times a week in a highly technologic, but also startlingly intimate hospital unit that sustains life.

Virtually all renal dialysis patients react to their dependency with varying degrees of ambivalence, varying both from one another, and within themselves over time. Almost all have episodes of significant depression, and the suicide rate for dialysis patients is many, many times normal. Suicide, however, represents only one form of self-destruction: dietary indiscretions, voluntary withdrawal from dialysis programs, accident-prone behavior—all of these have elements of suicidal equivalency. Because of the prevalence of such behavior and the kinds of feelings that promote them, the renal dialysis unit staff must be able continuously to confront such issues.

Despite this, most chronic renal disease patients seem to do reasonably well, and there is little evidence of gross emotional maladjustment. Most experience a variety of problems, however, which become facts of life for them and other individuals who care about and for them. Most have some degree of organic impairment of their intellectual functioning. Almost all have a decreased stress tolerance, both psychological and physiologic. Many have complicated social and economic problems and are involved with a number of social agencies. All must learn to interact reasonably comfortably with the complex and time-consuming demands of multiple professionals, both in and outside the hospital.

The disruptions inherent in family life as a consequence of the extraordinary time and emotional commitment the patient must make to the dialysis program result in changes in social life and internal struggles with regard to personal commitment. There are very few families who are not jealous of the time that this patient spends on the unit. Many families feel a sense of rivalry with the dialysis program staff in competing for the patient's love, time, and attention.

Virtually all patients must struggle with the facts of their dependency on the machine and on the program staff. Struggles concerning independence/dependence result in seesawing behavior about myriad small details. Dietary restrictions and dialysis schedules are not simply technical details, they are daily symbolic issues in which the patient must decide how much control over his or her own existence to relinquish to technologic experts. The balance is often precarious. At times of powerlessness and frustration, staff are often surprised and irritated to see regressive behavior, including crying, whining, and what staff regards as childish demands.

As they lie in their beds or recliners, watching the blood course through the tubes, many or most dialysis patients ponder a recurrent question, "Is it worth it for me to live in this fashion? To whom? Myself? My family?"

One measure of the psychological impact of the dialysis program can be found in the patient's changing sexual activity and enjoyment. As patients go from uremia to dialysis, whether the patient is male or female, the pattern is to be less sexually active and to gain less pleasure from what sexual activity does occur. The causation for this is uncertain, but issues of depression, dependency, and divided commitment must surely play a role. Many dialysis patients are reluctant to talk about such issues. Preservation of their self-esteem remains a crucial issue for most, and they therefore feel particularly vulnerable when talking about such personal issues.

In addition to the vexing psychological problems, dialysis patients also face many complicated physiologic problems, each of which has its persistent and pervasive effects on morale and personal coping styles. These include continuous bouts of feeling sick, being anemic and weak, and having intercurrent infections, clotting of shunts, and bony demineralization and consequent susceptibility to pathologic fractures.

A unique aspect of life for the dialysis patient, relevant to all in at least some period in the course of their illness, is the possibility of transplant. Transplant represents not only an escape from the rigors of dialysis, but a glimmering chance for rebirth. Unfortunately the patient's hopes of transplantation are often not realized, and, even if transplantation does occur, many face a failure of the graft. For those in whom successful transplantation does occur, the overall adaptation is good. Most transplant recipients have some ambivalence about the donor, although this is rarely a significant barrier to the exhilarating sense of being born again. If the donor was anonymous, many have a continuing curiosity about the person whose death made possible their own life. Many feel a sense of guilt and wonder if their own desire for transplant in some way led to the death of another. If the donor was a relative, most patients struggle with feelings of indebtedness and, occasionally, guilt at the relative's increased vulnerability by virtue of being left with only one kidney.

Dialysis program staff struggle with the same issues that the patient does. Staff become heavily involved with the patients in a manner that has few parallels in an acute care hospital. Working intensely and intimately with a small number of patients, many hours each week, for month after month, creates a genuine sense of intimacy. Staff and patients often become friends over the years they know one another, and it is almost impossible to remain objective and dispassionate in managing the details of daily care. It's almost like being responsible for the health care of a roommate or dear friend. Only pediatric wards have as many birthday parties for their patients as do dialysis units. Staff must struggle with problems of overidentification with the patient, conflicts between dependence and independence, and "unrealistic" expectations of the patient. Denial is at least as much a problem for staff as it is for patients. Staff need to focus on the positive aspects of what they are doing and find it difficult to look at the psychological toll that dialysis dependence often incurs. Staff need to believe that things are going well for the patient and often are reluctant to recognize small clues that things are not going well. Staff are constantly challenged to find a comfortable balance of concern and professional distance.

Relationships within the dialysis unit often get so complicated that useful guidelines are difficult to come by. Nonetheless, some general principles may be helpful. Anyone working on a renal care unit must be aware of the importance staff and patients have for one another. If you spend any extended time on such a program, be sure to look after your own needs as well as those of the patient. Avoid getting the two confused when you are struggling with patient-care decisions. It's as important for you to have a satisfying life outside the hospital as it is for the patient. Avoid confusing your needs with his or hers. The inevitable intimacy that develops between patients and staff on renal units can be useful to both, but rarely without considerable emotional pain. Be alert for intense relationships between patient and staff and discuss them openly. All this may be very tricky indeed; rely on consultation and outside help whenever necessary. However much we want to make major decisions for the patient, the burden rightfully belongs to the patient. Such a task is difficult, since we are likely to find ourselves caring so much about what happens to each individual patient.

We must remain sensitive to the complex moral issues involved in dialysis programs. Just as patients ask from time to time "Is it worth it?" staff are likely to come up with the same kinds of questions when the going gets rough, or a particularly valued patient dies or becomes self-destructive. At such times, individuals are likely to question the worth of what the physician is doing, and to struggle with issues of cost versus effectiveness. While each such episode represents a crisis of personal values, it must also be seen within the broader perspective of implementing social values. At a time when our whole society is struggling with issues of how best to allocate our medical resources, each person is entitled to a personal perspective. Avoid rancorous confrontations at a time when a staff member is struggling with such issues.

Oncology Wards

Oncology wards are units designed to prolong the process of dying. The dramatic and exciting instances of cancer cures, as in the case of Hodgkin's disease, still remain the exception rather than the rule. However, the possibility of the dramatic cure helps to sustain morale on such units. The principal human problems on oncology wards are mutual dependence between the patients and staff, anxiety in the face of death, depression at the inevitability of death, and denial. Patients tend to deny the inevitability of their prognosis, staff tend to deny their inability to alter significantly the patient's course, and everyone tends to deny the difficulty of their task. I point out the prevalence of these emotions with some trepidation. None of us likes to have our unpleasant emotions shoved in our face; such a confrontation usually results only in more unpleasant feelings. Like our patients, it's much easier for most of us to deny our anxiety or to transform it into something that has more instrumental value: anger, aloofness, withdrawal. The frustrating inability to deal with such emotions directly, however, often leads to either guilt or scapegoating. We blame the patient for not following the regimen we have outlined precisely, we blame family for their lack of support or their inadequacy, and our consultants for their foolish consistencies and narrow focus.

It's hard dealing with our inadequacies to alter the course of one patient; unquestionably, facing a wardful of individuals who are dying takes an emotional toll. The principal human problem of oncology wards is maintaining equanimity in constantly dealing with death and impending death.

Many are surprised by how much ambivalence they feel, but the ambivalence explains a lot about the behavior of both staff and patients. Compassion draws staff toward the patient, to provide aid and comfort even when treatment is discontinued, but the repugnance of impending death simultaneously drives staff away, to protect themselves from impending separation and loss. Similarly, patients are often extremely ambivalent about staff and the cancer ward itself, which comes to represent both fragile hope and inevitable demise.

What I am focusing on here are the reactions in yourself (and other persons working on the oncology ward) that will tend to impair your effectiveness and consequently the satisfaction you get from your work.

Customarily, staff members on such units go through a series of stages, each of which is predictable and has certain characteristics. The first stage is one of high expectations and technical fascination. The scientist in the physician comes to the fore. Subtle differences between various neoplastic processes get great attention, and involved protocols are worked out for various subtypes of disease. Treatments are often daring, using high-potency chemotherapeutic agents, high-dosage radiation, and invasive surgical techniques. The admitted dangers of such procedures and the well-known side effects are rationalized in the hopes that the high risk will be balanced by the chance for dramatic gains. Occasionally such hopes are realized, often enough to sustain some people in their work. Some oncologists manage to sustain such therapeutic optimism for a professional lifetime. However, a significant percentage cannot, and go through a second stage.

The second stage is distinguished by discontent, feelings of worthlessness, a sense of failure, self-doubt and doubts about the field, and a profound sense of loss. The earlier omnipotent hopes and dreams now seem to be cinematic fantasies. The tendency is to become morose, often blaming others for our own failures to meet our expectations. Our earlier teachers seem like false prophets, and it's easy to scapegoat them or others. Sometimes the decision is to stop working with cancer patients, and some think about leaving medicine entirely.

For those who are lucky, a third stage of balanced perspective and personal comfort becomes possible. The limitations of scientific medicine are understood but not allowed to dominate one's consciousness. Chemotherapy and radiotherapy and surgical procedures become tools, sometimes appropriate and sometimes not, rather than panaceas. The pervasive suffering and the inevitability of death becomes an opportunity for a humane and personal contribution rather than a testament to one's own inadequacy. The new goal is to provide "safe passage" for both patient and family. The dramatic successes are still welcomed when they occur, but the day-to-day satisfaction comes from more humble achievements.

Wherever you are in your own evolution, many of your colleagues will inevitably be at different stages in theirs. Be patient and accepting with them and yourself.

Bibliography

Abram HS: Survival by machine—the psychological stress of chronic hemodialysis. *Psychiatry in Med* 1:37–50, 1970

———: Psychiatric reflections on adaptation to repetitive dialysis. *Kidney Int* 6:67–72, 1974

Birnbaum ML: High tech—low touch? *Crit Care Med* 12:1006–1008, 1984

Blacher RS: The hidden psychosis of open heart surgery—With a note on the sense of awe. *JAMA* 222:305–308, 1972

Coody D: High expectations—nurses who work with children who might die. *Nurs Clin No Amer* 20:131–142, 1985

Denour AK: Adolescents adjustment to chronic hemodialysis. *Am J Psychiatry* 136:430–433, 1979

Dugan NL: The professionalization of feeling. *Pharos* Summer 1983, p 41

Friedman E: Slicing the pie thinner. *Hospitals* October 16 1982, pp 62–74

Hackett TP: The psychiatrist's view of the ICU—Vital signs stable but outlook guarded. *Psychiatr Ann* 6:467–474, 1976

Levy NB: The hemodialysis patient. *Hosp Physician* October 1975, pp 21–25

MacGregor FC: Surgery—the patient and the surgeon. *Clinics Plast Surg* 9:387–395, 1982

Miller RW: Doctors, Patients don't communicate. *FDA Consumer* July–August 1983, pp 6–7

Moynihan RT, Outlaw E: Nursing support groups in a cancer center. *J Psychosoc Oncology* 2:33–44, 1984

Pochedly C: Pediatric oncology—The painful specialty. *Hosp Physician,* (June) 1978, pp 32–34

Schnapner N, Cowley RA: Overview—Psychiatric sequelae to multiple trauma. *Am J Psychiatry* 133:883–889, 1976

Tyson J, et al.: Effect of nursing staff support groups on the quality of newborn intensive care. *Crit Care Med* 12:901–906, 1984

Weiner MF, Caldwell T, Tyson J: Stresses and coping in ICU nursing— why support groups fail. *Gen Hosp Psychiatry* 5:179–183, 1983

Yancik R: Coping with hospice work stress. *J Psychosoc Oncology* 2:19– 32, 1984

Younger SJ, et al.: ICU visiting policies. *Crit Care Med* 12:606–608, 1984

Zawicki BE: ICU physician's ethical role in distributing scarce resources. *Crit Care Med* 13:57–60, 1985

3

Psychiatric Emergencies

The Crisis Situation

There cannot be a crisis next week. My schedule is already full.
—Henry Kissinger

If all else fails, immortality can always be assured by spectacular error.
—John Kenneth Galbraith

The man who makes no mistakes does not usually make anything.
—E. J. Phelps

A psychiatric emergency is a severe emotional or behavioral "disturbance" in a patient, requiring immediate attention. However, in the sense that urgency is a subjective sensation, there is a psychological component in all emergencies. A crisis occurs because the event arises suddenly, or comes to the consciousness of staff or family suddenly. The crisis results from the disproportion between the stress and the resources available to cope with that stress. Events which constitute an emergency in one setting may not be regarded as an emergency in another setting. For example, a convulsion on a dermatology ward is almost always regarded as an emergency, whereas it is usually regarded as a routine occurrence on a neurology ward. Whenever an emergency occurs, it is always important to ask, For whom is this an emergency? For the patient? For family? For staff? Who is feeling the stress, and whose resources are being overwhelmed? The answer may not be the patient as often as you would think.

Because emergencies are defined in part by the resources available to cope with them, emergencies tend to occur when and where such resources are skimpiest. For instance, a given event is most likely to become an emergency when you are short-staffed, or are tied up with other things, and consultation is not readily available. If any of these conditions were not present, the event might not have escalated to emergency proportions in the first place. It is the nature of the beast that emergencies occur when you least want them to, and, in the hospital, particularly at night and on weekends.

Emergencies invariably carry with them a certain set of expectations:

1. that the crisis situation will be promptly relieved,
2. that a physician will take responsibility for seeing that this is so, and
3. that the focus of all treatment efforts will be on the patient who "caused" it in the first place.

If you fail to meet any of these expectations, you can expect considerable static. For instance, if the emergency occurs in x-ray and you simply tell the x-ray technician to handle the problem, he or she will not like it and you are likely to hear more about the matter from the hospital administration. If you change the focus of your ministrations from the patient to the staff and do so without any subtlety, the staff won't like it. "He's the patient," a staff member will say, "not I." You should therefore approach all emergencies with a knowledge of the kinds of expectations inherent in the situation, and balance these with a variety of problem-solving techniques. You needn't do exactly what the family or staff implicitly or explicitly ask, but you ignore their expectations entirely at your own peril.

Many staff members, family, and observing patients respond to a crisis in a predictable fashion: there is usually considerable adrenalin flowing. Emotionally, people become scared, angry, frustrated, and impatient. Of course, the fewer emotional reserves possessed by staff, the more likely an emergency is to occur in the first place. When staff is tired and overworked, everyone is more likely to respond insensitively, in an angry or belligerent fashion, and make errors.

While you and others will have an understandable reluctance to get involved in situations for which you lack any formal training, you will nonetheless be able to make a useful contribution if you keep in mind certain principles, potential resources, and a sense of priorities about the tasks to be undertaken.

Effective crisis resolution stems from pragmatic and creative problem solving, and the passage of time. Virtually all crises are time limited. You must have confidence that the emergency will soon pass, and you will be able to deal with the sequelae at greater leisure. However, whether those sequelae are pleasant or unpleasant may depend on how you manage the emergency itself.

Inevitably you will make errors. That is a natural cost of facing challenges for which you have not been specifically prepared, but, with experience, you will find your skills improving. Your primary role in any emergency situation is to convert chaos to order.

To achieve that goal you have three principal resources: yourself, the persons around you, and drugs. Medications are listed last because they should be thought of last. Your primary resources in emergencies are human resources.

The most important key to the effective use of self is a confident awareness that you can in fact help. If you have that awareness and let it show on the outside, people around you will be reassured by its mere presence. Focus on your behavior as well as what you say. Your manner should be calm, confident, and professional. Control your voice: keep the tone reassuring and modulate the volume so that you are neither shouting nor speaking so softly that the patient or others will have difficulty hearing. If you don't already know the patient, introduce yourself by name and professional title ("I am the physician on call this evening."). Ask the patient what his or her name is. Do not use the patient's first name unless he or she indicates that this is acceptable. In the event that you do use first names, stay away from diminutives: call the patient Tom or Thomas, rather than Tommy. You want to come across as someone who is respectful in manner and who is available as a stabilizing resource in a difficult situation. Avoid any comments that would tend to diminish the patient in his or her own eyes. If the patient seems to respond positively, you can further establish contact by touching. Generally, the patient in a crisis situation will feel more in control if he or she touches you rather than vice versa. Say, "Take hold of my hand," but don't push if the patient doesn't wish to, and allow him or her to let go at will. *Go very slowly* with touching when the patient appears frightened of you or is paranoid or potentially violent. In that event, maintain a respectful distance.

In addition to yourself, another line of resources for use in psychiatric emergencies is the people around you, including family, nursing staff, other patients, and other hospital or clinic personnel. Each person chosen to assist should assume a role similar to that you would assume yourself if you had the time and the inclination to spend it with the patient. The ideal person is someone who is stable, known to and liked by the patient, and calm, alert, and forthcoming by nature. The intent is to supply a reassuring and gentle restraining presence. Human beings are infinitely preferable to physical restraints. Not only are they more easily modified, but they are much less likely to seem punitive and therefore much less likely to have the paradoxical effect of increasing agitation rather than modulating it. Each individual chosen by you to spend some time with the patient should be instructed to be accept-

ing toward the patient's release of emotion. The idea is to help nudge
the patient in productive directions rather than confronting or directly
restraining.

A third resource, the use of medication, has a dual usefulness: a
specific chemotherapeutic effect (e.g., antianxiety or antipsychotic),
and a device for buying time. In the latter circumstance, the drug is
used to so sedate the patient that the emergency is attenuated. While
such a function is never listed as a formal indication for the use of any
given drug, it nonetheless remains a common reason for using psychochemotherapeutic agents in the clinical setting.

TASKS AND PRIORITIES

1. Your first task in any psychiatric emergency is to stabilize the
environment and obtain control. You must deescalate the emergency
from the crisis situation to one your staff can handle in stride. You
want to combat panic and to buy time so that important decisions can
be made with prudent consideration. First, you must gain everyone's
attention. If this doesn't happen by virtue of your simple presence, say
in a commanding voice, Hold it. What's going on? Draw attention
away from whatever is upsetting the assembled multitude and focus
decision-making powers upon yourself. If a great number of people
have accumulated, tell some of them to go away, "All right, there are
too many people here. Everyone not immediately involved with this
patient's care please leave the area." If there are only one or two
persons present, send someone to get more help. The effect is to have
a manageable number of people present and to centralize decision
making.

2. Assess the situation. For whom is this an emergency, and why?
Try to find a reliable informant. If you don't know the patient, and if
time allows, consult the medical record so you will have some detailed
information about this patient's background. If you can't consult the
chart, try to acquaint yourself with the patient's medical history by
asking some responsible person who knows the patient. Why is this
happening now? Regardless of the patient's strengths and weaknesses,
what is the stressful event that overwhelmed his or her coping powers?
On initial impression, are your efforts best focused upon the patient?
The family? The staff? Or on some other individuals?

3. Establish contact with and assess the patient. If you are not
already familiar with the patient, ask him or her for a brief history.
What is happening from the patient's point of view? Say, I would like
to help, but I don't know you and I don't know your circumstances.
What is happening? Help me to understand how things look from your

point of view. At the same time, perform a visual physical examination. Does the patient look toxic? Are there any gross neurologic signs? Does he or she look sick or well? Without formally putting the patient through a detailed mental-status exam, assess the level of the patient's intellectual functioning as discussed in chapter 5, Confusional States. Is there any evidence of organicity? What seem to be the psychological and environmental contributants to this emergency?

4. Sort out any urgent factors. Is there any immediate risk of the patient's hurting himself or herself or others? Where does the sense of urgency lie? Is the patient pressuring you to make a decision, or is the staff? Do you feel pressured yourself? Do you think involuntary detention is in order?

5. Assess resources. Does the patient have inner sources of strength that you can tap into? Almost everyone does. Don't write someone off simply because he or she is partially decompensated. Is there anyone on the ward among patients or staff whom this patient trusts? Ask the patient. Are there family or friends around who would be willing to assist? In your thinking and as you speak out loud, ask, "Who is there who can help *us?*" Let your thinking and your wording place you as an ally of the patient with the two of you seeking to find a solution together.

6. Begin treatment and/or ask for a consultation. Remember, you are treating the emergency rather than the underlying circumstances that perhaps led up to the emergency. Definitive treatment must await further evaluation. Mobilize human resources and use medication as you think best. Specific treatments will depend upon the precise nature of the problem; examples are included in the sections to follow.

7. Focus on the response of others. Remember that an emergency is seldom an emergency for the patient alone. If various members of hospital staff were very much caught up in it, they will need your support and an opportunity to talk about their experience. If you have neither time nor the inclination, see if co-workers or supervisors or consultants can fill this role. Don't forget the family. If they were present and knew about the emergency, they are most likely afraid for the patient and afraid for themselves. The emergency may well have arisen out of some family interaction, and they may have a great deal they wish to talk about. See to it that someone is available for them.

8. Follow through. Remember that you have thus far only treated the emergency, and not necessarily the basic conditions which spawned it. See that these are attended to. Be particularly sure to look after any organic factors that may have lowered the patient's ability to cope with stress. If in doubt, do a careful physical exam when the stability of the patient's condition allows you to do so.

The Psychotic Patient

Insanity in individuals is something rare—but in groups, parties, nations, and epics, it is the rule.

—Friedrich Nietzche

Why is it when we talk to God, we're said to be praying—but when God talks to us, we're schizophrenic?

—Lily Tomlin

The treatment of the acutely psychotic patient advocated here fits within the mainstream of American psychiatry. However, my definition of what constitutes psychosis is idiosyncratic and far more restricted than you will read in most medical texts. My own view is that the terms *psychoses* and *psychotic* are used far more often than they are warranted and largely serve as pejorative labels for behavior and people we find bewilderingly different, unattractive, and frightening.

Conventional definitions of psychosis emphasize impairment of reality testing, communication, and ability to relate to others, such that the individual in question is unable to meet the ordinary requirements of daily living.

I find all that distastefully fuzzy, subject to enormous personal distortion and consequently of little practical value. In struggling to understand how things look to persons of other cultures or even of differing experiences within my own culture, I find that objective reality too frequently blurs with cultural bias, and reality testing evades precise definition the more closely we examine it. Many statements by public figures or, indeed, even private remarks by ordinary individuals, suggest that much "communication" is designed to obfuscate rather than clarify. You can therefore measure impairment of communication only if you know a person's intent, and you can know *that* only if they tell you and you trust what they say. And how in God's name do you judge how one person "relates" to another? What precise standards can you use that would be equally applicable to so-called psychotics, your divorced colleagues, your friends who get tense and angry when talking to their parents or children, or you, for that matter, when you are struggling to "relate" to a demanding and critical patient?

My bias also stems, without doubt, from my own personal experiences and those of my friends and from the individuals I encounter in my environment (which happens to be San Francisco and Northern California). I know many people who have made unconventional choices and live highly individualized lives. Their minds and perceptions work well for them, or at least as well as they do for most people, and I continually learn from them. Yet I know that some of my psychiatric and other medical colleagues would label similar idiosyncratic life-styles as not merely weird or eccentric, but as psychotic. They do so without malicious intent but because such a tendency is fostered by convenient professional terminology and a cultural tendency to describe behavior in psychiatric terms.

With that background, let me proceed with my own definition of psychosis. A psychosis is a condition or state in which an individual experiences blatant hallucinosis or gross delusions, such that any reasonable person, layman or professional, when faced with the same information about the individual in question, would concur that hallucinations and/or delusions were present. Hallucinations are false sensory perceptions without apparent external stimuli, and delusions are persistent false beliefs which are not shared by an extended social or cultural group. Upon knowing these definitions, a layman should be able to discern their presence or absence. Though an inexperienced interviewer may be less able to elicit information concerning what is going on in the patient's mind, once having that information available he or she should be able to decide as well as any more experienced professional whether the patient's thought content constitutes hallucinations or delusions.

The able clinician can elicit information concerning hallucinations and delusions by observation and third-party reports, by careful interviewing, and by psychological testing.

A patient actively conversing with an unseen presence is probably hallucinating. A woman in an empty room recoiling from illusory monsters visible only to herself is probably hallucinating. A man who says he is the living embodiment of the spirit and flesh of Sir William Osler, Adolph Hitler, or Jesus Christ is probably delusional. In each case, there are potentially other explanations, however unlikely. The conversational isolate may be memorizing lines from a play in which he or she is to perform. The woman struggling with the monsters may be awakening from a vivid nightmare, prompted by a bad conscience, and will recognize her nightmare for what it was as soon as she is fully awake. The "delusional" patient may be on an extended metaphor for the sake of illustrating some obscure, but personally meaningful point, or he may just be putting you on. The best way to find out is to ask the patient about what you have observed or someone else has reported to you. However, you can never really know what goes on in someone else's mind. You can only interpret what you see and what you are told.

The second method for revealing the presence of hallucinations is via the patient interview. Ask the patient, "Do you see or hear things that other people think aren't there?" If the patient has never had hallucinations, he or she will either simply say no, or won't know what you're talking about. Patients who have hallucinations will understand the meaning of your question and usually either respond positively or become elusive. If the patient asks "What do you mean?", elaborate: "Do you ever have the feeling that some unseen presence is talking only to you?" One of the difficulties in eliciting information about "crazy" thinking is that you often have to sound pretty peculiar yourself in order to succeed. If you stumble over questions such as those I have outlined, don't be surprised. Most people do. However, overcoming your awkwardness with a patient who has experienced hallucinations will pay useful dividends.

Be careful about overinterpreting patients' responses. Some perfectly sane individuals will respond to what seems to them to be a peculiar question by becoming playful: "Ah, yes, doctor; I see beauty about me where others see only ugliness." If you are uncertain whether the patient is pulling your leg, explain why you are asking the question: "I know the question sounds peculiar, but I'm trying to find out whether you have ever had any hallucinatory experiences." Most individuals respond forthrightly to such a direct approach. If the patient gives some indication of having had hallucinations, ask what they were like: "Who was talking? What did the voices say? Were you told to do anything specific? How real were the voices? And how close did you come to acting upon what was said? What was seen? Was the experience frightening or pleasant? Are the hallucinations like old friends, to be looked forward to, or are they frightening?"

Picking up on the evidence of delusions during a patient interview can be a great deal more difficult. Many individuals can seem perfectly sane unless you tap directly into their delusional system. Even when all the information about the delusion is readily accessible, it is often difficult to get broad agreement that what one person considers a gross delusion is in fact a gross delusion to others. For instance, most of us would regard as delusional a person's belief that he or she spends part of each day on another planet. Similarly, we would regard as delusional a person's statement that his or her sexual energies are all controlled by beings from outer space. However, if the same person were to describe the same phenomena by saying "I really find how much I turn on depends upon my astrological sign and what's happening with the moon and stars," many of us would regard that as peculiar, but not necessarily crazy. In order to find out about a person's delusions, you have to be sensitive to clues that possible delusions exist, and then ask follow-up questions. All this information must be interpreted circumspectly. Most people's belief systems, whether derived from religion or the study of ethics or fantasy, get a little fuzzy around the roots, and have a sense of unreality about them to anyone who treasures a different belief system.

When you suspect that a person is genuinely delusional, but you have difficulty eliciting details by interview, consider psychological testing. Though rarely convenient in an emergency, projective testing, particularly in the hands of someone who is interested and capable, can be extraordinarily revealing in terms of picking up delusional systems. You will also have the advantage of a professional opinion other than your own in sorting out what may be some very complicated information.

Once you have ascertained the presence of hallucinations and/or delusions and decided that a psychosis exists, you must remember that the term describes a process or a state of being, not a person, even though certain persons may have a predisposition to psychosis. Most often, psychoses are time-limited, rather than enduring, even in patients for whom they are recurrent phenomena. Compare the relationship between schizophrenia and psychosis to that between diabetes and ketoacidosis. The first term in each pair describes a population (schizophrenics and diabetics) which is particularly prone respectively to the conditions (psychoses and ketoacidosis). However, at any given time, most diabetics do not exhibit ketoacidosis, and most schizophrenics do not exhibit psychoses. In addition, both ketoacidosis and psychoses occur in populations other than diabetics and schizophrenics.

There are several advantages to such a restricted definition of psychosis. First, you have only to deal with the notions of hallucinations and delusions; the more vague concepts of reality testing and ability to relate and communicate are irrelevant. The criteria are precise and readily comprehensible to a person of average intelligence even without specialized training. Second, this precision minimizes room for observer prejudice, and the application of the label therefore becomes somewhat less a simple function of the observer's bias. Third, the very restrictiveness of the definition favors false negatives over false positives. You may end up calling some people sane who could be labeled psychotic, but you are far less likely to label somebody psychotic whom others of us would regard as sane.

Once you have labeled somebody psychotic, particularly acutely psychotic, what do you do about it? You must, of course, take into account any feeling of crisis in the environment, and deal with that as suggested earlier in this chapter.

The cornerstone of treatment of acute psychosis is the prompt use of antipsychotic agents in sufficiently high dosage. The style of treatment is exactly the same as the approach used in digitalizing a patient with congestive heart failure, or giving colchicine to a person with acute gout. You give an initial dose to test for hypersensitivity or idiosyncratic reactions, and—if there are none—then continue to give the medication on a prearranged schedule until the desired therapeutic effect is achieved or toxic effects appear. If the patient has had the medication in the past and tolerated it without difficulty, you needn't be quite so cautious with the first dose.

Since drugs often obtund the patient and confuse the diagnostic picture, medication should be given only if the diagnostic picture is already clear, or the patient's behavior constitutes a significant hazard to himself or herself or to others, or represents an intolerable strain on family or staff. In the latter event, recognize that you are treating the patient when at least in part it is the family or staff who are in need of your assistance.

Once you have decided to give medication, the next decision to make is which agent to use. Assuming there are no known hypersensitivities or specific contraindications in your patient, the major considerations stem from how much sedation you decide is necessary or tolerable, and which kinds of side effects will be least troublesome in your particular patient. The most sedating antipsychotic medications are the aliphatic and piperadine phenothiazines, and the least sedating are the piperazine phenothiazines and the butyrophenones. I will give examples from each group shortly.

In general, stay away from tablets (which the patient can stick in the cheek or under the tongue instead of swallowing, and in any event are decomposed and absorbed slowly) and intravenous administration (in which the most serious adverse reactions are likely to occur). Instead, use oral liquid concentrate (perhaps mixed with juice or water) or intramuscular injection.

The following dosages represent reasonable amounts for an adult of medium weight and reasonably good overall health. Decrease the dosage with decreasing weight, extremes of age, debilitated condition, and especially in the presence of diseases of the liver, heart, or kidney.

You should develop reasonable comfort and facility in using one sedating and one nonsedating antipsychotic agent. The following merely represent two examples of the breed.

1. Chlorpromazine (THORAZINE). Begin with a dose of 50 to 100 mg intramuscularly or orally in a liquid concentrate (some people would say these doses are high), and repeat the dose every 30 to 60 minutes until you have reached a total of 600 mg. Some individuals have tolerated up to several grams per day, but you should proceed beyond my recommended maximum only with caution. Most of the side effects of chlorpromazine are bothersome rather than dangerous, including drowsiness and a variety of anticholinergic side effects such as dry mouth and blurred vision. The principal potentially serious side effect is postural hypotension, which may present a major problem if the patient is up and around, though is seldom a problem when the

patient is bedridden. Use this drug with great caution in the elderly. They need whatever cortex they have, and the sedating effect of chlorpromazine may obtund them sufficiently to add a component of delirium to their condition, making them appear more confused with medication than without.

2. Haloperidol (HALDOL). Give 5 to 10 mg intramuscularly or orally in a liquid concentrate, and repeat the dose every 30 to 60 minutes up to a maximum of 60 mg. Haloperidol has little sedating effect and is therefore to be preferred over chlorpromazine in elderly patients. The principal side effects are bothersome anticholinergic effects such as dry mouth and blurred vision. Extrapyramidal side effects are common but not universal and rarely represent a reason for discontinuing the drug. Simply treat these manifestations with an antiparkinsonian agent of your choice; e.g., biperidin, 2 mg (AKINETON); benztropine, from 1 to 2 mg (COGENTIN); or trihexyphenidyl, from 2 to 5 mg (ARTANE). When needed at all, these agents are usually necessary for the first few days of treatment only, along with the antipsychotic agent. Beware of their additive anticholinergic effect in vulnerable patients, however.

Once you have achieved an acceptable therapeutic effect with whatever drug you have used, add up the total amount of drug given and consider this total figure as your "digitalizing dose." Most patients do very well on a daily dose which equals from 50% to 75% of their digitalizing dose. Some patients need no antipsychotic medication at all after the acute episode is over. Most patients who do need to be maintained on medication can usually suffice with a single daily dose after the first few days.

Do not rely on drugs as the sole means of treatment. Protect the patient from harming himself or herself or others. If the hallucinations are frightening, he or she may resort to wild activity in a vain attempt to run away from them. Delusional instructions have led patients to jump out of windows, to pull apart operative incisions, and to ingest all manner of materials.

Whenever possible, attempt to "talk down" a psychotic patient. Counteract panic, disorientation, paranoia, suicidal depression, and a fear of loss of control. Tactics for approaching all of these problems are discussed in other parts of this book.

Be understanding of staff, family, and other patients who witness the psychotic outburst. Very few nonpsychotic individuals enjoy spending time with psychotics. Such contact can be upsetting and confusing, even to experienced clinicians. Be patient with the staff and let them know you understand when they are thrown off their stride by the emergency.

After the acute emergency is over, take some time to sort out contributing factors. Perceiving the psychosis, especially as defined here, is usually easy, but sorting out toxic or other organic contributions is sometimes more challenging. If you have any doubt, call in a consultant.

Checking for organic contributants need not alter your initial management of the psychosis per se. However, you will wish to treat the coexistent organic factors too, for example, by discontinuing prednisone or by initiating oxygen where hypoxia may be contributing to a psychotic delirium. Do a thorough physical and neurologic exam whenever the patient's behavior permits it, or immediately if the patient's physical condition shows obvious deterioration, such as in a subarachnoid hemorrhage.

The Suicidal Patient

> There is only one truly serious philosophical problem, and that is suicide.
> —Albert Camus

> Amid the miseries of life on earth, suicide is God's best gift to man.
> —Pliny the Elder

If the quotation by Pliny the Elder rankles a bit, you are certainly not alone. Most physicians reflect the values of a society that now maintains that suicide is both a manifestation of mental illness and a senseless tragedy. Suicide has been defined as a clinical problem. The historical and romantic view that suicide is a logical solution to unbearable stress seldom offers much consolation to a physician faced with a patient who is blatantly suicidal. Regardless of the patient's values and expectations, society expects us to act to protect the patient's life, our medical co-workers share that expectation, and we usually feel the same way.

This section avoids defining suicide in terms of any philosophic or psychopathological framework. Rather our approach is, Given that we have clinical responsibilities in the event of suicidal behavior on the part of patients in our care, what are the best practical approaches for discharging those responsibilities?

Genuine suicide attempts are rare in doctor's offices or general medical-surgical hospitals, and even these are seldom successful. However, when suicidal behavior does result in death, the results are devastating to medical personnel as well as to the patient's family and friends.

When suicide attempts do occur, they most commonly represent impulsive acts, associated with stress, anger, and loss of emotional support. They may have little relationship to the severity of the patient's physical illness. In fact, if a hospitalized patient is vulnerable to feeling suicidal, an attempt is especially likely to occur in anticipation of discharge from the hospital, at a time when major questions concerning the nature of the patient's physical illness have been resolved. Whenever possible, it is best to anticipate suicidal behavior rather than having to deal with it on an emergency basis.

Risk factors for suicide have been well worked out and offer some reliable guidelines. The patient who is most likely to commit suicide is a male, over the age of 45, who lives alone, or feels alone, and uses alcohol to excess. He is depressed, has a history of impulsive behavior (perhaps a previous suicide attempt), finds it difficult to request or accept help, and has suffered a recent loss. The latter may be a person (e.g., a spouse through death or divorce), a thing (e.g., a job or a place of residence), or a dream or fantasy (e.g., the hope for renewed good health via a kidney transplant).

Any patient with a history of previous suicide attempts should be assessed for a current suicidal potential. Some people's lives have been dominated by self-destructive behavior, including serious drug abuse and a history of accident proneness, and you should not assume they will take a sabbatical from such behavior simply because they are physically ill.

Nurses who work with the hospitalized patient are usually the first to recognize suicidal ideation. They may discover that a male patient, aged 50, had a father who committed suicide at the same age. They may pick up on nonverbal communication, such as the patient's giving all his possessions away. They may note an abrupt lessening in the depth of the patient's depression, when the patient's circumstances have stayed the same or gotten worse, and sense that the patient has resolved his depression by deciding to end his life.

Ultimately, the best way to assess the patient's suicidal potential is to ask the patient. You should certainly ask any patient who appears depressed, and you should ask any person who scores high on the risk factors enumerated above.

Most people, especially when depressed and as they grow older, think about suicide from time to time, especially with all of the media stressing that it is perfectly normal for people to think about suicide. How, then, do you separate the thinkers from the doers? Again, ask the patient. "How close have you come to killing yourself? Have you thought how you would do it? How imminent is the possibility?" In particular, it is useful to know if the patient has deferred the idea of suicide unless or until something happens.

How does the patient act when talking about suicide? Does he or she seem concerned? Matter-of-fact? Relieved? A good rule of thumb is this: so long as the patient worries about his or her suicide potential, I don't have to. If a patient admits to thinking about suicide regularly and is not concerned about being preoccupied in this way, that is the time for me to begin to worry.

In order to discuss the topic of suicide comfortably with patients and to deal successfully with imminent suicidal behavior, you have to understand your own feelings about the subject and have reached some measure of comfort with them. Medicine is dedicated to healing and saving lives, and therefore suicidal behavior often seems antithetical to the role most physicians see for themselves. Some physicians regard the expression of suicidal thoughts by patients as a direct affront: "Hell, he knows I'm responsible for him here in the hospital; the least he could do is wait to commit suicide until after he leaves the hospital." The response of some physicians may also be based upon a projection; i.e., How would I behave if I were in the patient's shoes? If I had cancer and my family walked out on me, would I respond with grim determination? Would I become hopeless? Would I act according to my ethical and religious upbringing? It is impossible to make an accurate prediction of what it would be like to be in the other fellow's shoes, but a recognition of our feelings and values is helpful for putting in perspective our responses to the patient.

Often the physician's response depends upon whether the suicidal thoughts and expressions are seen as "manipulative" or evidence of "true despair." The former often produces anger towards the patient, withdrawal from the patient, and occasionally punitive responses. The latter is much more likely to elicit an empathic readiness to help.

Whatever your perspective about the existential merits or tragedies inherent in suicidal behavior, you have to get a clear sense of the limits of your responsibility in the matter, the limits of others around you, and the limits related to the patient's own responsibility for self-determination. Once you decide that a patient is imminently suicidal, your approach will be based upon social policy as embodied in laws. A physician must act so as to comply with society's requirements; the benefit to the patient is often incidental. In almost all jurisdictions, you must seek a psychiatric evaluation and/or commit the patient.

If the danger of suicide is present but not imminent, if no psychiatric consultation is readily available, or if commitment is for some reason impractical, you must take a somewhat different approach. Your strategy is to protect the patient, to provide support, and to buy time.

Protection of the patient must be geared to the specific patient in question, the most likely method of suicide, and the characteristics of the environmental setting. The most common methods of suicide in a general medical–surgical hospital are ingestion, slashing, and jumping.

The latter is by far the most dangerous, its damage most difficult to salvage, assuming the patient has jumped from a significant height. Protecting the patient therefore involves having a responsible person present as an observer-protector, keeping the patient away from windows, and (where practical) removing the patient from the uppoer stories of the building. Whether or not you should search the patient for potential implements of self-destruction is a matter upon which there is no general agreement. My own preference is to not search the patient, but instead say, "I need to know if you have anything with which you may injure yourself. I don't want to search you. I want to be able to trust you, and have you be able to trust me. Do you have anything on your person or nearby with which you might injure yourself?" If the patient denies having such implements, but I don't believe the denial, I say: "I would just feel more comfortable if you show me that what you say is so. I would appreciate it if you open up your bedside stand, and show me that you have nothing in your pockets."

The next step must be based upon the understanding that emergencies occur when stresses overwhelm resources. You must therefore work to diminish stresses and augment resources. Try to find out what the precipitating stresses were. If the patient is currently in the hospital, was an operation or discharge scheduled? If so, cancel or postpone whatever was on the agenda. Sometimes the stresses are facts of life and cannot or should not be minimized. In that event, say: "You're right, those are terrible burdens and stresses. It's understandable that you are so upset. However, I hope you will believe that your ability to confront these problems will improve with time."

Focus on augmenting resources, both internal and external. Try and see what the patient feels and says and does in some positive light. If the patient says, "Life seems worthless to me; I don't want to live any more," respond by saying, "I understand; those are perfectly natural feelings under the circumstances; I'm glad you're expressing those feelings rather than keeping them inside." Also provide external support. If you can, give some of yourself: "I haven't got much time, but I'd like to sit here with you for just a little while to let you know that I care." Ask someone else to sit with the patient after you've gone, to monitor the patient's feelings, to provide support, and to look after the patient's safety. A companion, particularly someone whom the patient likes and trusts, is the most important resource you can provide. Oftentimes a friend or a member of the family can do this far better than medical personnel. Assess what resources are available, and be sure to utilize them.

The most important goal in most emergencies is to buy time, and to attentuate the crisis so that details can be dealt with calmly and thoughtfully and with more thorough understanding. In order to buy time, it is most useful to get a commitment from the patient that he or she is willing to stay alive for some period of time, for twenty minutes, a few hours, a day, whatever. Say, for example, "Another patient of mine is seriously ill and I must attend to him. Will you promise to stay alive until I come back?" In order for such a commitment to be meaningful, there must be an alliance between you and the patient. The personal appeal works only when you have a personal relationship with the patient, and he or she cares enough about anything to care about you and the relationship with you.

Ultimately, unless you are very sure of your own skill in handling such situations or unless you know your patient very well, you'll be well advised to request a psychiatric consultation. Often, psychiatric hospitalization is not only the most sensible alternative, it is mandated by law.

However, no matter what you do or don't do, you must always accept the possibility of failure. Most physicians, sooner or later, have one or more patients who commit suicide. That is always a grueling experience, and there is little to be done to remove the anguish from the situation. There is almost always a mixture of guilt over things not done, resentment directed at the patient and perhaps others around, and a personal sense of failure. If we were very involved with the patient, we feel a personal sense of loss. If we were not very involved with the patient, we may ruminate about Why didn't I do more?

If a patient of yours does commit suicide, consider conducting a psychological autopsy. Invite anyone else who may have been involved with the patient, and ask a psychiatric consultant to discuss the case with you. Like any other clinical conference, you will want to review the history, the patient's presentation for treatment, your examination, and the course of treatment. You will of course want to consider alternate approaches you might have taken, and you will want to learn from the case what you can. In many such situations, the most important lesson is that there was nothing else to do. The psychological autopsy, however, provides an opportunity for ventilation and mutual support, and those are useful in themselves. You must understand suicide as a representation of an individual's anguished inability to find his or her own sense of purpose and meaning. It is impossible to understand what goes on in the depths of someone's soul, particularly in retrospect, and it is therefore impossible to say with any assurance what should or should not have been done. Whatever else you do or do not do in a psychological autopsy, avoid trying to fix blame. If you start looking around for things or persons to blame, there is no end to what you will find. Ultimately, blaming demeans those doing the blaming as well as the blamed.

The Violent Patient

Violence is as American as cherry pie.

—H. Rap Brown

The lion and the calf shall lie down together, but the calf won't get much sleep.

—Woody Allen

I'm not sure how it was that violent behavior ever came to be defined as a medical or psychiatric problem, but it has. Many physicians and nurses who would never think of confronting a potentially violent person on city streets will decide to do so within a clinical setting. The gist of this particular section is that violence is a human responsibility rather than a medical responsibility, though your human potential for averting violent behavior will be enhanced by the special role that you enjoy in health care setting by virtue of your being a physician. As long as you can keep the potential for violence from erupting into actual physical confrontation, it makes sense to do so. However, blatant physical violence is a police matter, not a medical matter. Do not allow any omnipotent fantasies on your part to prevent you from recognizing that distinction.

Assaultive behavior is actually rare despite myths to the contrary. Though a patient may threaten harm to the family or others, and the situation may seem difficult and even dangerous, actual violence seldom ensues. Your responsibilities in the matter are to deescalate violence and avert physical confrontation whenever possible, and to recognize as early as possible situations beyond your capabilities.

We will discuss in the next chapter that prediction of violence is fraught with hazards. Nonetheless, you must take seriously any patient's threats that he or she intends to harm someone. The best indicators of violence are a past history of violent behavior and what the patient says, although you must recognize that the overwhelming majority of people who threaten to kill do not in fact do so.

Most violence derives from anger, and it would therefore be useful to review tactics for approaching the angry patient. Violence is usually also focal; that is, a potentially violent individual wants to hurt someone in particular and will not harm others unless they pose a direct threat. Sometimes violent behavior is simply symbolic of the patient's frustration and rage. There is no wish to hurt anyone, simply a wish to put one's fist through a door or break a chair for the momentary freedom from controls and the coexistent feeling of power and effectiveness. Again, individuals like this do not represent a danger to others, except for those who inadvertently get in the way. Violent behavior is almost always situation-specific behavior; that is, once the individual is removed from the person or situation that provoked the violent feelings in the first place, there need be little concern that the violence will spill over and harm those not directly involved.

Though violent behavior occasionally derives from pathologic intoxications, psychomotor seizures, postictal furor, and other pathologic states, violence is not usually a pathologic phenomenon.

A physician faced with a potentially violent patient has responsibility first as a human being and second as a physician. I won't preach to you about your human responsibility; your own view of that subject is certainly as valid as mine. As a physician in a clinical setting, like it or not, part of your role is as an agent of social control. You have a responsibility to use reasonable means to protect the patient, others, and yourself.

Effective treatment of the potentially assaultive patient depends upon an odd mixture of fear and trust. You will be afraid if you are dealing with a potentially violent patient and if you have any sense. If you are afraid, do not pretend that you are not. Don't be reluctant to say "Mister, you scare the hell out of me." Show that while you are afraid of physical assault, you can handle your feelings and express them openly.

This is a useful approach because you must assume that the patient is also afraid. Patients do not usually become violent in a clinical setting unless all other means of dealing with the situation as they see it have failed. If they become violent, they do so to make an impact and they know of no other means of achieving such a goal. In telling the patient you are afraid, you acknowledge that impact, obviating a resort to violence. In acknowledging your fear in a calm and confident manner, you also help the patient have confidence in you as a potential resource. If you were simply to crumble before his or her eyes, you would be of no potential assistance at all. However, if you were to take the opposite approach and become confrontive and potentially violent yourself, you add to the patient's fear and frustration, deprive the patient of a measure of control in the situation and, in many cases, add to the likelihood of violence. To reduce that likelihood, you must help the patient have trust—either in you as a person, or in the situation— such that he or she can be confident that events will evolve in a comfortable manner without the need for violence.

Avoid behavior that the patient may interpret as threatening: rapid movements, clenched fists, or anything else that may be interpreted as a direct physical confrontation. If you can do so with any comfort at all, try sitting down. Say: "I told you, you scare the hell out of me, but I'm not interested in any physical confrontation with you, and I'm going to sit down to prove it."

Try to avoid meeting with the patient in a small room with only one exit. If the patient is afraid, he or she will become more so if you block the exit. If *you* are afraid, you will become more so if the *patient* blocks the exit. It is best to get both of you in a place where there is room to move and where neither of you feels threatened by the other's location in the room.

Set limits, but do so in a nonpunitive fashion. Let the patient understand that you are in command of yourself, but you have no desire to oppress him or her. Allow the patient to have a feeling of control too, with some sense of an opportunity to make meaningful decisions. Say: "I am a physician. I am here to help you, but I need your cooperation in order to do it. If you become violent and hurt someone, the issue will become a police matter and you and I will no longer be able to work things out ourselves. We cannot permit violence here. I need your help so that the two of us can work things out together. Will you help me?"

Explain in a matter-of-fact way everything you do, especially if the patient is paranoid.

If violence ensues anyway, don't be a hero. Again, try to avoid a physical confrontation. Say in a loud, clear voice: "Stop that! That kind of behavior simply will not be tolerated here!" Get other people nearby, but not oppressively so. If the patient feels suffocated by numerous people around, he or she may become more violent. The obvious presence of hospital security officers or police within the patient's view not only will tend to subdue the patient but will help allay your fears and make you a more effective agent of control. However, you must speak clearly and confidently and authoritatively if you wish to continue in control of the situation instead of transferring that responsibility to the police officers.

If physical force is absolutely necessary, a good rule is one person for each limb, plus one person. Each individual involved should be reasonably strong, in good health, calm, nonpunitive, and (it is hoped) experienced in dealing with similar patients. If you do not have enough force to physically subdue the patient, you will do far better with one small woman who appears nonthreatening to the patient than with two medium-sized and combative men whom a male patient thinks he just might be able to tackle.

After the immediate threat of violence is over, assess the matter in greater detail and more carefully. What circumstances led up to the episode? Does the patient constitute a continuing threat to others? If in doubt, ask for psychiatric consultation.

Bibliography

Anderson WH, Kuehnle JC, Catanzano DM: Rapid treatment of acute psychosis. *Am J Psychiatry* 133:1076–1078, 1976

Donlon PT, Tupin JP: Rapid "digitalization" of decompensated schizophrenic patients with antipsychotic agents. *Am J Psychiatry* 131:310–312, 1974

Donlon PT, Hopkin J, Tupin JP: Overview—efficacy and safety of the rapid neuroleptization method with injectable haloperidol. *Am J Psychiatry* 136:273–278, 1979

Dubin WR, Hanke N, Nickens HW: *Psychiatric Emergencies*. New York, Churchill Livingstone, 1984

Fernando S, Storm V: Suicide among psychiatric patients of a district general hospital. *Psychological Med* 14:661–672, 1984

Gift TE, Strauss JS, Young Y: Hysterical psychosis—an empirical approach. *Am J Psychiatry* 142:345–347, 1985

Gorton JG, Partridge R: *Practice and Management of Psychiatric Emergency Care*. St. Louis, Mosby, 1982

Hanke N, *Handbook of Emergency Psychiatry*. Lexington, MA, Collamore Press, 1984

Lowenthal U: Suicide, the other side—the factor of reality among suicidal motivations. *Arch Gen Psychiatry* 33:838–842, 1976

Reich P, Kelly MJ: Suicide attempts by hospitalized medical and surgical patients. *N Engl J Med* 294:298–301, 1976

Ripley HS: Suicide in general hospitals. *West J Med* 130:408–410, 1979

Rofman ES, Askinazi C, Fant E: The prediction of dangerous behavior in emergency civil commitment. *Am J Psychiatry* 137:1061–1064, 1980

Slaby, AE, Lieb J, Tancredi LR: *Handbook of Psychiatric Emergencies* (2nd ed) New York, Medical Examination Publishing, 1981

Stevenson I: Do we need a new word to supplement "hallucination"? *Am J Psychiatry* 140:1609–1611, 1983

Urbaitis JC: *Psychiatric Emergencies*. Norwalk, CT, Appleton-Century-Crofts, 1983

Walker JI: *Psychiatric Emergencies*. Philadelphia, Lippincott, 1983

Wexler DB: Seclusion and restraint—lessons from law, psychiatry and psychology. *Intl J Law Psychiatry* 5:285–294, 1982

Yesavage JA, Werner PD, Becker JMT, et al: Short-term civil commitment and the violent patient. *Am J Psychiatry* 139:1145–1149, 1982

4

The Patient's Right
to Self-Determination

Procedure is the essence of the law; the substantive result is usually not as important to lawyers as whether it was reached by the correct mechanism.
—Maurice DeG. Ford

All honour to those who have the courage of their convictions. I include in their numbers the patients who have gone out of hospital against my advice. I have seen them pioneer the modern treatment of . . . many diseases. I would pay special tribute to the casualties; but the funny thing is I can't remember any.
—Anonymous

What facts are relevant when the patient's right to self-determination is in doubt, and how do you assess the patient in such circumstances? What are the legal criteria for depriving a patient of the right to self-determination? What are the reasonable alternatives to taking such formal legal steps? Beyond the legal definitions, it's helpful to develop one's own personal philosophy with regard to these troublesome problems, because, as a practical matter, one's own values, sense of responsibility, and motivation will influence what happens to the patient almost as much as any specific legal strictures. Finally, because the matter is so complex and abounds with heavy moral, legal, and philosophical overtones, I hope we all can try to be reasonably accepting of philosophies that may differ from our own.

Often, when treatment of the nonconsenting patient becomes an issue, physicians feel caught on the horns of a dilemma: assault versus negligence. You are damned if you treat the patient and damned if you don't. Fortunately there are very few situations in which these concerns are necessary.

Often in such circumstances, the physician caring for a patient refusing treatment decides to request psychiatric consultation. In my experience, the psychiatric consultant in such a situation is asked to arrange one of four possible outcomes. The preferred result is usually that the psychiatrist will help the patient overcome his fears, so that the patient will accept the treatment the physician would like to render—perhaps because the psychiatrist is expected to be more understanding and have more time to devote to the process than the doctor requesting the consultation. Often the implied message is: "This patient is obviously a nut; you can talk to nuts; you convince him!" An alternative goal is to declare the patient incompetent "so we can do what we have to do" despite the patient's objections. A third is to declare the patient competent "so we won't get sued for not treating." The accurate implication here is that refusal of treatment by an informed and competent adult relieves the physician of responsibility for not performing a specific treatment. Finally, psychiatric consultants in such circumstances are sometimes asked "to get him (or her) out," either voluntarily by getting the patient to leave, or involuntarily by commitment, "so we won't have to struggle with the problem any longer."

In choosing an alternative that would limit the patient's right to self-determination, I encourage you to ask, Who cares? The family? The physicians? The social workers? The nurses? This question is neither facetious nor fractious. There are many professional and cultural biases that influence our thinking and push us towards certain conclusions.

Some harsh and stereotypic examples of this are the following: in requesting a court-ordered operation, "it's obviously because the surgeons want to cut." In initiating commitment procedures for a confused old man, "it's just because the social workers want to mother the patient." In questioning an older woman's competency to manage her own affairs, "it's because the family wants to steal the old lady's money."

Fortunately, there are more sanguine perspectives on "what's in it" for the person who cares. Better feelings result all around when one can find laudable components to other people's motivations. It is a fact, fortunate or not, that health professionals tend to equate human health and human welfare. A person's welfare therefore is best looked after by ensuring that health is optimum. Some believe that the most fundamental right of the patient is that of adequate treatment, and therefore this should take precedence over an absolute right to liberty. That's not my view, but I can understand it without needing to attribute malice to a person who holds that perspective. An overall cultural perspective that tends to influence the matters discussed in this chapter is the tendency to value doing something active rather than doing nothing. Intervening, albeit against the patient's will, is therefore seen as preferable to doing nothing on the patient's behalf (except respect the right to self-determination).

Though I will generalize about legal criteria concerning issues of self-determination, statutory law varies considerably from state to state, and courts at various levels will interpret even these laws still more broadly. Obviously each physician must be acquainted with the circumstances in local jurisdictions. In general, courts afford enormous weight to predictability. Can the court know for certain what would happen if it fails to act? Once you enter the judicial arena, the patient's medical record will become the key document, and you must rigorously detail all information that is relevant to the issue at hand. You must be absolutely clear about the medical facts in the case, as well as the natural history of the patient's disorder, and how that history would be affected by all treatment alternatives, including nontreatment.

As a practical matter, if in doubt, turn to an attorney for advice, but don't be surprised if the attorney hasn't researched the matter any more thoroughly than you have. Frequently, your most important source of guidance will be your own philosophy about the nature of your relationship with your patient and the relative responsibilities each of you carries for the patient's ultimate welfare.

In contrast to outright depriving a patient of constitutional liberties, a much more insidious infringement upon the patient's rights to self-determination stems from ambiguous and nebulous decision-making processes. That is, the patient simply does what he or she is told without realizing that there are any decisions to be made. Usually, the decisions are obscured by local policies, and often enough we don't think about alternatives that might be available to patients in other locales. For example, you diagnose a patient as having a specific neoplasm and automatically place the patient on the treatment protocol used at your hospital. The nature of the protocol may depend more heavily on the relative clout carried by your departments of oncology, radiotherapy, and surgery than on any objective assessment of the literature. Often, individuals passing through the system (for example, patients and house staff) have little or no knowledge of such decision-making processes. No wonder some patients seem paranoid.

At another level, a patient sees you in your office for what looks like a strep throat. The doctor up the block would automatically order a throat culture, and the doctor across the street would ignore the laboratory's possible contribution and simply prescribe penicillin. What would you do? What percentage of physicians would present the two alternatives to the patient with a brief outline of their pros and cons, and leave the decision to the patient? Not many, I'll bet.

Informed Consent

An understanding of the term *informed consent* is crucial to an understanding of the other issues discussed in this chapter. The importance is not only legal—for instance, getting the patient to sign the appropriate slip of paper—but also philosophic and ethical, appreciating the patient's role as an active participant in his or her health care and destiny generally. Treatment must proceed only with the agreement of the person being treated. The key elements are the patient's right to self-determination and your respect for that right.

Informed consent obviously has two principal components: information and consent. The physician is required to give the patient sufficient information so the patient can make an intelligent decision. This includes the basic facts of the patient's condition, as well as the relative advantages and risks of the treatment being suggested and alternate forms of treatment, including nontreatment. Any potential complications must be explained in lay terms, and at the very least, should give the patient some rough idea of the risk of death or serious bodily harm. The more elective the treatment or procedure, or the more novel or experimental, the greater the doctor's duty to inform the patient.

The physician is excused from the duty to inform when: (1) the risks are minor and generally known (e.g., drawing blood), (2) the patient already knows or should know (e.g., the patient facing surgery is an ICU nurse), or (3) the information would so alarm the patient as to constitute bad medical practice. The latter, however, called "therapeutic privilege," is a very fuzzy exception and one on which you should not act lightly. When you withhold information "for the patient's own good," the risks and the reasons for withholding should be disclosed to the closest relative, and a note explaining the use of therapeutic privilege should be placed in the medical record.

The "consent" portion of informed consent requires that the patient's agreement with treatment must be competent, voluntary, and understanding. Here is where psychiatry and psychiatrists come in. While *voluntary* and *understanding* are terms which can reasonably be assessed by a layman (though with perhaps varying interpretations), *competence* is based upon a legal determination which relies heavily on psychiatric evaluation.

There are three major exceptions to the requirement for informed consent: minors, unconscious patients with emergency requirements, and the mentally incompetent.

When possible, the patient should be informed well enough in advance so that he or she has a chance to weigh the information in a reasonable fashion and consider the alternatives.

It must be understood that consent, once freely given, may also be freely withdrawn. Once withdrawn, the fact of the previous consent is no longer relevant.

While the doctrine of informed consent is a compelling one, I think it would be a mistake to concentrate on the legalisms to the neglect of the human interaction involved. Often, it is not so much what you tell the patient as how you tell the patient. If you are a persuasive person and you approach a frightened and dependent patient in an empathetic manner, you can get him or her to sign almost anything. Under the circumstances, your respect for the spirit of informed consent seems more important than simply adhering to the requirements of the law.

It is also true that standards about informed consent vary considerably from one state to another. As of 1983, about one-third of the states have established judicial standards for informed consent (the most "liberal" self-determination standards are found in California); whereas in the other two-thirds, a patient who asserts that a doctor gave inadequate information must *prove* that the information given was inadequate when compared to the standard of the medical community.

However, the key point is that there is a growing belief that it is the prerogative of the patient and not the physician, to determine in what direction the patient's best interests lie. Loss of liberty is the most severe penalty a civilized society can inflict upon an individual. Every safeguard must be given to the citizen at risk—in this case, the patient. One has to be a patient oneself, in a situation where patient and physician disagree, to appreciate this to the core of one's being.

Fortunately the courts have been paying increased attention to the patient's right to self-determination. Many physicians become defensive in face of the courts' decisions, because the implication is that patients cannot trust health care facilities, including their doctors. At least part of this stems from the increased complexity and bureaucratization of sophisticated technologic treatment. This defensiveness by physicians is fortunately balanced by an increased respect for patients' right to determine their own medical destiny. Physicians are coming to value this right as much as they desire to treat any given condition in any specific manner.

The facts are these: Any competent adult has an absolute right to refuse treatment. Any competent adult has an absolute right to refuse to be examined by any particular individual. Any competent adult has an absolute right to refuse to participate in teaching activities. The latter is incorporated into the Patient's Bill of Rights that serves as a set of guiding principles for all JCAH-approved (Joint Commission on Accreditation of Hospitals) hospitals.

As much as such rights are respected and valued, they impose certain hardships on the health care givers. Many physicians feel legally vulnerable when they fail to treat disease in the manner which they feel is most advisable. However, this concern is usually disproportionate to the risks as long as the physician operates within the doctrine of informed consent and documents that he or she has done so. There is also the frustration of having to stand by and watch a patient persist in what we regard as self-destructive behavior. That frustration can only be balanced by a respect for the patient's right to self-determination.

There are other possibilities. One is to "use the system" to compel the patient to accept the treatment that you think is best; and, as we shall see, this can be acceptable in certain narrowly defined situations. Another approach is to find alternatives to judicial intervention that will help the patient come closer to getting the kind of treatment you recommend.

We have multiple alternatives.

MANAGERIAL

Though this is rarely a first choice, you may sometimes choose, together with the patient's family, to make certain basic decisions for the patient in his or her behalf. This approach is more likely to be used in a situation where there is an ongoing relationship between the doctor, the patient, and the family; and much less useful in the complex medical center where doctor and patient are new to one another. But there are of course exceptions, and this option may sometimes be taken.

ADVERSARY

The adversary position, as used in legal process, merely means that each party will present the strongest possible case for one's own position. A more widely used meaning of the term, the one used here, refers to each party approaching the other as an opponent or enemy. When doctor and patient are in direct conflict, both may sometimes gain the satisfactions that accrue with righteous indignation. Direct conflict has the further advantage (if it's one you seek) of impelling the patient to precipitously leave your care. However, it just as frequently results in complaints, lawsuits, and a sense of failure on the part of all concerned. Each party views the other as being in error or malicious, and one or the other usually loses face. Certainly as a general policy, adversary relationships are a poor foundation for a professional life based upon mutual respect. As a practical matter, approaching one patient in an adversary fashion is usually communicated to other patients as well (on the ward, if the conflict occurs in a hospital setting, or in the waiting room or other examining rooms of your office or clinic), and it seldom produces much lasting satisfaction for any of the parties involved.

SHAM VOLUNTARINESS

It is sometimes possible to get a patient to voluntarily accept a preferred course of treatment simply by leaving him or her no alternative. A classic example is the following: "If you don't go into the hospital voluntarily, I am afraid I will have to sign commitment papers on you." We can talk the patient into accepting one procedure by using scare tactics to outline risks associated with alternate procedures. We can frighten impressionable or dependent patients into doing what we want by making clear our disapproval of the alternatives. We can threaten to withdraw from the case if we don't get our way, or we can bludgeon the patient and family with guilt-inducing tactics: "Of course, it's your decision, but I can't imagine that many parents who truly loved their children would choose a course other than the one I'm suggesting."

COLLABORATIVE

Ultimately, if we are to work together with the patient, we have to find shared premises. If you can't get the patient to agree with you, find something on which you can agree with the patient. Do whatever you can to maintain a therapeutic alliance. Seek to understand and respect the patient's reservations. You may be able to reach him or her more successfully by giving additional information, but also consider conveying that information in a *different* manner that the patient will find more comfortable. You may wish to enlist such allies as family, friends, ministers, and other medical personnel. Say "Though I don't think I would choose the same course in your place, I of course don't know, and I respect your right to choose for yourself." Let your manner say, "Given our differences, how can I help?"

Competence and Incompetence

The issue of competency raises the question of who will or will not be allowed to live as a responsible and free human being.

Incompetence may rarely be inferred, despite the fact that the patient is diagnosed as having a psychotic disorder, or is on phenothiazines, or even if the patient is confined to a mental institution against his or her will. Generally we talk about competence as though it were a global phenomenon—either a person is competent or incompetent. Adults are assumed to be competent to make decisions regarding their own welfare, but when competency is questioned, the questions are usually directed at a selected area, such as competence to care for one's own financial affairs or to execute a will (testamentary capacity). It may sometimes be useful to document present competence by examination, e.g., to witness that the patient is of sound mind at the time that he or she is executing a will. Certain types of competency are not assumed, but are subject to determination by a governmental or quasi-governmental body: competency to practice medicine, to drive a car, to handle radioactive materials, etc.

Competency and incompetency may be selective. For example, a patient may be unable to handle financial affairs, but may be quite capable of deciding which medical treatment is in his or her best interest.

The assessment of competency may be very much affected by the mesh of examiner and subject. For example, if you have traveled in a foreign country, you know how easy it is to appear incompetent to persons whose language you don't speak. The examiner's exam may be flawed by personality conflicts, social or cultural differences—or simply by hostility of the patient toward the whole process.

The basic criteria for determining competency, however, are identical, regardless of the specific act being considered. The individual in question must have sufficient intellectual capacity to: (1) understand the simple nature and purpose of the act itself in lay terms—"My consenting to medical care means that you can't do it unless I say okay"; (2) comprehend the basic facts of the case—"You say I have this disease even though the doctor I saw before said I had another disease"; (3) recognize alternative ways of acting—"The choices are an operation or radiotherapy or both or neither."

Though we are talking about competency and incompetency in a medical setting, declaring a person incompetent in any respect is a judicial process which depends upon expert opinion, usually submitted as documents. In our culture, the expert opinion usually comes from the psychiatrist, though often the opinion of others, especially other physicians, will suffice. In general, most psychiatrists and other physicians find the role of declaring someone incompetent distasteful. There is an implied arrogance and presumption in one person's sitting in judgment of another's right to self-determination. Nonetheless, there *are* individuals who are grossly disabled and unable to make sound judgments for themselves. Where one draws that line depends upon personal judgment as well as the facts of the case. Just as there are hanging judges, there are psychiatrists and other physicians who are more or less likely than their fellows to find a patient incompetent.

In making a determination of competency, any psychiatrist whose assistance you ask must satisfactorily perform a series of tasks.

1. Determine the nature and degree of the patient's impairment.
2. Make a judgment concerning the specific competence in question.
3. Put that judgment in writing.

4. Advise you how to proceed in providing the patient with medical care in a manner consistent with the law.

The psychiatrist therefore must have a comprehensive knowledge of the relevant law *in your state*. I personally have found such knowledge extremely hard to come by. Mostly it is tucked away in nooks and crannies of civil code in ways that make it inaccessible to many lawyers.

The process of determining the "nature and degree of impairment" depends upon both an adequate history and examination. In practice, a formal diagnosis tends to make little difference; describing and documenting the impairment is what is important. It is customary in competency exams to review the patient's history with special attention to general level of functioning, reasoning capacity, and emotional stability, with special effort at documenting episodes of decreased functioning (e.g., confusion). It is further customary to examine in the patient those attributes of intelligence that are crucial to judgment and decision making. These include (1) perception (sensory impairment, language skills); (2) cognition (attention, concentration, memory sufficient to process data, thought processes logical though not necessarily correct); and (3) defense mechanisms (denial, paranoid projection).

In my experience, all such information, while giving a fuller view of the patient as a person, is superfluous to the specific issue at hand and sometimes leads to unwise decisions. The essentials are: Does the patient understand what he or she is being asked to do? Does he or she have a basic comprehension necessary to make a decision? And does he or she have a reasonable understanding of possible alternative modes of action?

One persistent problem in determining competency is the fluctuating nature of intellectual capacity, especially in elderly persons who are physically ill. They may be perfectly adept at one time, marginal at another, and clearly impaired at a third. How does one decide in circumstances where a patient has clearly lucid intervals? I don't know, except that I never label a person incompetent unless he or she is persistently so; and, if in doubt, I opt for the patient's right for self-determination. Whenever competency is determined in nonemergency situations, more than one evaluation session should take place, and the history should be obtained from more than one person.

I must reemphasize that the psychiatric judgment of incompetency is *never* the sole requirement for depriving someone of the right to self-determination. The latter requires a formal judgment by appropriate judicial authority that can decide for itself how much weight to lend to the expert's opinion. As a practical matter, as we will discuss later in more detail, a finding of incompetence by the psychiatrist or perhaps any physician, may be sufficient to render life-saving treatment against the patient's will in emergency situations.

Refusing Treatment

A necessary corollary to the rule of informed consent is that the patient has a right to refuse treatment. Freedom is only meaningful if it allows people to take actions that others or even they themselves may later regard as foolish mistakes. The patient's basis for refusal of treatment may be rational or seemingly irrational. It may be based on fear, a contentious personality, a desire to frustrate medically oriented relatives, or even paranoid or delusional thinking. In most jurisdictions, the patient has a right to be as idiosyncratic or eccentric as he or she wishes.

It therefore stands to reason that refusal of treatment by an informed, competent adult relieves the physician of responsibility for not treating. However, if the patient is clearly incompetent (e.g., insane or delirious), the physician may properly treat the patient without consent in an emergency situation. The key elements here are "competence" and "informed consent" and "emergency situation." There are emergency treatment provisions in most states, but "emergency" is defined differently and procedures vary from jurisdiction to jurisdiction. Unless you know that your state law has a different interpretation, you will do best to read "clearly life saving" in place of "emergency." In a clear emergency, a judge can usually give a court order for treatment by telephone.

The right to refuse treatment is rooted in common law which holds that unauthorized medical treatment in nonemergency situations constitutes assault and/or battery. Therefore any physician who, for example, operates without consent is subject not only to civil proceedings under malpractice law, but also criminal proceedings. Since consent is the key, it matters not at all whether the treatment was skillful or even helpful to the patient.

There are a few exceptions to the patient's nearly total right to refuse care. There is a tradition in the common law that, if the patient is grossly incompetent, the consent by a relative is generally accepted. "Grossly" means that any fool can see it.

In clearly life-saving situations, the physician may act based upon several considerations—(1) no individual has a constitutional right to choose death at his or her own hand; (2) no individual has a right to authorize his or her own death at the hands of a second party, either by omission or commission; and (3) no one can be held legally at risk for preventing a suicide.

In the case of parents refusing treatment for minors, parents generally have considerable freedom where there is no serious risk of life. If there is a serious risk of life and medical and surgical treatment are available, feasible, and necessary, the parents probably have no right to withhold care. However, you still need to get a court order to treat a child against the parents' will, and you should consult your attorney in this regard.

A patient's refusal to accept treatment is not equivalent to demanding mistreatment. The patient's refusal usually refers to a specific treatment, and it is rarely necessary to stop *all* treatment. When the patient refuses one kind of treatment, request consent for alternative treatments, even though they may be less desirable from your point of view. It is only when the patient refuses any and all treatment that you may wash your hands of responsibility, given that you have made reasonable attempts to inform the patient of the risks involved and have made reasonable attempts to persuade him or her to accept what you regard as appropriate care.

Your duty is to refrain from unauthorized treatment, but to provide the best possible medical care within the limitations imposed by the patient's refusal of specific treatments.

It is useful to remember that refusal of treatment is simply a step on a continuum of impaired collaboration between doctor and patient. As such, it is best dealt with by anticipation and prophylaxis. Be alert for early signs of disgruntlement on your patient's part. Try regularly to assess your patient's satisfaction with the way treatment is progressing. Try regularly to make sure that you and your patient are working on common ground and not working toward inconsistent goals.

In summary, you can treat an individual against his or her will *only* in life-saving situations with a reasonable probability of success, and then you should limit the treatment to that necessary to save the patient's life. In emergency situations, perhaps we worry too much. There is no case in which a physician has not been upheld for saving life in an emergency situation. Philosophically too, it seems prudent to err (if we must) in the direction of life, in order to preserve the individual's future right to decide what is best for himself or herself.

Discharges Against Medical Advice

The threat to leave the hospital against medical advice (AMA) is usually the culmination of a sequence of events that has not produced a response which the patient sees as reasonable or appropriate. It is one possible consequence of a physician's insistence upon a mode of treatment which the patient refuses.

Any patients of sound mind can leave the hospital at any time they wish. To keep them against their will leaves one vulnerable to prosecution for false imprisonment. The hospital can request the patient to sign an AMA discharge form, but the patient has no obligation to sign as a precondition for release. The only (and rare) instance in which a competent adult can be held in a hospital against his or her will because of medical illness has to do with contagious disease laws in some states.

Why do patients threaten to or actually leave the hospital AMA? The answer has been sought in the psychodynamics of the patient, the psychopathology of the patient, disease-related factors, and staff-related factors. For my money, there are three consistent themes to look for with each AMA patient: communication, control, and sequestered information.

The patient, by his or her actions, is yelling, "Listen to me!" in the belief that he or she will not be heard as well by taking less precipitous action. The reason the patient is having difficulty being heard may relate to his or her own style or inarticulateness, or it may be that you or your staff is furiously busy or not particularly interested in the patient, or some other factors.

The issue of *control* surfaces as the patient's bid for equality or supremacy in what he or she sees as a power struggle with the physician. Such a bid reemphasizes the fact that he or she can relate to the physician as an equal, and need not simply do as told. I think it is revealing that one category of patients who have a particularly high incidence of AMA discharges are physician-patients. Physicians, even more than the average patient, dislike the one-down-position inherent in the traditional doctor-patient relationship. The point here is simply that AMA discharges are much more likely to become an issue when you have a patient who is used to being—or needs to be—in control. Stereotypic examples include adolescents in the midst of rebellion, hard-driving executives, rigorously independent entrepreneurs—but of course the realities extend beyond the stereotypes. Anyone who has exited AMA in the past is probably likely to do so again.

By sequestered information, I refer to facts in the patient's life that the patient has not chosen to share with the physician. Often, the patient must simply balance competing priorities, matters of time pressures, money, external responsibilities, and even such compelling habits as alcohol, drugs, or tobacco. There may also be considerable external pressures from the family, job, or others on the patient to return to life outside the hospital. We can know about these factors only if the patient chooses to tell us, and we can of course help by making ourselves accessible and asking directly what kinds of pressures are drawing him or her away from the care we think is so important. At least one study has concluded that a significant subset of against medical advice (AMA) discharges is composed of patients who enter the hospital never intending to stay more than a few days. Doctor and patient approach hospitalization with profoundly different expectations: the doctor gearing up for definitive diagnosis and treatments, the patient viewing the hospital as a temporary way station for symptomatic relief.

Whatever the factors, and however much we psychopathologize the etiology of AMA discharges, the fact is that AMA discharges can be therapeutic to the patients. What studies have been done indicate that the majority of AMA patients have few regrets, and there are few significant adverse effects relative to controls. Careful review of the papers on this subject, and my own experience, suggest that the major detriment of AMA discharges is to the morale of the staff and to the relationship between the patient and the specific physician involved. A single AMA discharge needn't be a cause for alarm, but a pattern of AMA discharges suggests that the physician involved should take a good look at himself or herself and at the specific hospital unit, to see what each is doing that may be contributing to such behavior.

With regard to treatment, as with the patient who refuses care, the treatment of choice is to anticipate the problem and prevent it. Emphasis on the collaborative approach to patient care is the most important aspect of prevention. Specifically, the physician should anticipate the patient's request to "listen to me" and encourage the patient to talk freely about any concerns regarding medical care. The physician should also seek to share control of the patient's treatment through an approach that emphasizes bargaining and compromise in the face of disagreement between doctor and patient. There will always be aspects of the patient's personal life which will remain unknown to you, and you therefore cannot totally prevent "sequestered information" becoming a potential barrier. However, if you present yourself as a caring and accessible person, the patient is increasingly likely to tell you of important pressures and stresses when they become germane to his or her hospital management.

Finally, if a patient of yours does leave your care, attempt to remain an ally of that patient. Seek to understand the patient's motivation, emphasize your respect for the patient's right to decide what is best, and say that you hope he or she will feel comfortable in seeking care from you in the future. Encourage him or her to call and let you know how things go, and you will have turned a potentially angry situation into a reasonable, amicable, and medically prudent one.

Commitment

Civil commitment refers to the process of hospitalizing a patient against his or her will, usually for reasons of mental illness. The traditional purposes of civil commitment are threefold: (1) benevolent coercion (protecting people from harming themselves or providing care and treatment for those who need it but wouldn't accept it); (2) protecting society (protecting people from harming others); and (3) convenience (getting nuisances or bothersome, eccentric people off the streets).

Involuntary commitment has declined rapidly over the past several decades. Voluntary psychiatric hospital admissions now outnumber involuntary admissions. The reasons have largely to do with legal agitation and trends toward availability of outpatient treatment as alternatives to hospitalization.

States vary considerably in their requirements for civil commitment. You simply have to know the criteria in your own area. Often they are sufficiently ambiguous so that a patient can be involuntarily confined if he or she is apparently psychotic or seriously depressed or grossly confused. In general, a physician who has personally and recently examined a patient runs no legal risk in signing commitment papers so long as there is no evidence that the physician acts maliciously (e.g., the physican had better not be having an affair with the spouse at the same time that he or she signs the commitment papers on the patient). The physician's vulnerability is further decreased if the patient is sufficiently alone or legally naive or impoverished to have no ready access to legal redress. In a manner parallel to criminal incarcerations, civil commitments are largely a phenomenon of the socially disadvantaged.

The states typically separate emergency commitment from long-term commitment procedures. Emergency commitments are generally geared to the convenience of institutions and rarely provide time and safeguards for thorough examination of facts. The general pattern of emergency detention statutes is to allow an institution to hospitalize an individual for from one to 30 days for the purposes of evaluation, with the amount of treatment allowed or required remaining unclear. The petition for detention generally requires evidence or statements suggesting committability, which in many states is simply a diagnosable mental illness and the need for treatment. This petition customarily must be signed by one or more physicians, or occasionally by a non-physician, such as a psychologist, a nurse, or a police officer. Sometimes the order must be signed by a judge of a court of record, or by a physician who is court appointed and working as an agent of the state, sometimes in an officially designated hospital.

As a practical matter, to me it makes little sense to commit a person for a brief stay unless he or she will be there long enough to make some difference in the condition. Therefore, it is seldom advisable (especially from the patient's point of view) to submit the patient to emergency detention unless he or she is likely to fulfill the criteria for sustained detention, or unless the problem is likely to be short-lived, as in the probable toxic psychosis or with situational violence.

However, procedures that make little sense when viewed from one perspective suddenly become very sensible when viewed from another. A prime reason for writing up emergency detention papers in an emergency room setting is simply that it is the easiest, quickest, and least liability-linked option open to the physician. In effect, it removes the responsibility for the difficult decision (i.e., what is really the best disposition for this person) from the doctor in the emergency department and shifts it to some psychiatric detention center. The popularity of this procedure is generally due, not to any nastiness or sloth on the part of the emergency room doctor, but rather, to the onerous and impractical nature of the alternatives: making numerous phone calls to mobilize a reliable support system for the patient; interviewing and sorting through the conflicting stories of various significant others; and/ or prying a reluctant psychiatric consultant to come take care of a difficult and sometimes unpleasant patient who often has no way to pay a consultant's fee. All this while kids with croup, adults in cardiac failure, and miscellaneous trauma victims cry out for attention in the background.

If you do arrange for emergency detention, it's useful to know what will happen to the patient upon admittance to the detention center. Many, of course, are let go after a very brief stay. The facilities are too crowded, the need for detention does not remain apparent, et cetera. Statutes concerning sustained detention usually allow for an institution to hold patients against their will for anywhere from 15 days to 6 months and may be indeterminate. The procedures are complicated, usually requiring evidence from at least two physicians and necessitating formal court proceedings. In the past, sustained detentions have often been handled informally, with judge and physician chatting in the judge's chambers and the disposition decided in a gentlemanly fashion, but with the patient's participation not at all guaranteed. Increasingly, sustained commitment procedures have been subject to constitutional safeguards and increasing attentions to the rights of the patient, as well as the requirement that the patient be notified of these safeguards and rights. Over the years ahead, some or all of the following may be required in some jurisdictions: (1) reasonable notice that commitment procedures are under way; (2) the right of the patient to respond to those proceedings; (3) the right of the patient to legal counsel during the proceedings; (4) the right to jury trial for extended detention; (5) Fifth Amendment protection against self-incrimination; and (6) proof of meeting commitment criteria beyond a reasonable doubt.

As a practical matter, however, for the physician confronted with a potentially suicidal patient, it is easiest to consider alternatives to commitment when the patient is someone you know well, when friends and relatives are involved and reliable, and when psychiatric outpatient treatment is easily accessible and skilled.

Once you have decided on commitment, make sure that the medical record thoroughly documents the circumstances that require commitment, and that it is written as though it will be subject to careful scrutiny and criticism in a court of law (although it is far more likely that not a soul will ever read it after the week is over). The receiving facility should be notified, and you should confirm that they will accept the patient. Copies of documents should, of course, be sent and transportation needs arranged. Ideally, the decision for commitment should be made in conjunction with friends and relatives; at the very least, they need to be informed. Don't neglect to tell the patient your plan either, though if you anticipate a spirited objection, it's sometimes useful to wait until ambulance personnel and/or police are present. In discussing your decision with the patient—either before it is made or afterward—it is often helpful to say, "As a physician, I am responsible to you for your physical health. In addition, the law requires that I make some judgments about your safety. Unless I am convinced that you are not a danger, to yourself or others, or gravely disabled, I am requiried by law to see that you are held for evaluation at an appropriate facility against your will if necessary."

DANGEROUSNESS TO SELF

Few jurisdictions describe very precisely the nature of the harm a patient may do to himself or herself or its likelihood or imminence. For instance, whether dangerousness to self constitutes potential suicide or self-mutilating behavior or unwise financial judgments is seldom outlined with precision. There is a philosophic problem too in that dangerousness to self could conceivably be extended to include such risk-taking behavior as ski jumping, motorcycle racing, or even smoking three packs of cigarettes per day. Nor do the statutes require that the persons signing commitment papers weigh the likelihood of dangerousness to self against the known and very real risks of involuntary hospitalization, which include such things as loss of self-esteem, stigmatization, loss of job, separation from family, and the potential brutalization that may derive from confinement and certain forms of somatic therapy. The tendency is to define the criteria more narrowly to the danger of imminent suicidal behavior. If you cannot assure yourself that other safe alternatives exist for the patient, then proceed with commitment.

DANGEROUSNESS TO OTHERS

This area is subject to a whole range of philosophic and practical problems. The philosophic ones center mostly on the problem of definition. There are many different kinds of acts that are dangerous to society but are not included in the civil commitment laws; e.g., such acts of commission as air pollution and teaching kids corrupt values, and such acts of omission as failure to vote. Neither is it clear why only the "mentally ill'' should be subject to special commitment procedures on the basis of dangerousness to others, since the base rate for violent behavior is no different for the mentally ill than for the general population.

The practical problems arise in that it is very difficult to predict dangerousness or even violent behavior. Despite the impression you may have from reading your daily paper, violent events are rare events, and it is extremely difficult to predict rare occurrences. Is it better to overpredict or underpredict? And, better for whom?

Even individuals with great experience and savvy have terrible track records for accuracy in predicting dangerous acts. There are no adequate criteria applicable for a broad spectrum of persons—not diagnostic categories, not psychological testing, not even intuition. There is no reason to believe that the more information you have about a person the more accurate the prediction. Violent behavior in general is at least as much a function of the social context as of the specific person.

There are people in whom anyone can predict violence: those with a consistent history of violent behavior, and those who say with conviction that they plan to kill or maim someone. However, such predictions are not the sole province of health professionals, and there is no clear relationship between such behavior and mental illness.

In general, health professionals will overpredict violent behavior, and as a natural corollary, will overcommit individuals because of potential violent behavior. They will do so because (1) while violence is a rare event that is situation specific, it is devastating when it occurs, and no health professional wants to carry a thus-burdened conscience; (2) it is impossible to get feedback on false-positive patients because, once a person is confined, there is no way to determine whether he or she would have been violent if not confined; (3) regardless of the validity of the prediction of violence, it is always possible to rationalize commitment as a means of getting a needy person into treatment; (4) there are really no adverse consequences to a maker of false-positive predictions. Physicians participating in commitment proceedings need have little fear of liability so long as they have personally examined the patient within the required time period, have complied with procedural requirements of their state, and are operating in good faith (i.e., without malicious intent or to achieve personal gain).

Once you decide that a patient is dangerous and have said so in the medical record, then, what you must do may be a matter of law. For instance, right or wrong, once you decide that a person is truly dangerous, you may be required to commit the individual and/or notify any potential victims. The law in this regard is in flux, and you must contact your attorney or another reliable source for current information. When examining a patient, if you are in doubt concerning potential dangerousness, ask for a second opinion before you put any definite statements in the medical record.

GRAVE DISABILITY

The inability to care for one's self is variously defined in the different states. In California, grave disability is defined as "inability to provide for basic personal needs of food, clothing, or shelter." Still, within that narrow definition, there is considerable room for individual interpretation. For instance, under those guidelines some physicians would assess the appropriateness of dress and the appropriateness of distribution of finances for various basic needs. Given that approach, would a person qualify for grave disability if he or she were practicing selective nudity, or fasting because of political conscience? The law is rarely as precise as you might believe.

Whatever you call it and however you define it, there is no question that some individuals are temporarily or permanently gravely disabled. Some can be cared for at home, and many forms of assistance are available to those who imaginatively seek them out: self-help groups for the elderly, volunteer organizations, mutual-aid living situations, granny sitters, visiting nurses, home health-care workers, church groups, and so forth.

The borderline cases are always agonizing problems for the physician, other medical personnel and family. We talk about death with dignity, yet in commitment we deprive fragile, elderly people of what little self-respect and dignity they have managed to hold on to. Still, there is no dignity in withering away alone, being unaware of the most basic bodily needs or the means to satisfy them. Ultimately, despite the unattractiveness of the task, there will be some patients for whom you will need to institute commitment proceedings. For most, you will need the assistance of your psychiatric consultant or social worker.

While guardianship as a legal instrument is separate from commitment, many individuals who have legal guardians because of mental illness have a history of involuntary confinement. Most people who are committed, however, do not end up having guardians.

Most states have some procedure to appoint a guardian for an individual who becomes incompetent to handle his or her own affairs, either by reason of "insanity," disease, or just old age. The guardianship, whatever it is called, may be limited. For example, a financial guardian makes decisions and acts for the patient in a limited sphere—paying rent, giving the patient an allowance, investing capital, etc. Or the guardianship may be general, in which case the guardian may make a broad range of decisions covering what the patient may do, where he or she may go, whether he or she may marry, etc.

The court-designated guardian may be a person—perhaps a relative—or an institution such as a bank or a particular bureau of the county government. Finding sensitive and able persons to fill such a role is no easy task, even if there were reasonable financial compensation, which usually there is not.

Procedures vary enormously from one state to another, but sometimes temporary orders for guardianship can be obtained in a few days. Extended guardianship is increasingly subject to all the requirements of due process mentioned earlier for commitment procedures, and may take months or even years.

The right of the guardian to authorize medical treatment against the patient's will is not at all clear. In general, except in emergency situations, you should respect the patient as an individual, as you would any other patient, and you should refrain from treatment without a specific court order.

Bibliography

Annas GJ: *The Rights of Hospital Patients*. New York, Avon Books, 1975

Applebaum PS, Roth LH: Clinical issues in the assessment of competency. *Am J Psychiatry* 138:1462–1467, 1981

Barton GM, Scheer N: A comparison of patients discharged against medical advice with a matched control group. *Am J Psychiatry* 131:1217–1220, 1974

Birns H, Levien JS: Dangerousness–legal determinations and clinical speculations. *Psychiatric Quarterly* 52:108–131, 1980

Brody EB: Patients' rights—a cultural challenge to western psychiatry. *Am J Psychiatry* 142:58–62, 1985

Ford MD: The psychiatrist's double bind—the right to refuse medication. *Am J Psychiatry* 137:332–338, 1980

Hall GE: Liability of committing physician. *JAMA* 209:325–326, 1969

Hiday VA: Are lawyers enemies of psychiatrists—a survey of civil commitment counsel and judges. *Am J Psychiatry* 140:323–326, 1983

Lipsett PD, Lelos D: Decision makers in law and psychiatry and the involuntary civil commitment process. *Comm Ment Health J* 17:114–122, 1981

Long JP, Marin A: Profile of patients signing against medical advice. *J Fam Pract* 15:551–556, 1982

Miller RD, Fiddleman PB: Emergency involuntary commitment—a look at the decision-making process. *Hosp Comm Psychiatry* 34:249–254, 1983

Munetz MR, Lidz CW, Meisel A: Informed consent and incompetent medical patients. *J Fam Pract* 20:273–279, 1985

Peszke MA, Affleck GG, Wintrob RM: Perceived statutory applicability versus clinical desirability of emergency involuntary hospitalization. *Am J Psychiatry* 137:476–480, 1980

Pierce GL, Durham ML, Fisher WH: The impact of broadened civil commitment standards on admissions to state mental hospitals. *Am J Psychiatry* 142:104–107, 1985

Rosenfeld S: Race differences in involuntary hospitalization. *J Health Soc Behavior* 25:14–23, 1984

Rubin LC, Mills MJ: Behavioral precipitants to civil commitment. *Am J Psychiatry* 140:603–606, 1983

Rubsamen DS: Discussion. *Prof Liability Newsletter* 14(11):4, 1983

Schopp RF, Quattrocchi MR: Tarasoff, the doctrine of special relationships and the therapist's duty to warn. *J Psychiatry and Law* (Spring) 1984 pp 13–27

Spensley J, Werme PH: Conservatorship—an involuntary legal status for 'gravely disabled' mentally disordered persons, *West J Medical* 130:476–484, 1979

Starkman MN, Youngs DD: Psychiatric consultation with patients who refuse medical care. *Int J Psychiatry Med* 5:115–123, 1974

Steadman HJ: The right not to be a false positive—problems in the application of the dangerousness standard. *Psychiatric Q,* 52:84–98, 1980

Steinglass P, Grantham, CE, Hertzman M: Predicting which patients will be discharged against medical advice—A pilot study. *Am J Psychiatry* 137:1385–1389, 1980

Wilbert DE, et al.: Determination of grave disability. *J Nerv Ment Dis* 162:35–39, 1976

Wise TN: Psychiatric management of patients who threaten to sign out against medical advice. *Int J Psychiatry Med* 5:153–160, 1974

5

Confusional States

I must be getting absent minded. Whenever I complain that things aren't what they used to be, I always forget to include myself.
—George Burns

Do not go gentle into that good night, Old age should burn and rave at close of day; Rage, rage against the dying of the light.
—Dylan Thomas

This chapter concerns the spectrum of confusional disorders, how to anticipate them when possible, recognize them when they occur, and treat them effectively, particularly in the hospital setting.

We will be dealing explicitly with what are regarded as the "organic" psychiatric syndromes. Sharp distinctions between organic and so-called functional psychiatric disorders are not only misleading but useless. Patients tend to ignore dogma and texts, and a "touch" of confusion, with both physiologic and psychosocial components, is common, especially in the hospital.

Most confused patients are not recognized as confused by the doctors caring for them. Patients tend to conceal their defects whenever they can and to be labeled only if they attract attention to themselves by disturbing people around them. However, chance favors the prepared mind, and if you look for subclinical cases of confusion, you will find them.

I believe confusion to be among the most common of psychiatric disorders, and the most treatable. The reason for the universality of this condition is the sensitivity of cortical function to changes in physiologic and psychologic homeostasis. The brain is likely to be the first organ to show subtle signs of impairment in anemia, hypoxia, fever, anaesthesia, sleeplessness, and toxemia.

In particular, confusion is the response of the elderly brain to stress.

Because of this, the astute clinician can use confusion as a sensitive
indicator. You may be able to follow the patient's overall medical
condition more closely by monitoring the patient's mental status than
by following the temperature sheet or laboratory data.

Most clinicians tend to think of confusion in terms of two proto-
types: delirium tremens in the alcoholic and dementia in the elderly.
Since neither example is an attractive one, physicians are seldom very
interested in confusion per se. Often there is an unexpressed attitude
that "either they'll get over it or they won't, and either way there isn't
a whole hell of a lot for me to do." As a consequence, there's a
tendency for everyone to abdicate responsibility for the confused patient.

The confusional states represent conditions in which there is an
impairment of intellectual "grasp," a decreased ability to understand
the meaning of words, things, and events, and the relationship among
them. Confusion is also described as a clouding of consciousness, with
consciousness being a state in which such functions as thinking, perception, memory, attention, concentration, and judgment can occur.
Like most things, confusion is seldom an either/or phenomenon. Its
manifestations can run the gamut from misinterpretations to delusions,
from anxiety to panic, from fear of helpless dependence on strangers to
frank paranoia.

The terminology that has grown up around the confusional states is
as confused as the patients are. There are, of course, the lumpers and
the splitters, those who are interested in similarities and those who are
interested in differences. My general bias is that it is most useful to
concentrate on the similarities, and only emphasize the differences
when they become extreme and represent clearly distinct patterns.

The official terminology does not refer to the confusional states per
se, but tends to lump them under what has been called the organic brain
syndromes or organic mental disorders. Neurologists tend to be unen-
thusiastic about this classification because it is anatomically imprecise
and could conceivably include all brain disease above the tentorium. I
am not enthusiastic about that label because while organicity is almost
always present in the confusional states, it is usually only part of the
picture, and (as we shall see) not always located within the central
nervous system. Other terms used for clinical examples of the confusional states include confusional psychosis, encephalopathy, toxic psychosis, dementia, pseudodementia, delirium, organic hallucinosis, and
senile decay.

I will use these various terms to represent points on the confusional
spectrum when I believe a distinction should be made; otherwise, confusion will be used as a generic term which includes all of the more
specific terminology. For example, delirium and dementia are useful

terms to describe prototypic conditions, and will therefore be described in some detail. Clinically, however, there is considerable blurring of theoretic distinctions. For instance, delirium is not qualitatively different when it is superimposed on dementia, as it often is.

Delirium is usually defined as a potentially reversible condition with recognizable onset, characterized by impaired level of intellectual functioning and clouding of consciousness, customarily attributed to metabolic or toxic causes. The process is most usefully viewed as a dynamic equilibrium, which varies along with the other factors that play a contributory role. In the prodrome, there are typically brief lapses of awareness, with a tendency to misperceive external stimuli and with problems in attention and concentration. Usually the patient feels considerable fatigue, with a tendency towards drowsiness, impaired task performance, and intrusive thoughts. Fine motor movements are usually impaired, and electroencephalography often reveals diffuse slowing. The patient may or may not have any complaints at this stage. In frank delirium, perceptual difficulties are obvious and the patient is overtly confused. Hallucinations are so common that it requires no professional skill to discern them. In contrast to the auditory hallucinations of so-called functional psychoses, the hallucinations of delirium are usually visual, although occasionally they can be olfactory, tactile, or even auditory. The patient is usually extraordinarily restless, manifests a hollow-eyed suspicious stare, is frequently grossly paranoid and delusional. The patient's perceptions are usually vivid and rich in detail, and it appears to the external observer that the patient is living through a nightmare with his or her eyes open.

Dementia is customarily defined as a chronic, irreversible condition, characterized by gross and diffuse impairment of intellectual function, caused by structural disease of the cerebral cortex. Such global impairment affects not only intelligence, but is also associated with a disruption of normal personality and behavior patterns. The definition as stated is correct in its bare outline and in extreme cases. Practically speaking, there are few cases which are so irreversible that the clinical manifestations cannot be ameliorated by changing how we interact with the patient and by altering the environment.

Many patients have so-called reversible dementias (e.g., from meningiomas, pernicious anemia, myxedema, etc.) which respond dramatically to treatment of the underlying problem. Other causes of "dementia" that are reversible when appropriately treated include: Wernicke's encephalopathy, normal pressure hydrocephalus, internal carotid stenosis, and space-occupying lesions in so-called silent areas of the brain, which therefore produce no focal neurologic signs (e.g., frontal lobe abscesses, tumors, or subdural hematomas).

Typical manifestations of dementia include major gaps in knowledge and intelligence, a monotonous clinical picture in which the patient presents a vacant, vacuous appearance, an impoverishment of psychic life, and a deterioration of personality which borders on a caricature of the patient's premorbid personality. It would almost seem that all the patient's worst traits become more prominent. Though the degree of impairment is highly variable, there is less diurnal variation than with delirium. However, the degree of the patient's deficit may be intimately tied in with other aspects of health as well as social and psychological variables. For instance, the patient may appear grossly demented with a pneumonia in your hospital, yet function perfectly adequately at home and in daily activities after the pneumonia has resolved.

It seems to me most useful to see delirium and dementia as symptom clusters characteristic of different stages of the confusion continuum, each of which can fluctuate in severity. Each represents a dynamic process, with forces of disorganization battling organizing, homeostatic mechanisms. It is easy to see dementia as the end stage in which this dynamic battle has been lost, but unless the patient is a vegetable, gains are always possible. Delirium represents an unstable equilibrium and dementia a more stable, but seldom petrified, equilibrium. The issue of curability is a red herring, almost everything on the confusion spectrum is treatable, if not reversible.

The Patient's View

To understand the behavior of the confused patient, think of how *we* would feel and respond in the event that we lost that most treasured possession, mental acuity. Given an awareness of a significant loss, most of us would be terribly upset and attempt to minimize the severity of the impairment. We would tend to retreat to familiar circumstances and avoid getting into new or challenging situations that were beyond impaired ability. We would probably feel inadequate, vulnerable, depressed, and fearful that the loss would be permanent or get worse. In unavoidable social situations, many of us would attempt to conceal impairment from others, both by distancing behavior, such as aloofness or crusty irritability, and by structuring the conversation along familiar lines. Understandably, many confused persons—who don't surrender despairingly and passively to their condition—have similar feelings, and their behavior correspondingly is designed to hide debility and structure social interactions. For example, the elderly withdraw into daily rituals and the privacy of their homes, and the alcoholic with an encephalopathy confabulates to conceal gaps in memory and information which careful interrogation would uncover.

How the patient experiences his or her deficit depends upon the level of awareness (i.e., insight), the rapidity and severity of the process, and what the person was like before all this happened.

Nonetheless, we can make certain generalizations. In delirium, thinking becomes progressively more difficult; ideas, words, and perceptions take on a puzzling aspect. Logical, coherent thinking becomes an unbearable task as the patient becomes increasingly tired, yet unable to sleep. Often, the hospitalized patient is aware of pain. If the patient is in the hospital, the repetitive awakenings which are a part of hospitalized life foster an increased irritability. The patient is aware of pain, but little else has as much reality. As the patient thrashes about in bed, he or she becomes highly responsive to both internal and external stimuli, though hardly aware that they have occurred. Interacting with the external world becomes increasingly difficult, and dream life becomes correspondingly more important. The dreams are often frightening and astonishingly vivid, frequently focusing on monsters, pain, destruction, and death. Because daydreaming and nightdreaming tend to occur constantly, the patient has difficulty discerning where dreams leave off and the external world begins. The uncertainty is terrifying and very, very lonely. The patient, without perceiving it, desperately needs someone to help sort out what is real and what is not. Patients become malleable and suggestible; they are too tired and uncertain to be otherwise. All in all, delirium is a terrifying experience.

The classic demented patient experiences his or her condition much differently, but there are similar aspects. Dementia is usually a much more slowly evolving process than delirium, and the demented person therefore has more time to adapt to disability than does the delirious person. Since dementia is principally a phenomenon of the older age group, the patient's perspective on what is happening is closely tied in with personal views of aging. Many regard the condition as an inevitable consequence of old age, though most are aware that the condition does not affect all aging individuals equally. Gradually the patient's interests narrow, and a certain intolerance to change develops. An increasing percentage of the time one's mind is vacant and featureless, and there is difficulty in connecting one thought with another. Most patients are aware of their deficiencies, know that they handle new situations poorly and integrate new information and facts only with great concentration and energy expenditure. If the patient is embarrassed and reticent, he or she may sit quietly on the sidelines, hiding confusion behind a vacuous grin, an affable and self-deprecating manner. For the patient who is more aggressive, particularly one who took active pride in previous intellect, there are usually more vigorous attempts to conceal deficits. These efforts may take the form of confabulation, maneuvering conversation and activities to familiar ground, or irritability when challenged. For either individual, there is considerable possibility of being overwhelmed by depression and apathy. Where the environment has become bewildering and frightening, misperceptions easily become distortions, and anxiety can rapidly escalate to panic.

Whether the patient is demented or delirious, the condition is likely to be worse at night, when one is more isolated, when sensory input is limited to auditory cues, and counterbalancing influences (such as familiar persons and things) are less readily perceived or not present at all. At night in particular, increased anxiety further impairs cognitive function, resulting in an anxiety spiral which may culminate in frank delusions and hallucinations.

Effect on Care Givers

Since delirium occurs most commonly and dementia almost exclusively in the elderly, views of the confused patient will be intimately tied in with views of older people in general, particularly those in our own families. Often there is a great deal of ambivalence: a mixture of respect and condescension.

Usually taking care of confused patients is extraordinarily taxing. As the hospitalized patient becomes more confused, he or she often becomes louder, moaning and chanting apparent drivel, calling out continually for people who aren't there, upsetting staff and other patients. The inclination to cover such an individual with a mound of red, yellow, and blue sedatives is almost overwhelming.

The same is frequently true for confused outpatients. The patient is brought in by relatives or nursing home personnel who are upset by the patient's behavior and seeming misbehavior and who very much want the doctor to "do something" which will make the patient more manageable.

Many physicians are reluctant to embarrass such patients by a thorough assessment, especially if the physician is by nature respectful of elderly individuals. The thinking is, "I'll only embarrass both of us by asking what day it is." However, we do such patients no favor by avoiding careful assessment. Through thoughtful and careful conversation with the patients, we can save them from many tests, an admission to or an extended stay in the hospital, and the possibility of missing conditions which are contributory to confusion.

There is a further tendency to blame the patient for the condition, and many physicians have a tendency to diagnose such patients as psychotic or attach a psychiatric label with particular emphasis on personality disorder or previous alcohol abuse. What we see before us is a doddering old fool, often someone with whom we have had no previous relationship, whose previous strengths and virtues and achievements are completely unknown to us. Consequently it is often difficult to treat the person as respectfully as we might if the patient's admirable qualities were clearly displayed before us.

Physicians are often puzzled by rapid fluctuations in states of consciousness with such patients. We have a tendency to think that others who examine the patient at different times are either sloppy or idiots. You see a hospitalized patient at night; he or she is clearly out in left field, but the hospital notes make no mention of this. Did the people in charge of this patient's care not do a thorough workup? One must be very careful of divisive behavior with one's colleagues under such circumstances.

Part of the physician's response is determined by the nature of how the patient becomes our responsibility. The patient often presents as a crisis; of course, the more severe the dementia, the more vulnerable the patient is to an acute confusional episode. The more demented the patient, the more difficult it is to pin down the precipitants of whatever it is that has brought the patient to medical attention.

The physician is often left with a confused, usually uncooperative, unkempt, unattractive patient vulnerable to being regarded as a dump: "We have to take care of the old man because everyone else shirked their responsibilities."

While that assessment is sometimes accurate, it is proffered as the sole explanation far more often than is commensurate with the situation. Elderly confused patients present as crises for some predictable and understandable reasons: (1) they become more confused with flare-ups of old physical problems or the beginnings of new ones; e.g., transient ischemic attacks, congestive heart failure, uremia, etc; (2) they become more confused as a consequence of environmental change; e.g., loss of a primary support person or relocation to a new living situation; or (3) the "enough is enough" phenomenon sets in, and a more-or-less loving and caring family becomes finally taxed to their limit with the patient's incontinence, wandering in the streets, or disrobing in public.

Generally, it is most useful to seek to empathetically understand such precipitants. It will make us less angry and resentful, we will work better with the patient and family, and will enjoy the process more.

Whether or not stress overwhelms the orderly and effective functioning of the cerebral cortex depends upon (1) the amount of cortex a person has and how well it usually functions, (2) the degree and type of stress, and (3) counterbalancing forces that bolster an individual's resistance to stress. Virtually anybody's cortex can be overwhelmed with sufficient assault, and therefore anybody can become confused with sufficient stress. Typically, a child's cortex reacts to the stress of fever with convulsions; the elderly person's brain typically reacts to hypoxia and toxins with confusion.

Most people run their cortex lazily most of the time, using only a small portion of what they have. How they function under stress depends on how much additional cortex they can call into use and how well they have learned to use it. The concept of cortical reserve capacity therefore makes a great deal of sense to me.

The average healthy young adult has considerable cortical reserve capacity, and therefore can respond effectively to a wide variety of demands on the cortical function. Even when the specific demands of a situation exceed the person's ability to respond as requested (e.g., ten people asking questions all at the same time), the cortex can frequently sort out the variables (e.g., "There is more input than I can process effectively"), and respond so as to reduce the stress (e.g., "All right, everybody, please badger me sequentially and not in concert").

A person may function satisfactorily (e.g., without clinical dementia) when the external demands are minimal and routine, but nonetheless be functioning with little cortical reserve to meet contingencies. Such a person leads a marginal cortical existence, and may easily decompensate with stress. Remove the stress, and there is a return, gradual or abrupt, to base line. Because there is "normal" function under ordinary circumstances, we would not label the person demented. The episode of confusion, because of its reversibility, is likely to be seen as a delirium-like occurrence, but it only occurs because subclinical and perhaps irreversible cortical disease has left no cortical reserve capacity.

The situation is very similar to that of a chronic lung patient or heart patient who does well in ordinary daily activities, but decompensates (e.g., becomes dyspneic) when challenged. The challenge may take many forms—infectious (e.g., pneumonia), metabolic (e.g., water overload), psychologic (e.g., panic), or environmental (e.g., smog). Each of these challenges is as likely to precipitate confusion in a person with limited cortical reserve capacity as it is likely to produce dyspnea in a person with limited respiratory reserve capacity.

To keep the relative considerations easily accessbile, I use a mnemonic device called the "five A's" (Table 5.1). Each A symbolizes a category of considerations, which can be graded 0, 1, or 2 depending on the degree of importance to the patient in question. The Five A's scale can therefore range from 0 to 10 points. I would expect any patient scoring 10 points to be grossly confused; the patient scoring 5 points usually has confusional episodes, sometimes clinically apparent and sometimes not. Any patient who is grossly confused deserves an evaluation of each of the five A categories. They are:

1. *Age.* Under 55, 0; 55–65, 1 point, over 65, 2 points. Shade the numbers to fit your prejudices, and follow the age of the person's spirt more closely than the chronologic age.

Table 5.1 The Five A's of Confusional Syndromes

1. AGE
   normal wear and tear on cortical neurons
   adjust score as necessary if age of the spirit differs from age of the body

2. ALCOHOL
   catchall for likely intracranial diseases
   include presenile dementias, tumors, infections, trauma, cerebral arteriosclerosis, etc.
   include distant disease likely to seed into brain, such as subacute bacterial endocarditis, carcinoma of the breast, lung neoplasma, etc.

3. ALONENESS
   catchall for social and sensory deprivation
   include anything that tends to impair orientation, such as monotony, sudden changes in living circumstances (e.g., transfers from one ward to another), foreign language or culture, deafness, glaucoma, cataracts, isolation because of infectious disease, etc.

4. ANESTHESIA
   catchall for metabolic and toxic abnormalities
   watch for hypoxia, fever, drugs that impair intellectual grasp (especially barbiturates), hypotension, dehydration, uremia, nutritional impairment, anemia, electrolyte abnormalities, endocrinopathies, etc.
   watch especially for the effect of prolonged surgical procedures

5. AGONY
   catchall for psychologic stress
   include anxiety, pain, fear of death, sleep deprivation, fatigue, depression, apathy, fear of disability and disfigurement, etc.

2. *Alcohol.* This is a catchall category for intracranial disease, because in our society alcohol is the single most important cause of destroyed intracranial neurons. Give anyone with a history of delirium tremens 2 points, and any good, solid cocktail-circuit drinker 1 point. Figure in any previous history of head trauma or craniotomy as you think best.

3. *Aloneness.* Any patient who has no friends, no relatives, and is confined to bed but does not indulge in such sedentary activities as reading or watching television gets a good, solid 2 points. The patient with plenty of visitors who is able to get out of bed and whose mind is always occupied gets 0 points. Figure everyone else in between.

4. *Anesthesia.* Include any iatrogenic factors that cloud mentation. This point can't be overemphasized. Any patient on eight or more systemic drugs gets 2 points, regardless of the identity of the specific agents. Remember that many elderly individuals live on the brink of cerebral hypoxia; presumptive evidence of hypoxia, fever, impaired nutrition, toxins, or toxemia is worth a portion of a point. If the problem is clinically manifest, the patient gets a full point; if it becomes a serious problem the patient gets 2 points.

5. *Agony*. Assess all types of suffering. Figure the point score according to your own rough assessment.

One phenomenon of medical life deserves special attention because it happens so frequently and involves so many of the five A's, and that is surgical operation. I believe that the incidence of postoperative confusion, ranging from mild and transient to severe and prolonged, is extremely common, especially in the elderly.

I'll state flatly that any patient over 65 years of age with a history of serious alcohol abuse who undergoes a lengthy surgical procedure (anesthesia time over 4 hours), with consequent pain and suffering, is absolutely certain to undergo postoperative confusion. It's easy to minimize such hazards, but if the confusion is blatant and the manifestations include pulling out IVs, nasogastric or chest tubes, you will wish you had anticipated the problem.

Surgical procedures are exhausting for patients, a fact which most of us don't appreciate fully until we ourselves are operated upon. Even a quick and uncomplicated appendectomy will leave a patient with reduced energy for almost three weeks. If the person is not a healthy young adult to start off with, the recovery time will be even greater. Surgical procedures requiring three to four hours will keep healthy young adults below average energy for as long as two to three months.

The metabolic depletion inherent in surgical procedures and the energy requirements of healing are considerable.

Usually the second through the fifth postop days are the worst, especially with major chest or abdominal surgery. Watch for postoperative confusion/delirium/psychoses at that time! That is when the combination of pain, fragmentary sleep, chaotic hospital routine, and metabolic depletion usually reaches the critical level for the patient.

Remember, virtually everyone will go bananas when deprived of restful sleep for a sufficient period of time. Experimental studies have shown that approximately 100 hours of wakefulness are the most that anyone can take. Fragmentary sleep is not enough; the body must have rest.

Remember too that virtually everyone will lose contact with reality after sensory deprivation of sufficient intensity and duration. Very, very few healthy and motivated subjects can tolerate sensory deprivation experiments for more than 72 hours. Sensory deprivation is a peculiar phenomenon that takes many forms; it involves not only a diminishment in the absolute intensity of stimuli, but may involve simply an absence in variation of stimuli. For individuals in a state of sensory deprivation, the visual world becomes a pale blur, the auditory world becomes a monotonous drone, and the tactile world seems a cocoon; the world is imposed upon them and they are powerless to change the nature of the sensory input.

Assessment

You know more than you think you do.

—Benjamin Spock

The above quotation is the opening line from the revolutionary *Common Sense Book of Baby and Child Care,* and, as it was designed to reassure parents in dealing with children, its use here is designed to reassure you in dealing with the other end of the age spectrum.

While the following comments are relevant to any patient, the type of examination described is particularly directed toward a patient whom you have recognized as confused or at risk for being confused, and this is most frequently the hospitalized patient. *Every* older patient should be assessed for acute or chronic confusion. No special skills are required, and you should certainly be able to perform a screening examination without any difficulty. It should be sufficiently short so that you won't skip it, sufficiently simple so that you can do it yourself, and possess enough face validity so that you will believe the results once you've got them.

The test is designed to assess disorientation and decreased intellectual grasp which form the substrate of confusion. However, a good exam is designed to identify the patient's strengths as well as defects. Whether defects are a product of normal aging or pathologic process may matter little as far as the examination is concerned. We need to know the patient's baseline performance in order to adequately test for cognitive slippage as the treatment course progresses. Serial findings are crucial; mentation changes so much in the confused patient that a single examination is seldom enough.

PRELIMINARY ASSESSMENT

The preliminary assessment involves three parts—discussion with the patient, information from friends, relatives, and significant others, and observations of the nursing staff if the patient is hospitalized.

The patient interview

Assessment of the patient depends upon five questions which we ask of ourselves, not the patient. We can gather the needed information during the process of small talk with the patient; a detailed interrogation is seldom necessary. This "small-talk" examination is extremely useful because it is usually comfortable both for the doctor and the patient, yet is productive with careful listening. The questions to ask of ourselves are as follows:

1. Is the patient a good historian? By the time you have finished your history and physical exam, you will certainly come to some con-

clusion about this. If you are tempted to write "unreliable" or "poor historian" at the top of the write-up, that implies some important clues about the patient's mental status. In particular, it implies that either the patient is confused or is a setup for confusion.

2. What is the patient's knowledge of present circumstances? Does the patient know how he or she got to your office or to the hospital? Does the patient know who referred him or her or understand the reason for seeing you? If this is not your first meeting, does the patient recall previous ones? If you answer no to one or more of these questions, raise your index of suspicion.

3. What has the patient learned since arrival? Can he or she describe the nurse who took vital signs? Was the waiting room empty or full? If the patient is hospitalized, has the patient learned the name of roommates? Does the patient know where the bathroom is? Where the nursing station is? Has he or she figured out how to raise or lower the bed or turn on the TV set? (You may disregard negative answers to the latter questions if you yourself have not yet figured out how to raise or lower the hospital beds.)

4. How does the patient keep his or her mind occupied? It may require some ingenuity to assess maximum functioning. Try to get the patient talking about a subject of mutual interest so you will be able to assess accuracy. Try to get comments in some detail. If he or she watches television, ask what channel a favorite program is on. If he or she writes letters, ask how much postage is required for first class mail (this requires a mind that is alert to rapidly changing current events). Ask about hobbies, foods, or places to visit.

5. How good is the patient's short-term memory? You may well have formed some preliminary opinions about this in the course of your other questions, but focus on the question specifically for a moment. Before leaving the patient's bedside, say, "Please feel free to call upon me if you need me. By the way, do you remember my name?" In fairness, make sure that you have carefully and clearly enunciated your name to the patient when you first met. Make sure that he or she can't read your name tag while you're asking the question. Since many persons have difficulty remembering names after brief encounters, a person who does remember your name seldom requires further assessment of short-term memory. If the patient doesn't recall your name, you can assess memory in a more stilted fashion by asking the patient to repeat an address or phrase after from two to five minutes.

Friends or relatives
Talk to friends or relatives, or have someone else do so for you. Not only will you get an additional viewpoint on the patient's history, but it

is an opportunity to ask questions you feel uncomfortable asking the patient.

If you can't get the answer from other sources, you may well have to ask the patient directly. Other sources may be hard to come by, as an increasing number of elderly patients live alone, without family nearby, and whose friends have been gradually dying off. In that event, a social worker (if not harried beyond endurance already) may be able to contact neighbors or a landlord. Useful information concerns the patient's level of competence—work history, life achievements, relationships with others, and ability to care for himself or herself. Look in particular for recent personality changes, confusional episodes (particularly at night), recent falls or trauma, or any history suggestive of withdrawal phenomena from alcohol or other drugs.

Observations by nursing staff

These are particularly important because confusional episodes, particularly at the beginning, are characteristically spotty in nature. Initial episodes are usually a matter of a few minutes, apparent lapses in the normal level of acuity, which you simply have to be there to see. Since nursing staff are around the patient 24 hours a day and physicians are with the patient on an intermittent basis, nursing staff are far more likely to pick up these lapses. That is especially so because confusional episodes characteristically begin at night after the sun goes down (the so-called sundowner's syndrome), and therefore it is the night nurse who most often is the first person to spot the condition. We may be inclined to doubt the nurse's report when the patient looks great the following morning, but we must not do so. Pay attention to reports of nocturnal restlessness, apparent nightmarish behavior, and the like. Ask nursing staff to watch for these kinds of events. They are often forerunners of full-blown confusional episodes.

If the assessment thus far indicates any cause for concern, you will want to examine the patient more carefully. Possible additional techniques include a careful mental status exam, a detailed neurologic exam, and such special studies as psychological testing, electroencephalogram, and other neurodiagnostic tests. While we are talking specifically about confusion, information about other aspects of the patient's medical condition (including other complaints or significant physical or laboratory findings) will need to be integrated into our understanding.

MENTAL STATUS EXAMINATION

In order to evaluate the mental status exam, we must conceptualize disease as a whole person process, and see the mental status exam as a means of assessing the disease as well as the person with the disease.

The mental status exam is a contrived and ritualized way for one human being to assess the intellect and personality of another. Therein lie both its advantages and disadvantages. The advantages are that it is a convenient bedside technique, a simple verbal form of psychological testing; it provides an organized outline for persons needing a convenient assist to memory. It is logical in that it proceeds from the superficial and general to the more specific; it is apparently comprehensive; and it provides a shared clinical language for conveying assessments to colleagues (e.g., how the patient performed on proverbs and serial sevens). Its disadvantages are that it lacks the virtues of detailed psychological testing, and therefore may mislead us into thinking that we have assessed aspects of the patient's mentation which we have not; it is not truly comprehensive; there is no standardized administration of examination items (with consequent lack of standardized interpretation); and there is no numerical score to objectify results. There are standardized mental status exams ranging from ten-point inventories to long computer-scored tests of obstacle-course proportions, but generally these are poor compromises between the bedside mental status exam and genuine psychological testing.

Nonetheless, the mental status exam is the quickest and handiest tool available for serial analyses of the patient's level of consciousness and intellectual grasp, so it pays to be able to perform one. Doing the job thoroughly will provide a detailed picture of the patient's intellect, and clues as to the nature and the location of specific pathologic processes.

The precise order of the exam doesn't matter as long as all bases are covered and it proceeds comfortably. Follow the same general approach you use in sizing up people in general, whether poker opponents or at a party. However, remember that your purpose in the clinical setting is unique and specific: assessment of the patient's intellect and personality for signs which indicate treatable impairment or potential problems in the patient's ability to cooperate in treatment.

The following approach proceeds from the obvious to the subtle, from the superficial to the less readily accessible.

Appearance

Evaluate the patient's general physical condition, the care taken with appearance, dress, and grooming. Watch especially for such characteristic concomitants of dementia as shuffling gait, a posture characterized by an overall tendency to flexion (i.e., the patient bent forward with both arms and legs slightly flexed). Examine the facial expression, checking the level of alertness, looking for apprehensiveness, an air of bewilderment, or a vacuous expression. Be alert for a distracted picking at clothing or sheets, which is characteristic of the confused patient.

Speech

Aside from what the patient says, assess the manner of speaking. Is the patient appropriately responsive? Does he or she answer your questions directly, or go off on tangents? Is the speed of reaction within the range of normal? Are responses pondered unduly? Does the patient seem to be paying reasonable attention to interaction with you, and is there any difficulty in concentrating? Do you have difficulty following what the patient says? If so, is that the patient's problem or your problem?

Content

Listen to the patient's ideas and words. Does he or she obsess about any one particular subject? Does this patient seem able to discuss intelligently a broad range of subjects? Do you have any reason to believe that the patient may be having hallucinations or delusions? If in doubt, ask the patient, "Do you ever see or hear things which you think are not really there, or which other people are unable to see or hear?" If the patient seems at all suspicious or paranoid, ask if he or she ever has the feeling of being watched or picked on. If you get an affirmative response to any of these questions, ask for more detail.

Emotional state

Does the patient's emotional state remain reasonably uniform throughout the examination? Are emotional changes appropriate in response to what is happening, or does the patient undergo major emotional shifts without apparent stimulus? Emotional lability is an important concomitant of confusion for many individuals. Did the responses appear superficial, apathetic, blunted, or exaggerated? Watch, as always, for signs of anxiety and depression.

Insight

Does the patient understand what it means to be sick and to be seeing a physician? Is he or she capable of understanding? Ask the patient, "What is your understanding of why you are here? What are your expectations in this circumstance?" Do not be content with superficial answers; see how detailed a comprehension the patient has of his or her plight.

Sensorium

Assessment of the sensorium can range from the superficial to a truly comprehensive survey of cortical function which examines memory in detail, problem solving, language and arithmetic ability, abstract thinking and logic, and appreciation of complicated visual-spatial relationships. If you are uncomfortable asking the patient about the following material, feel free to introduce it by saying, "I'm going to ask you what you may regard as some silly questions. Please bear with me and answer as best you can. If you are in doubt, guess. Your answers will help me understand you better, and put me in a position to be of more assistance to you."

1. *Orientation.* Since disorientation is the key to many confusional states, inquiring about orientation is crucially important. Record the patient's responses verbatim in your write-up. Ask: "What is today's date? What day of the week? What month? What year?" (Being off a day or two is seldom significant, unless it represents a persistent pattern.) "What is the name and location of this place?"

2. *Concentration.* There are a variety of ways of testing concentration, and the most important consideration is choosing one *you* feel comfortable using. Ask the patient to count backwards from 100. Alternatively, ask him to perform serial sevens ("Please subtract 7 from 100, then subtract 7 from that answer, and continue to subtract 7 from each answer until I tell you to stop"). Try to make the test appropriate to the patient's interests or ethnicity: if the patient has trouble with numbers, ask him or her for detailed steps in cleaning a carburetor or making an apple pie.

3. *Short-term Memory.* Any test of memory is automatically a test of concentration, and there are a variety of ways to approach it. One convenient method is to have the patient repeat after you a series of digits forward, and then a series of digits backward. Say, "I'm going to tell you some numbers, and when I stop, I want you to repeat them." Start off with three digits and work up to seven, changing the series each time you increase the number of digits. If you want to make it easy on yourself, you can give the patient portions of phone numbers which you know by heart. However, that gives you an unfair advantage, and it may be more reasonable to make up a series of numbers and see if you can remember them as well as you are asking the patient to. You score this test by adding up the length of the series the patient is able to reproduce forward and backwards. Anyone with healthy mental function should be able to repeat six digits forward and then backward; many middle-aged adults can do eight or more. Some experts believe that a difference of more than three between the number of digits reproduced forward and the number of digits reproduced backwards represents significant impairment. Again, many individuals who perform poorly with numbers can repeat every item on a grocery list, or every record on the current "Top 20."

4. *General Knowledge.* Ask the patient a series of questions to which virtually everyone should know the answer. You can stop asking questions when you feel you have a good assessment of the patient's general knowledge. In a given individual that may require a lot of questions; in others, you will have gotten a good idea of general knowledge from the small talk that you have already performed. Ask, for instance, "What is the name of the current president? Tell me, in order, the presidents before him. Who is the vice-president? How many weeks are there in a year? How many days are there this month? What day is Christmas?" Most individuals can remember most of the presidents who served during their own lifetimes, but you needn't have an 80-year-old person complete the list all the way to Theodore Roosevelt. We're interested in a rough measure, not ability to reproduce detailed lists.

5. *Simple Arithmetic.* The patient's ability to do simple arithmetic is indicative of one's ability to manage transactions of everyday life. At the most basic level, you can ask questions like: "How much is 3 and 6? How must is 12 and 9?" At a slightly more sophisticated but nonetheless more revealing level, ask: "How much does a loaf of bread cost? How much change would you get back from a dollar? How much is your social security check? How much is your rent? How much money do you have left from your check after you have paid your rent?"

In general, I find that testing the patient for simile and proverb interpretation provides results that are useful primarily when they are patently bizarre. Ordinary individuals vary considerably in the concreteness or abstractness of their responses, so I include this area in mental status examinations only if I believe a patient is delusional and refusing to talk about it. In such a circumstance, proverb interpretation, if the patient is willing to do it, might give some clue about what is going on in the patient's mind.

NEUROLOGIC EXAMINATION

You will, of course, do your usual neurologic exam in the same way that you would with any patient for whom you suspect possible intracranial pathology. Aside from looking for localizing findings, there are a number of neurologic signs that indicate diffuse impairment. Look for them in any patient who is confused or potentially confused.

Paratonic rigidity

Also called *gegenhalten,* or involuntary resistance, this is a finding of increased tone with passive manipulation of the patient's extremities during exam. This finding is most dramatic if you manipulate the extremities rapidly, while simultaneously urging the patient to relax. This is a sign of diffuse cortical impairment.

Asterixis

Also known as *liver flap,* this is a coarse tremor at the wrist in the patient whose arms are fully outstretched, with the hands hyperextended at the wrists. Though customarily associated with liver disease, it is sometimes seen in uremia, gram-negative sepsis, chronic pulmonary disease, and other metabolic disorders. Any patient who demonstrates asterixis is a likely candidate for delirium.

Grasp reflex

This medical sign, like the one that follows, is a primitive reflex which indicates profound regression to an infantile level. Together, the reflexes are sometimes referred to as frontal lobe signs, but their presence is usually indicative of diffuse cerebral impairment. Though associated with dementia and therefore structural damage, the reflexes often come and go depending on the patient's overall status. The grasp reflex is elicited by stroking the palm of the metacarpal phalangeal joints or laterally from the hypothenar eminence. A positive response is when the patient grasps the finger and increases the hold as you pull your finger away.

Oral rooting reflexes

Variously called the *suck-and-snout* reflexes, these clinical signs have the same significance as the grasp reflex. To elicit the suck reflex, insert a fingertip or straw or similar implement between the patient's lips. A positive response is when the patient demonstrates a persistent, strong sucking motion. The snout reflex is elicited by gentle stroking of the patient's lip from the nasolabial fold laterally, with either a finger or a tongue depressor or similar implement. A positive response is when the patient's lips protrude as if seeking to suck, with the patient tending to follow the direction of the stimulus.

PSYCHOLOGICAL TESTING

The process and results of careful testing by gifted clinical psychologists are a joy to behold. While psychological testing is not unfailing in revealing brain disease, it is sometimes astonishing in the precision with which it can localize cortical lesions. Defects can be enormously subtle and simply undetectable by any other means. To pick up such nuances requires a meticulous approach, and the one doing the testing must be interested, experienced, and able. To achieve high levels of precision a reasonably cooperative patient is also required, although psychologists who enjoy doing testing are often very good at achieving such cooperation. Rapport is especially likely if you help the patient have positive expectations concerning the testing itself. Unfortunately, in this country, psychological testing has tended to occupy a less glamorous position than psychotherapy in most psychology training programs, and many psychologists regard psychological testing as drudge work. Therefore, when you find gifted psychologists who enjoy testing, let them know how much you appreciate them. They deserve all the support and encouragement they can get.

SPECIAL NEURODIAGNOSTIC EXAMS

There are numerous laboratory and other studies you may wish to order to pursue the possibility of specific diseases in any given patient. A discussion of the indications, techniques, and interpretation of such studies is more appropriate to a general medicine or neurology text than here.

Treatment

Helping the confused patient, especially in the hospital, depends upon a team effort, ideally including sympathetic nurses, an attentive family, and a good doctor-patient relationship. All must be allies in helping the patient overcome stress. Each must recognize the patient's impaired adaptability and do the utmost to be patient and understanding. Treatment is directed at the symptom itself, as well as any etiologic factors. Each step is useful not only in the hospital, but also at home, where concerned relatives are trying to make a difficult situation more tolerable.

Where possible, anticipate confusion before it occurs. Watch for the patient at risk. Review the five A's, and watch for their presence in your patients.

Orienting approaches

Since the core of the confusion experience is disorientation, use all means at your disposal to assist the patient with orientation and encourage others working with the patient to do the same.

1. Call the person by name. This has the double advantage of not only helping to orient the patient, but also helping to orient you with regard to who the patient is. Whether you call the patient by first or last name is a matter of mutual preference and will depend upon such matters as social class, ethnicity, and discrepancies in age. In general, older patients appreciate being addressed as Mr., Mrs., or

Miss, especially by younger strangers, even when those strangers happen to be physicians.

2. Identify yourself and your function vis–à–vis the patients each time you see them, unless they clearly know or recognize you. Name tags are obviously helpful in this regard. Remember that although the patient knows who you are on one occasion he or she may not remember later.

3. Help orient the patient as to time. A clock and calendar in the room can be extremely useful. Additional helpful devices include current newspapers, magazines, a radio, or television.

4. Keep a pad of paper or notebook at the patient's bedside and within easy reach for the patient. Encourage the patient to write down important names, the room number, pending laboratory tests, etc. When the patient repeatedly asks the staff a question, see that the answer is written down and remind the patient to look up the notation when the question is repeated.

5. Help the patient identify his or her room. Put a piece of colored tape or the patient's name on the door. Encourage the keeping of personal items inside the room—pictures of family, items of clothing, and the like.

6. Guard against nighttime confusion. Put a night-light in the room. Encourage the night staff to introduce themselves to the patient. Use your ingenuity. Some patients will be assisted by a sign in the room that says, "You are in Memorial Hospital, Ward 4B. Today's date is. . . ."

Style of communication

Keep communication simple and straightforward. Speak slowly and clearly. Avoid presenting many thoughts at once. Allow time for the patient to absorb what you are saying, to integrate new information with what he or she knows already, and to ask questions. Above all, be patient. However, be careful of your manner: don't talk down to the patient as if to a child.

Respect feistiness. A bit of cantankerousness means the patient still has pride, which is perhaps his or her most valuable asset. You have to be comfortable enough with yourself not to become defensive if feistiness takes the form of deriding everyone else.

Try to avoid direct conflict. Attempt to direct the patient's wanderings, rather than to prevent them. Instead of tying the patient into a chair, put a piece of tape on the patient's back: "My name is thus and so, please help me find my way back to Ward 4B."

Confusion as a symptom

Continually reassure the patient and the family that confusion is an understandable symptom of what is happening with the patient's general overall condition, and this symptom will improve as the overall condition improves. Emphasize the positive prognosis. The patient and family need to know that the patient is not irreversibly crazy.

The staff must remember to see the behavioral manifestations of confusion as an attempt by the patient to cope with severe stress. Help them to accept it as such and not to see the patient's behavior as mere obstreperousness. Help them to understand the fluctuations in the patient's awareness as a product of a dynamic equilibrium, a battle between the forces of awareness and the forces assaulting the patient's awareness.

For yourself, recognize the value of confusion as a symptom, and remember to look for subclinical deterioration of the patient's physiologic functioning whenever confusion becomes more pronounced.

Constancy of staff
Wherever possible, see that the confused or potentially confused have consistency of staff during their hospitalization. Avoid transferring them from one ward to another. At times of house staff rotation, make a special effort to ensure that the new house staff introduce themselves to the patient. Encourage nursing staff to keep personnel assignments constant during such changeovers.

Support for retained functions
Give unreserved praise for small accomplishments and avoid petty criticisms of oversights and failures.

Attend to such potential hazards as unnecessary obstacles in the room. Be alert to such small but important details as grab bars in the bathroom and side rails on the bed.

Keep the patient in the best possible physiologic condition by careful attention to nutrition.

Support the patient's confidence by focusing on areas of the patient's life where he or she has functioned effectively. This may require interest, persistence, and ingenuity on your part. You must find areas of mutual interest with the patient in order to do this task well.

Do whatever you can to remove obstacles to restful sleep. Decrease the frequency of monitoring vital signs at night. Rearrange audio monitoring devices so there aren't constant noises at the patient's bedside.

Attention to sensory deprivation
Make sure the patient has glasses and hearing aids available if he or she needs them. Request large-type books if necessary and consider a radio or TV in the room an essential part of your treatment. Write an order requesting a volunteer to read to, or write letters for, the patient. Encourage nursing staff to find a garrulous roommate for the patient, and help that roommate to understand the patient's needs and confu-

sion. See that the intercom is kept in working order, and make sure the patient knows how to use it. Do whatever can be done to avoid monotony of color, immobilization in bed, and the nerve-racking drone of equipment. Touch the patient when you are talking to him or her. Move the patient into a chair near the nursing station. Call in a "granny sitter" to keep the patient company. Ask occupational therapy for diversionary materials and activities. If the food menu is beyond help, encourage friends and relatives to bring in interesting things to eat. Hell, bring the patient a dill pickle yourself.

Treatment of concomitant medical disorders
Obviously.

Medications
The first task with medications is to decrease the total number of medications and size of dosages. Many elderly patients with complicated medical disorders are on a dozen or more medications. Scrutinize the list and seek to eliminate any that can impair the patient's adaptability to stress, especially those with sedative properties. Avoid barbiturates like the plague.

If the patient appears to need nighttime sedation, remember that most will respond to nonpharmacologic treatment or mild measures such as a glass of warm milk, a glass of wine, or a shot of whiskey. Some need small doses of chloral hydrate or a short-acting benzodiazepine. Seek sedation that does not produce clouding.

There is considerable disagreement about the specifics of drugs to be used with the elderly confused patient. Clearly, there is room here for your own idiosyncracies. When tranquilizers are needed, my first choice is a major tranquilizer that does not produce sedation and concomitant grogginess. Of the phenothiazines, I customarily choose trifluoperazine (STELAZINE), from 2 to 5 mg b.i.d., either orally or parenterally, and increase the dosage to 10 mg b.i.d. if necessary. For a nonphenothiazine, a butyrophenone—e.g., haloperidol (HALDOL), in the same dosage—is equally useful. Both have the advantage of causing no significant cardiac side effects. Taper the medicines when intercurrent stresses have subsided. Parkinsonian side effects are frequent with these drugs, but less serious than other side effects of other major tranquilizers. Such patients also customarily respond to a day or so of antiparkinsonian drugs, e.g., trihexyphenidyl (ARTANE) and benztropine (COGENTIN). However, if the latter are necessary, beware of increased anticholinergic activity, and beware of such potential problems as ileus or urinary retention.

For delirium associated with alcohol withdrawal, benzodiazepines are probably the most widely used agents. These are given in high doses. An example is chlordiazepoxide (LIBRIUM) from 50 to 100 mg in an intramuscular injection, every four hours, which can be reduced to four times a day, whenever the patient is stable, and then tapered. Remember that *delirium tremens* is a complicated medical condition and a potentially hazardous one, and requires more comprehensive treatment than simply the use of tranquilizers.

Adequate convalescence

Be wary of discharging your patient prematurely. Make sure his or her condition is stable, and see that adequate discharge plans are made. Careful discharge planning for the potentially confused elderly requires thoughtful consideration of alternatives and the investment of considerable time in investigating them. Don't demand that the social worker do this in a single day. Get the social worker involved early in the patient's hospital course. Often, there are a wide variety of self-help groups, family-support groups, and other resources which can substantially lighten the burden of the patient's care.

Bibliography

Arie T: Dementia in the elderly—diagnosis and assessment. *Brit Med J* 4:540–543, 1973

Bower HM: The differential diagnosis of dementia. *Med J Aust* 2:623–262, 1971

Cath SH: The institutionalization of a parent—the nadir of life. *J Geriatr Psychiatr* 5:25–45, 1972

Engel GL, Romano J: Delirium, a syndrome of cerebral insufficiency. *J Chronic Dis* 9:260–277, 1959

Grassian S: Psychopathological effects of solitary confinement. *Am J Psychiatry* 140:1450–1454, 1983

Heston LL, White JA: *Dementia—A Practical Guide to Alzheimer's Disease and Related Illnesses.* New York, W.H. Freeman, 1983

Johns MW, Large AA, Masterton JP, et al.: Sleep and delirium after open heart surgery. *Br J Surg* 61:377–381, 1974

Katz MN et al.: Delirium in surgical patients under intensive care. *Arch Surg* 104:310–313, 1972

Kerstein MED, Isenberg S: Dealing with the confused elderly patient. *Hosp Community Psychiatry* 25:160–161, 1974

Lipowski ZJ: Delirium, clouding of consciousness and confusion. *J Nerv Ment Dis* 145:227–277, 1967

Lipowski ZJ: Transient cognitive disorders in the elderly. *Am J Psychiatry* 140:1426–1436, 1983

Massie MJ, Holland J, Glass E: Delirium in terminally ill cancer patients. *Am J Psychiatry* 140:1048–1050, 1983

Mayeux R, Rosen W: *The Dementias—Advances in Neurology, Vol 38.* New York, Raven Press, 1983

Morse RM: Postoperative delirium—Syndrome of multiple causation. *Psychosomatics* 11:164–168, 1970

Perez EL, Silverman M: Delirium—the often-overlooked diagnosis. *Intl J Psychiatry in Med* 14:181–192, 1984

Raber P: The dementia dilemma. *Geriatrics* 38(8):121–124, 1983

Reich P, et al.: Unrecognized organic mental disorders in survivors of cardiac arrest. *Am J Psychiatry* 140:1194–1197, 1983

Ruskin PE: Geropsychiatric consultation in a university hospital. *Am J Psychiatry* 142:333–336, 1985

Trzepacz PT, Teague GB, Lipowski ZJ: Delirium and other organic mental disorders in a general hospital. *Gen Hosp Psychiatry* 7:101–106, 1985

6

Emotional Aspects
of Major Disease
Categories

During your illness I suppose you did a lot of thinking about your situation. That is what these illnesses are for, you know—these mysterious ailments that take us out of life but do not kill us. They are signals that our life is going the wrong way and intervals for reflection.
—Robertson Davies

This chapter deals with people rather than diseases. One could study the emotional aspects of virtually every condition from epididymitis to deviated nasal septum, and sometimes in looking through the literature I am compelled to think that people already have.

Precise distinctions between the categories discussed here and those discussed elsewhere in this book are more arbitrary than real. An example is a 40-year-old banker, a bright and capable human being with an impish sense of humor, who has progressive diabetic peripheral vascular disease and retinopathy. Most of the time he copes valiantly, but intermittently he slides into depression and indulges in irritable dependency. When he feels best and is most effective in his family and job, he is denying his inevitable physical deterioration for all he is worth. Every now and then, when he feels really comfortable with someone he trusts, he can talk about what it is like to contemplate his increasing disability, to envision the natural course of what is eventually a terminal illness, and to ruminate about killing himself with an insulin overdose before he loses all self-esteem and becomes hopelessly dependent on all around him.

To file this man under any single chapter or section of this book is obviously more a reflection of our own need for simplicity and order than any natural properties of our patient. To label him a depressive or quarrelsome patient or a dependent personality is to fail to understand the nature of illness. As with so many patients, our understanding of him must transcend simple categorization.

Almost all the disorders to be discussed are complicated, so that any patient with a given condition is likely to have contact with multiple physicians, nurses, counselors, social workers, technicians, and rehabilitation personnel. In most complex medical centers, coordinating all these people and services is extremely difficult, even when one person takes the responsibility for doing so, which in my experience represents the exception rather than the rule. All this fragmentation of services presents numerous obstacles for even the motivated patient; it's easy to see how the discouraged patient, with flagging motivation, tends through simple inertia to remain in the sick role.

Our goals for these patients include helping them to function optimally, a task much easier to label than to define or achieve. Indeed, no one—healthy or ill—functions "optimally" all the time; and most of us function well below capacity much of the time. Demanding more of the sick or injured than we do of ourselves generally leads only to frustration for both ourselves and the patients, though the nobility of the intent is difficult to dispute.

So much of improved function depends upon treasured trifles which cannot all be anticipated or placed on a protocol; e.g., the extra quarter-inch on a stump prosthesis that eliminates pelvic tilt, reduces low back pain, and makes ambulation tolerable, or the smuggled aspirin at the hospitalized patient's bedside for self-medication when the overworked nurses can't bring analgesics punctually. Some of the details the patients can learn from us, some from other patients, some they can only discover by themselves. What is important is that we help establish an atmosphere in which such exchange of information and such discoveries are facilitated. How do we accomplish that? No one can do it alone, but an empathetic understanding of what it is really like for one human being to suffer from a certain type of affliction is a reasonable point from which to proceed.

At the same time, we need to remind ourselves that these same afflictions have emotional impact upon *us,* and we need to integrate into any formulation an understanding of our own reactions.

Feelings are contagious—whether grief, resignation, bitterness, or the like—a fact that often leads to some deeply rooted instinctual responses. Withdrawal is among the most primitive of these, and, while it has obvious self-preservation value for the health professional, most of us can develop more constructive responses as we grow in clinical experience. We vary in our expectations of, and responses to, the cardiac patient versus the alcoholic, the facially disfigured versus the chronic lung patient. Usually, we are most comfortable with patients who make the fewest emotional demands upon us, but we take care of them all, and (we hope) with a manner that enhances our own self-respect as well as that of the patient.

The Grossly Disabled

> . . . [B]ecoming less helpless is negative and is not equivalent to becoming more capable. Not being as bad off as the next man is different from being better off than he. Most crucial of all, not being a burden is different from being a help; and not getting worse seldom offers the same kind of satisfaction as getting better. The problem is not merely one of "positive thinking"; it is one of conflict of interest. . . . Many severely disabled patients prefer to remain in the hospital for precisely the reason that they feel themselves to be less burdensome there than they would be at home, especially if they can pay for their own institutional care.
>
> —F. C. Shontz

Being significantly disabled is to have the small details of daily living (such as dressing, eating, getting about the house) become major challenges. Activities other than those that can be managed as a routine— however complicated—may require enormous planning and psychic energy; e.g., visiting a friend or going to the store. Actual or potential helplessness pervades all of life. Whether a person is disabled from birth or from events in later life, the disabled person has segments of personality and life-style different from that of the nondisabled. Despite the fact that physical disability is not linked in any clear way to any particular psychological behavior, there is no question that disability often has dramatic consequences.

Severe disability means a decreased ability to cope with the physical demands of living, as well as diminished social functioning and impaired ability to carry on usual adult roles with family and friends. Whether such disability results from muscular dystrophy, multiple sclerosis, or paraplegia, the disability itself must be viewed as a dynamic rather than a static state. It is crucial to see the course of the disease and the course of the patient's adaptation to disease or injury, as subject to a natural evolution. At various stages, the patient can be expected to exhibit regression, dependence, interdependence, flight from dependence, or therapeutic nihilism, and we must be able to view these as part of a natural process.

There is general agreement that adaptation does not depend solely on the type and severity of the physical handicap per se. Variables include the full gamut of personality styles, the nature and amount of support and reinforcement in the environment, and the implicit and explicit expectations of the patients and those around them. For instance, if the disability is dramatically visible, people will tend to expect less of the patient than if the disability is not so apparent, and consequently patients may come to see themselves in the same way.

REACTIONS TO DISABLEMENT

The disabled, like all of us, have a desire for social approval; and, again like so many of us, much of their own self-esteem is dependent upon the esteem in which they are held by others. Much of the behavior of the disabled is designed to achieve seeming conformity to the dominant standards of behavior established by the well persons around them. Some disabled persons go to extraordinary lengths to demonstrate and explain how hard they work, how they are really "normal."

Yet most invalids are aware that they frighten and arouse uneasiness in others. If others don't expect you to be "normal," how do you respond? Do you go to elaborate lengths to prove yourself? Do you say "to hell with it," and give up trying? Do you learn to set your own standards, and live with them comfortably? Obviously, that depends a great deal upon the individual involved. It requires considerable personal security and comfort on the part of the disabled to be neither angered nor insecure in the presence of obvious discomfort on the part of the nondisabled.

In addition to the ordinary diverse roles that all human beings have to fill, the disabled person must juggle some additional kinds of expectations. The disabled person is, of course, a patient and is consequently often expected to be dependent, passive, and compliant; being defined as "sick," the patient is in consequence inextricably bound to the health-care system. Second, the patient is labeled "handicapped" and viewed as impaired and imperfect. He or she is not expected to function at a "normal" level, and these lowered expectations affect not only specific motor and sensory tasks, but also psychological, interpersonal, and economic functioning. Third, this handicapped patient is a helped person. He or she must expect to receive more help than a nondisabled person, from acquaintances and strangers alike, even when it isn't needed or wanted. Fourth, the disabled person is an explainer, one who must continually explain his or her performance level, not only because other people are curious, but also because they are uncertain what he or she can and cannot do. Any new social encounter is likely to include questions about the etiology of the disability, how the disabled person copes, et cetera.

Often we physicians tend to have low expectations for disabled persons, and consider any improvement or slowing of inexorable deterioration as evidence of success. Patients are seldom as sanguine about small increments of improvement as the physicians. They tend to adhere to the standards of society as a whole, measuring themselves by what "normals" can do rather than comparing themselves with other "handicapped" persons. Many will be unable to work at their predisability levels, and will feel disappointed and frustrated as a consequence. Most will feel restricted socially, unable to operate independently in terms of carrying out ordinary daily activities. Only a portion will be completely happy with their medical care and its consequences.

TREATMENT ATTITUDES

Successful treatment of disabled individuals depends first upon understanding our own emotional reactions in their presence, and second upon recognizing that the behavior of the disabled is more like than different from the nondisabled. Strive to be helpful without demeaning. Ask yourself, What are my goals for myself in working with this patient? Our goals need to be realistic for us, just as the patient's goals need to be realistic for him or her.

Ultimately, these patients must learn to make the transition from seeing themselves as sick, to seeing themselves as different. They must do so without losing their own sense of humanity, retaining the knowledge that however different they may be, they still share more similarities than differences with the nondisabled.

Mourning the loss of one's previous self is a frequent, if not necessary, step to adaptation. Some experts think that the lack of significant depression and mourning in the face of disability is sufficiently unusual as to constitute a potential cause for concern on the part of the physician. However, an important exception exists when the specific source of disability is a consequence of a long illness and concomitant suffering which was relieved by operation; e.g., amputation after a long and painful osteomyelitis or vascular disease.

Setting realistic treatment goals for the severely disabled may be difficult. One goal that is commonly mentioned is "minimal dependence on a paid attendant," but often that's a goal set for the patient by physicians and other health personnel. It is important to note the contrast between the values of such a goal to the patient and to society as a whole. In some instances relative self-sufficiency may have few rewards. Why should a patient leave a safe and secure hospital bed, where he or she is looked after by generally caring persons, for what may be a lonely and arduous existence in a single room in an unattractive and dangerous part of the city? The person saves money for society in doing so, but his or her own existence is likely to be more marginal.

Productivity and inner comfort, both of which are highly valued in our society, are not necessarily any more correlated in the handicapped than in anyone else. For example, which of the following has adapted better, and by whose standards: a cerebral palsy victim who drives himself, dragging his body on metal crutches to work each day, using every bit of physical and emotional energy he has, or a person with a similar disability who stays home, lives off of disability payments, and piddles around with various projects and activities of interest only to himself, but which nonetheless give him pleasure and a sense of personal growth?

Attempts to diminish dependency may be more a reflection of the values of the health care givers than of the patients. Still, ambivalence is common in both doctors and patients concerning dependency. Dependency may be frightening, but it has its appealing aspects too. On the other hand, in our culture it is a rare person who can be blatantly dependent without feeling guilty. Dependency implies subservience and inferiority and is often associated with hostility, perhaps subtly expressed, but aimed at the person or institution upon whom the handicapped person must depend.

Both doctor and patient should recognize that disability is an enormously frustrating condition. Learning to *use* frustration spells the difference between effective coping and unnecessary degrees of disability. Frustration should therefore not only be acknowledged, but perhaps even welcomed. When you see it in your patient say to yourself and perhaps to him, "Good. The frustration feels lousy, but it's a sign that you are struggling and in those struggles you will find new achievements and new meaning for yourself." As patients struggle with basic adjustments to disability, they may be intolerant of having to adjust to further demands put on them by yourself and others. They may be critical of you, clinic routine, rotations of house staff, staff inconsistency, and so on. Try to understand this intolerance and not take it personally.

Besides yourself, many resources are available to the disabled person. Among the most important are fellow patients. If your patient does not know anyone who has a similar disability, help him or her find someone. Often, the social worker or the physical therapist can provide useful referrals. Fellow patients can help provide not only technical information about coping with specific disabilities, but also modeling behavior, mutual support groups, and a potential new social matrix for spouses and family members who themselves are struggling with the implications of disability. As disabled persons become more familiar with their conditions, they may also be able to give suggestions and support to the newly disabled, and being able to give to someone else is gratifying for virtually everyone.

Thousands of other resources are available to the disabled, and many may be accessible within your specific community and relevant for any given patient. These resources are gold mines of technical information, financial support, transportation, counseling for families, et cetera. Getting your patient in touch with these groups is an important part of treatment. For most of us, patients or not, one's level of achievement is not only a function of personal motivation, but is also partially dependent on the attitudes and behavior of the people in our environment.

That is why patients are often reluctant to leave the hospital. There they feel generally accepted by other patients and sometimes by the hospital staff, whereas at home they may be regarded with resentment or even disgust. Most patients find it helpful to be able to talk about this paradox. Help them to understand that wishing to cling to the hospital is understandable and normal and needn't be a source of guilt. At the same time, if they wish to grow and evolve, sooner or later they will have to face the challenges of the outside environment.

The Disfigured Patient

We all of us want to make a good impression. The worse we are and the uglier, the more anxious we are to appear good and beautiful.
—Luigi Pirandello

Most of God's children are, in fact, barely presentable. The most common error made in matters of appearance is the belief that one should disdain the superficial and let the true beauty of one's soul shine through.
—Fran Lebowitz

What constitutes disfigurement is a matter of personal definition, comfort, and discomfort, both for the patients and for the people around them. Disfigurement can run the gamut from cleft lip to acne scars to hemimandibulectomy for carcinoma. In many respects, the problems faced by patients with each of these conditions differ only in degree and frequency from what we all encounter. While the discussion that follows is therefore relevant to persons with small facial scars or ptosis of one lid, most of the material will focus on the dramatically disfigured; e.g., the patient with a severe facial burn or with extensive orofacial surgery. (To a lesser extent the discussion is also relevant for patients with any highly visible injury or disorder, such as amputation of the hand or Parkinson's disease.)

REACTIONS TO DISFIGUREMENT

Despite the now extensive surgical experience with restoration of badly disfigured faces, the literature cites few examples of ideal psychosocial rehabilitation. If the patient's face appears stomach-turning from third degree burns or heroic surgery, his appearance is likely to remain discomforting to himself and others for the rest of his life. Many, many patients lose heart with the numerous hospitalizations and procedures necessary to produce modest cosmetic gains, in what basically is a horrenderoma. The tendency is to withdraw from medical care, and I have been unable to find much information about what happens to dramatically disfigured persons after that. My own assessment is that most are probably destroyed by social ostracism, loss of employment, dwindling finances, and shattered self-esteem. If a person's face is truly repellent, it becomes such a barrier to communication that comfortable social contacts become a virtual impossibility. Patients with second and third degree burns over 75% of their bodies now have a chance for life as a consequence of magnificent technologic achievements, but the quality of that life in fact may be so gruesome by generally accepted standards that the experience of medical care may be extremely difficult for the patients and for everyone concerned.

An ethic of our society is that everyone should be treated equally. In actuality, treating the severely disfigured equally may be extraordinarily difficult. The face is the most crucial part of our body in representing who we are to others. As the physician's first focus in a mental status exam is the patient's facial appearance, so also does the average person look at another's face in assessing what kind of person one is talking to. The face is widely viewed as the mirror of the personality. Consequently, in comparison with the rest of the body, the face gets lavish attention from us, from the beauty industry, and from journalistic photography. Advertising campaigns and heavy cultural emphasis on attractive appearances far outweigh any comments you or I could make regarding "what a lovely person you are on the inside." The indisputable reality is that looks *do* count in our culture, and research has amply documented that physically attractive persons tend to be viewed by themselves and others as "better" than less attractive persons.

Most of us feel terribly uncomfortable with the facially disfigured individual and as a consequence avoid him or her. Families usually feel similar discomfort and greater embarrassment and guilt in addition. Families therefore need enormous support themselves if they are to be able to provide support to the patient.

People in contact with the facially disfigured manifest their discomfort in various ways, often with stares or studied avoidance, sometimes with comments or questions, subtle or overt discrimination, and often with frank horror and uneasy humor. Jokes about scarfaces, harelips, and the like are legion.

How do disfigured persons view themselves? Without exception, the physical pain pales by comparison with the emotional pain. Most feel a sense of shame and a terrible self-consciousness. They know that other people are uncomfortable with them, and feel always on a stage. They continually calculate the impression that they make upon others, and ask, Is this a person who is comfortable with me? Most alternate between cowering and attempts at bravado.

While other patients can gain from mutual support groups, there are no groups for the facially disfigured: they simply don't want to look at one another. They desire to forget conflicts with the need to adjust to reality. Almost all have a strong desire to be seen as persons separate from their disfigurement, not in spite of or because of it—"I know my face looks horrible, but there's more to me than that." However, most find it difficult to convince themselves, and impossible to convince the staring people they meet in doctors' offices, hospital corridors, or on the streets. Those who probably do best are older and middle-aged individuals with solid achievements and skills which lend themselves to sheltered employment. If the patient is employed at all, he or she usually hides away (and is hidden) in back rooms away from the public. The disfigured tend to be offered, and to seek out, menial jobs.

How do physicians and nurses manage to work with such patients? Most have fairly conventional views regarding physical attractiveness and repulsiveness, but do their best to exhibit at least a superficial acceptance. In the hospital, stresses are greatest on the nursing staff, who have the most patient contact and the least authority for major decision making. Whether the disfigurement is caused by burn, trauma, or radical surgery, there are likely to be problems with tracheostomy and respiratory care, feedings and secretions, isolation needs, and often smell and immobility. Therefore, such patients often have enormous needs for additional staff time, energy, and physical effort. In addition, staff have to cope with the guilt they feel at their discomfort with the patient. The emotional reaction often includes feelings of Why doesn't she just just go away, or die? However, the patient often has nowhere else to go, and few patients escape thinking actively about suicide.

As is true of so many other conditions discussed in this chapter, persons who are facially disfigured customarily have contact with many health professionals including the ophthalmologist, orthodontist, plastic surgeon, otorhinolaryngologist, speech therapist, and prosthodontist. The multiplicity of health-care providers provides an agony of multiple social contacts for the patient, but also brings an opportunity to practice gauging the impact of one's appearance upon others. He or she soon learns that brief and businesslike contacts go tolerably well with individuals who are empathetic and interested, but that prolonged or more personal contact is difficult even for professionals used to dealing with the disfigured.

Mastectomy patients, ostomy patients, and others with a concealable disfigurement represent a much more private disfiguration, but the sense of mutilation nonetheless may be substantial. The emotional suffering of these patients may far outweigh the physical tribulations of surgery. The potential for grief is often greatest in terms of marital and sexual relationships; almost all patients worry about whether their spouse or significant other will be able to accept and survive the inevitable psychic shock waves.

TREATMENT ATTITUDES

How can we, as physicians, treat such patients most effectively? How directly should we discuss their physical appearance with them? Alternatives include (1) not discussing the matter unless the patients bring it up, (2) asking the patients about it if they seem to want to discuss it, (3) setting aside some time for specifically discussing the issue, (4) working it into a discussion gradually, or (5) discussing it with the patients if they wish but not dwelling on it.

Useful rules to go by are 1) respecting the patients' wishes in beginning, continuing, and ending conversations, and 2) providing a comfortable and accepting manner which will facilitate such conversations. In general, try to let specific discussions about physical appearance evolve as a natural part of your relationship with patients as their doctor. Let them know that you perceive them as people separate from their disfigurement, and try to convey this feeling by actions rather than words.

At a superficial level, you can talk about a patient's disfigurement as a visible part of personal history. You can liken it to "wisdom lines" on the face of the elderly, or the pride duelists used to take in visible scars. (This approach is generally useful only when the patient's disfigurement is the consequence of some activity in which he or she can take some pride or comfort, e.g., action by a fireman in the line of duty.)

One of the most important things that a physician can do is to come to terms with personal feelings of embarrassment. Do not demand full comfort in either yourself or the disfigured person. If you seek that as a goal, you are unlikely to find it, and you'll only end up feeling guilty. Expect and accept ambivalent feelings and behavior in everyone associated with the patient. Help the patient to understand such reactions.

Whatever you do, refrain from avoidance behavior. Try to be accessible and ready to listen, on the patient's terms. If you feel too uncomfortable to fill this role, make sure that someone else is available to do so.

Tell newly disfigured patients that they can expect to be shyer with strangers, hesitant in social situations, and more sensitive to rejection than is the average person. Tell them that with effort, patience, and understanding, they can expect to find satisfaction in working with familiar people, in family life, and in private kinds of recreation. If the patient has been involved in a stable family relationship prior to disfigurement, he or she can reasonably hope for it to continue. If the relationship was shaky to begin with, encourage the patient not to blame its dissolution on disfigurement. Both you and the patient must avoid attributing all of the patient's negative experiences to appearance.

Expect and acknowledge problems in the spouse, too. Emphasize that a period of adjustment is perfectly normal, and resumed sexual activity may take some time and adaptation for both of them. The patient may believe it is cheating one's spouse to continue their relationship, and may lose all sexual desire. One or the other may require covering or complete darkness to perform satisfactorily. To the extent the spouse is able and willing, involve him or her in major treatment decisions. Make sure that emotional support is available the first time the spouse views the disfigurement. Do not be surprised if the patient or spouse scapegoat you or members of the surgical team, deflecting helpless rage against fate (or one another) onto a handy and sometimes socially sanctioned medical target. Ironically, some studies show that among patients with breast cancer and subsequent disfiguring surgery, those who have the longest survival rates show the worst attitudes toward their physicians and are the most vocal in expressing their unhappiness about their condition and its treatment.

Consider referral to a cosmetician or make-up artist. Such individuals are not easy to find and are seldom a part of the normal health-care referral network, but when skilled—they can give an enormous morale boost to your patient.

Consider referral to local mental health resources, but don't refer randomly. Make certain that the person to whom you are referring the patient has experience and comfort in working with the severely disfigured. If you have confidence in the mental health services available, this confidence is likely to be transmitted to the patient, with profitable consequences.

Terminal Illness

> *If I am killed, I can die but once; but to live in constant dread of it, is to die over and over again.*
> —Abraham Lincoln

When there is someone in a family who has long been ill, and hopelessly ill, there come terrible moments when all those close to him timidly, secretly, at the bottom of their hearts wish for his death.
—Anton Chekhov

If you believe that the subject of the dying patient has been worked to death, we are in agreement. Nonetheless, most physicians have to deal regularly with the issue of death and dying, so the issue is clearly relevant to effective clinical practice. In addition, since our job is usually to support life and fight the possibility of death, we may (paradoxically) have more difficulty in discussing the matter objectively and comfortably than individuals who have had far less experience in the area.

There are as many ways to die as there are to live. Sudden death is the exception rather than the rule; more often, life continues while one is dying. Thus, the issue is not how to die, but rather how to live with the knowledge that death is imminent. Most individuals cope with this terminal portion of their life in much the way they have coped with other major stresses, i.e., most people die in character—angry people rebel, passive individuals remain acquiescent.

The issues of death and dying become manifest when either the doctor or the patient develops the assumption, spoken or unspoken, that the doctor-patient relationship will end in the patient's death, and that the physician can do nothing to significantly alter the time frame in which this will occur.

I believe our primary job is to not make the task any more difficult. I frequently have the feeling that the person who is dying, especially one who has gone through a prolonged course with repeated hospitalizations and therapeutic procedures, is more comfortable with the idea of impending death than those of us in professional attendance.

A reasonable goal for both doctor and patient during terminal care is death without regrets—"I did what I wanted to and what I thought was right."

The first major challenge with the terminally ill is discussing prognosis. While most physicians, nurses, and patients dread the process and moment of disclosure, truth is commonly a prerequisite for continuing mutually respectful relations. While you or the family can make a conscious decision about what you will or will not tell the patient, and you can conduct yourself accordingly in your relatively brief contacts, you must remember that especially the hospitalized patient has extensive contact with nursing staff and technicians. Much can be revealed inadvertently. It is almost impossible for the physician and family to keep all hospital personnel, from the nurse's aide to the x-ray technician, explicitly informed about what the patient has and has not been told. The patient almost always knows more than is explicitly discussed.

The rules are: don't run from the topic, and handle it naturally. It's not so much what you say, but how you say it. Adjust the *rate* of what you say according to the patient's needs, not your own.

It is most useful to think of disclosure as a hierarchy of truth which you ascend at a rate consistent with the patient's ability to cope. If you are sure of your instincts and have a good batting average with them, you can proceed along the hierarchy at a rate dictated by your clinical savvy. If you have any doubts, ask the patient what he or she knows or doesn't know and what he or she wishes to know. All this will be much, much easier if you routinely ask all your patients for their assessment of their own health state. Ask the patient, "What do *you* think is wrong with you? What does that diagnosis mean in practical terms of how it will affect your life? Do you expect to be disabled by this condition? Do you expect to die from it? What sort of time frame do you see for yourself?"

If at any level of the hierarchy, the patient's facts are in error, you can correct them. If at any level, the patient expresses ignorance, you can either give the information directly, if you think that is what he or she would like and is ready for, or if in doubt, say, "Well then, why don't I just let you ask me whatever questions you wish and I will respond as directly as I can." This latter approach allows you to regulate what you say precisely by the patient's spoken wishes. You will have to be alert to unspoken questions, but the approach nonetheless provides a reasonable general guideline. When you have answered a patient's specific question, ask, "Now what does that mean to you?" If the patient's response suggests blatant denial, do not force the issue. Further confrontation will only lead to more denial. Instead, say, "Well, we can talk about this more tomorrow or whenever you wish. I want you to feel free to ask me questions as they occur to you."

There are multiple ways of softening the blow when discussing a terminal prognosis. You can hedge on terminology: if the patient asks, "Is it cancer?" you can say, "Well, we call it an astrocytoma." If the patient asks what that means, explain it. Then ask for his or her understanding of what it is that you have said, and decide how to proceed upon that information. You can hedge on the certainty of the diagnosis. "Well, we *think* it may be cancer." If the patient is relieved by your uncertainty, you know that you will have to give him or her more time to absorb the information. If the patient wants to know the degree of certainty versus uncertainty, give it. You can hedge about prognosis: "The five-year survival rates are 25%." If the patient hears that to mean that he or she will survive five years, leave well enough alone. If you are asked, "Yes, but what does that mean in my particular case?", answer.

You can further soften the blow by emphasizing the role of chance. "The odds are thus and so, but one never knows. I've known people who've lived much longer." Or you can try to change the patient's focus from the issue of dying to something more manageable such as symptom control. "Of course everybody dies, but in your case we should be able to control the pain fairly well and you should be fairly comfortable."

Dying is a process, and a dynamic one at that, psychologically as well as physiologically. The process of adjustment is best seen as an evolution or a continuum which, for the convenience of our orderly minds, can be labeled as a series of stages.

Different authors have emphasized different kinds of labels for these stages, and you can freely conceptualize the process in any manner that makes sense to you. The important thing is to understand the diversity of potential responses, and to understand that each potential reaction serves a function for the patient. No response is pathologic per se; you can assume that any response manifested by the patient is serving a function for him or her. Therefore do not ask, Is this reaction helping or hurting the patient? Instead, ask, What function is this reaction serving for this patient at this time?

The dominant emotion at any given time is highly variable with the patient, the nature of the disease, the manner in which the prognosis is disclosed, the amount and type of resources available to the patient, the time frame, and, of course, the expectations and perspectives of the staff. Often, denial is a prominent early manifestation, though the type of denial varies, and denial in general becomes less prominent as the illness persists. Denial in fact is a key process: so long as a person is alive at one moment, one must function as though one will live the next. Various degress of depression, withdrawal, regression, and feelings of intense loneliness are common. Many patients express considerable anxiety, not only about death but also about the process of dying and whether they will be able to "perform" up to the level of their expectations. You should expect anger from a patient who is facing death, and you must see it as a natural emotion under the circumstances and not take it personally.

Acceptance of impending death ultimately depends upon acceptance of life as it has been lived. A person must accept who he or she is and isn't, what he or she has achieved and hasn't, relationships with loved ones, and the likely manner of death and its location. That's a lot of acceptance for any one person to achieve and most individuals fall short of total calm and happy acceptance. Acceptance may be either passive and take the form of calm resignation, or active, such as "putting one's affairs in order," "setting things right with God," feverishly making up for things undone, or studiously developing a philosophy concerning life and death. Occasionally, attempts at mastery over the dying process may take the form of self-destructive behavior. It is almost as though the patient says, "If I'm going to die, at least I can determine the manner in which I will go." Occasionally, patients fight their impending death with doctor-shopping, attempts at intensive living, and experiments with unorthodox therapies. It is difficult to say with assurance that any one activity or response is necessarily more meaningful or appropriate for any given patient than any other.

Most of the literature about death and dying does a thorough job of explaining the stages described so briefly above. However, it's important to understand that not only the patient goes through such stages. The people around the patient must go through a similar evolution in achieving their own acceptance of the patient's impending death. That's as true for the physicians and nurses who come to care about the patient as it is for friends and family. One can view death as a battle lost or as a way of meeting one's inevitable destiny. Major interpersonal problems develop when the patient and those around him or her are not going through the same stages at the same time: e.g., when the patient has accepted his or her fate, the spouse is overcome with depression and anger and the doctors and nurses are fighting death with a flurry of treatments.

The nature of the hospital milieu of course has its own effect upon relationships between staff, the hospitalized patient, and the family. Some wards are geared up for death, they face the problem regularly, and have their own protocol for doing so. The character of interactions will vary with whether dying is fast or slow, expected or unexpected, whether the patient is young or old, alert or comatose, aware or unaware, and alone or with a family.

The simple act of providing physical care to the patient may be emotionally draining if the patient is emaciated, disfigured, incontinent, confused, or emanates offensive odors. If family or staff has not frankly spoken with the patient about impending death, spending time with him or her can be very difficult, as considerable emotional energy must go into keeping "secret" information hidden, avoiding the appearance of lying, and coping with a sense of duplicity.

The principle difficulties for staff caring for dying patients occur when (1) there is disagreement about the amount of information to tell the patient, (2) the patient and staff are in disagreement regarding how much of a palliative nature should be done, or (3) the patient decides to die in a way the staff regards as lacking in dignity (i.e., exhibiting demanding, angry, or regressive behavior).

The challenge of deciding what *not* to do follows the challenge of deciding how much to make explicit. It is only by frank discussion of such matters with the patient and family that all the important individuals can hope to work together and in comfort on the difficult adjustment.

Once physician and family have agreed that "there is nothing further medically to be done," a period sometimes called the "Death Watch" ensues. It is appropriate to ask at this time if the patient would prefer to die at home. At the very least, when death is inevitable and imminent, each of us should do what we can to secure dignity and privacy for the patient and family. Having the relatives watch their loved one die amidst a clutter of noisy machinery, tubes, and apparatuses in the middle of a brightly lit intensive care unit hardly does much to make the moment of death peaceful and calmly accepted. Insofar as possible, do what you can to see that the patient will not die alone. Make certain that there is a place for family in the patient's room and for reserves in the waiting area. When patient and family accept that death is imminent, there often seems to be little for them to talk about. Conversations become stilted. After a social greeting, the most treasured contribution visitors can make to a dying patient is a comfortably silent presence. If visitors don't know that, it is often helpful for you or someone else to tell them.

If the patient is a Roman Catholic, either you or the family or hospital staff will want to see that the patient has access to last rites. Though Catholics who have last rites are usually comforted, the patient should of course have the opportunity to decline. Just as so many other things, the effect of last rites depends very much upon the manner in which they are administered and by whom. If the priest who administers the sacrament is calm and kind and good at his work, both patient and family will be reassured. But like physicians, priests also vary in their skills and their comfort with death, so the administration of the sacrament may occasionally seem more traumatic than helpful.

There are several points that are worth emphasizing in the care of the dying patient. In any prolonged hospitalization, the nurses and other hospital staff may form very strong attachments to the patient and the patient's family, and may therefore have to work through their own series of stages in the acceptance of death. Don't be surprised at intercurrent anger or denial, nor should you be unduly upset if these natural phenomena lead to some turmoil on the ward.

It is usually a worthwhile experience for physicians to work intensively with at least one dying patient. To be really close with one such patient, to empathize to the core, is a frightening but important developmental step for most of us. However, no doctor can mourn all patients, especially if he or she works in an arena where death or terminal illness are common. If you have many patients who face death, you will need your own personal support systems. Collegial support is clearly very important, but, beyond hearty pats on the back and reassurance that "you did the right thing," most of us need someone to open up to from time to time. Few of us have the emotional sustenance to manage all by ourselves the feelings generated by many such patients, and most of us are reluctant to take too much of the emotionally draining aspect of our work home with us at night. It's helpful to find a social worker, clergyman, psychiatrist, or colleague with whom we can talk about our reactions on a more intimate level. Once we have done so, not only can we manage more on our own, but we will have more tolerance for the needs of our patients and colleagues as well. Bottling it up inside will only lead to trouble.

If you can remain a calm and stabilizing source of support for your patient, there's no question that he or she is more likely to be able to adjust well to fate. Ask your patient, "With whom can you talk about this?" If you have neither the time nor the energy, see that the patient has access to someone who does.

Always recommend to your patient that spouses and family members know about the impending death. Some patients will want you to keep it a secret. Help the patient understand that everyone dreads the moment of disclosure, but things almost always go better once everyone knows. However, respect the patient's choice. Make a note in the medical record if you are uncomfortable with that choice, but respect it anyhow.

Treat regression in the patient with gentle, but firm limit-setting. Remember that it is common for patients facing death to focus on details and symptoms at the expense of facing the full implications of death itself. To that extent, minor complaints about pain, the food, and hospital staff are one adaptive response for the patient, and should be respected as such.

Whenever you emphasize a hopeful side of a patient's prognosis, ask yourself, Is this for the patient or am I doing this for myself? The fact that you need to emphasize hope for yourself does not necessarily make it wrong; you simply should know whose needs you're serving.

After a patient dies, many people may need an opportunity for acceptance, including the family, the staff, and yourself. It is useful to provide individuals with privacy for this purpose. You can tell family and others that after a death, survivors commonly go through a series of steps similar to those outlined for the patient before they come to full acceptance of the patient's death. Grieving takes some time, and feelings of resentment and guilt are common. Tell the family, "This will be a rough time for you," offer mild sedation if necessary, and suggest counseling with a minister or psychotherapist if things seem especially difficult.

The Chronic Disease Patient

The two greatest influences on my life have been my parents and asthma.

—Stanley Siegel

Prolonged illness requires that the person afflicted make fundamental changes in daily life-style, expectations of oneself, the degree of one's own involvement in personal health care, and one's hopes and dreams for the future. For almost all, total independence of physicians is impossible, but neither is it sensible to rely totally on the physician for management of every aspect of daily life. The goal is control, not cure; the patient must be an active participant with the physician and other resource people in effecting a maximum degree of control over his or her own health.

Chronicity may be defined by either permanency of disease and irreversibility of pathologic processes, or by residual disability and needs for extended care and observation.

Obviously there is considerable overlap in considerations relevant to the disabled patient and the chronically ill patient.

Chronic disease is not randomly distributed in our population; it is concentrated in the elderly. Also, the older the patient, the more likely that the spouse, friends, and other potential sources of support will also have chronic disease. It is often difficult to distinguish between limitations imposed by illness and those imposed as a natural consequence of increasing age. Young physicians certainly have difficulty in this regard, but so do patients; sometimes both fail to discern illness because they attribute impairments to aging.

Chronic disease is usefully viewed as a major life crisis which continues far beyond the time span shared by a physician who has only transient contact with the patient.

Chronically ill persons are commonly preoccupied in thoughts and conversation with what may seem to others as subtle nuances of their bodily function: rest, food, and elimination. To the outsider, these concerns may approach the hypochondriacal. When viewed empathetically, these same concerns represent an understandable reaction of someone whose life is undergoing fundamental change because of changing bodily processes. As with the dying patient, this narrowness of focus helps to concentrate attention on problems that are potentially manageable and curable in a way in which the basic disease process is not.

People with chronic illnesses tend to regard themselves as flawed and inferior not just in body, but also as persons. Such comments as

"I'm falling apart," "I'm not the man I used to be," and "I can't cut the mustard anymore," are usual. The chronically ill person is compelled to accept life on new terms and synthesize that part of him or her that is healthy with that part that is not. The patient with a chronic illness has to accept the notion that previous self-concepts are no longer appropriate. In that sense, the adaptation to chronic illness has many parallels with a person's adaptation to terminal illness. Frequently such adaptation involves multiple stages and a natural evolution through depression and various degrees of denial and anger to some degree of effective acceptance. All are a part of a natural process, and needn't cause concern in the physician simply by virtue of their presence.

Physicians and other health professionals also have to shift gears a bit and not approach the chronic patient with the same expectations with which we approach an acute patient. The patient necessarily performs differently, needs a different kind of relationship with physicians, and offers different kinds of rewards. Physicians who persistently get their psychic rewards only from curing people will inevitably be frustrated with the chronic patient and will tend to regard patients with chronic disease as turkeys or crocks or hypochondriacs. There is a further tendency to regard the sick, elderly patient as childlike or regressive. While this is one approach to categorizing and describing behavior, it commonly does little to enhance respect for the patient in his or her struggle with the changes going on within the self. Relationships with chronically ill elderly persons are commonly influenced by the physician's feelings about the elderly in general, especially with parents and grandparents. Some of us tend to respond with overconcern and overinvolvement, others with anger, rejection, and withdrawal.

Chronic disease should be perceived as a condition in dynamic equilibrium. The job of maintaining that equilibrium, and fostering modest gains rather than modest losses belongs both to the doctor and the patient. In acute medicine, treatment may be seen simplistically as doing something *to* the patient; all the patient has to do is consent. When a patient has a chronic condition, the undesirable consequences of this simplistic notion are more readily seen.

The role of the physician can be as complex as one wishes to see it, and therefore offers many different kinds of opportunities for professional satisfaction. Among these are long-term control of disease, limiting disability, fostering retraining and rehabilitating as necessary, helping to limit disruption of social and family life, and assisting in psychological readjustment to life on new terms.

Aside from frustration of the need to cure, the single most common dissatisfaction that physicians have with the chronically ill is injured pride in having a layman be a coequal in the management of a case. We physicians in general do not like to be told what to do, especially by patients. However, once we understand and accept a mutual interdependence of the patient and the health care team, the opportunities for satisfaction are considerable. It helps if you view yourself as teacher or consultant, and view the patient as a student or co-worker. We can then take pride in the patient's developing mastery and control. It also helps if we are willing to have the patient teach us something occasionally. Think of all the experience the patient with chronic disease has had in using and judging medical care. There is no question that many have a valuable perspective to contribute to us as physicians.

In approaching a patient with a chronic condition, it helps for the physician to exhibit a little humility. Say, "I expect any patient with a chronic or recurring condition to know as much or more about their own health as I do. How can I help you most?" Patients will commonly demur on this one knowing that physicians like them to do so, and reply, "That's what I came to you to find out." However, if you persist, you will find that most have a very clear idea of what they think will help them and what won't and what they want from you and what they don't. If you regard their requests as unreasonable, be prepared to bargain, but attempt first to understand why they feel as they do and grant that they may know something that you do not.

Control of disease in any patient with a complicated chronic condition requires teamwork; a single professional can't do it all. Instructing the patient and family in simple diagnosis and treatment, and the rationale behind them, frees the patient from daily dependence on you. However, physicians frequently feel too pressed for time to do an adequate job in this area. Even with the time, many physicians don't feel comfortable in the role of patient-educator. If that is true of you, patients can nonetheless profit from access to and assistance from other professionals who are interested in patient-teaching. Some nurses and dieticians are particularly good at this. There is an increasing amount of patient-education reading material available, but it is often difficult and time consuming to find good resources which are specifically relevant to your patient. There are some things which a patient is likely to learn only from you. For example, consider the man with chronic congestive heart failure who requires digoxin at near-toxic levels. If this patient can listen to his own lung fields for rales and check his pulse for irregularities, he will be a far more able partner in adjusting his digoxin levels than if he stayed on a rigid dosage scale until he developed frank failure or premature ventricular contractions or bigeminy.

Once you begin to view the patient as your co-worker, the opportunities for collaboration are endless. It also can be fun; it takes a good deal of responsibility off your shoulders and puts it where it belongs— on the person most intimately involved: the patient.

The Alcoholic Patient

[I]t is part of the doctor's function to make it possible for his patients to go on doing the pleasant things that are bad for them—laughing too much, eating too much, drinking too much—without killing themselves any sooner than is necessary.
—Rene Dubos

If we take habitual drunkards as a class, their heads and their hearts will bear an advantageous comparison with those of any other class.
—Abraham Lincoln

In part because it is defined as a disease, something that afflicts the innocent, many well-meaning individuals call for sympathy and under-standing toward alcoholism and alcoholics. However, the dominant cultural attitude remains quite different. At a distance, alcohol excess is regarded with amusement and even tacit approval. Probably the single most common theme of published cartoons in this country is the obviously inebriated individual doing or saying something that most of us would regard as outrageous but somehow fitting. At close range, however, the alcoholic is much more likely to be regarded with disdain.

I won't formally define alcoholism; we are not concerned here with objective reality, but rather with the kind of relationship problems which tend to evolve when a physician decides, on whatever basis, that a patient is an alcoholic. Typical empiric criteria for physicians are the following: a problem drinker is "anyone who consumes significantly more alcohol than I do" and an alcoholic is "anyone who obviously suffers—physically, socially, economically—as a consequence."

The emphasis here is not on alcoholism per se or even the personal-ity structure commonly attributed to the alcoholic, but rather on the interpersonal problems you are likely to have once you have defined a patient as a "typical alcoholic."

For most physicians, our stereotypes about alcoholics are derived from our experiences in three places: the Veterans Administration Hospitals (with their revolving-door cirrhotics, liver failure and esophogeal varices patients), various County Hospitals (filled with down-and-outers, with their missed cervical spine injuries and sub-durals, their alcoholic ketoacidosis and strange, resistant pneumonias caused by bizarre, opportunistic bacteria), and emergency rooms (where alcoholics blur with the drunks who cause so much human grief: the beat-up kids and spouses, the auto accidents and fights, the combative and abusive behavior with emergency room personnel). Each alcoholic brings with him the curse of ultimate failure: his own failure as a person, and our own therapeutic failure as we try to patch him up—often against his resistance—so he can go out and cause more grief for himself and others.

Under the circumstances, my assumption is that if you didn't like alcoholics before you picked up this book, your attitudes are unlikely to change with anything I say here. Since it is well documented that most physicians do *not* like working with alcoholics, the following is an appropriate question: Given a basic antipathy to the alcoholic, how can I nonetheless treat my alcoholic patients in the most humane way possible, and how can I find reasonable satisfaction in doing so?

Why do physicians find relating to such patients so difficult? There are two general explanations.

The first may be termed the "rat-hole theory of treatment." This explanation emphasizes that the patient takes up a good deal of time, that treatment is unrewarding, the patient's misery is self-induced and shows blatant disregard for his or her own body, the patient is noncompliant and resists meaningful comprehensive treatment. In effect, the physician asks, Since there is nothing I can do to alter the course of the condition except give occasional palliative treatment, why get involved? While this view is consistent with the fact that physicians generally are less enthusiastic about providing palliative treatment for chronic conditions than in giving other kinds of medical care, it still doesn't account for the anger and disdain which alcoholic patients can arouse in so many physicians. I think this first explanation therefore has to be augmented with a second, more personal explanation.

This is the For Whom the Bell Tolls Theory, and make no mistake about it, the bell tolls for us. There is a certain type of alcoholic with whom physicians stereotypically have the least patience, and with whom most doctor-patient management problems are likely to arise. This is usually someone of advancing middle years, with a previous good work history and evidence of early high aspirations, who has succumbed to life's pressures, feeling that family and occupational goals are unrealized. In essence, this is someone who showed early promise, but in effect says, "To hell with it—I'd rather drink." This alcoholic patient is so upsetting because he symbolizes a personal threat. I urge you to withhold immediate agreement or disagreement with what I say next; simply file it away in your mind, think about it, and perhaps discuss it with friends. Alcoholism represents a personal threat to physicians on two levels: the general problem of the superego running amuck, and the more specific problem of alcohol as agent of release.

The stereotype of the medical student cum physician is easily recognizable as conscientious, ambitious, single-minded, achievement-oriented, with a head crammed with data (all compulsively organized) and a body always running to beat the clock and to meet the demands of patients and profession. These character traits represent adaptive responses to the demands of our occupation. They are crucial for getting us through our rigorous training, and necessary for mastery of the incredible detail required in the practice of modern scientific medicine. They keep us pressing on, putting in the long and difficult hours, often delaying gratification interminably in the process.

However, behind the compulsive façade there is often a personality that, under stress, comes close to saying "the hell with it" and quitting. When things get rough it is sometimes our superego, or social pressure, or the lack of acceptable alternatives that keeps us going. We alternately resent and are grateful to all three, and the stereotypic alcoholic brings our ambivalence into broad relief.

Alcoholism is specifically threatening to physicians because so many physicians drink, often beyond the point of moderation. Where 70% of Americans generally imbibe alcohol, 90% of physicians do so. Probably half of those who drink consume moderate to heavy amounts of alcohol, that is, several drinks several times per week. Study after study has revealed that alcoholism is relatively common among physicians, even among physicians preselected for psychological well-being. Anyone who is involved in hospital staff credentialing committees knows that excess drinking is highly correlated with impaired performance among physicians and represents an important source of morbidity.

I'm not interested in rubbing anyone's nose in these disagreeable facts. The question is, Given reality, what do we do about them?

It's important for all of us to recognize that we can't rectify alcoholism (any more than any other bad habit) without getting the person out of the milieu that helps to perpetuate it. And that is not easy in our society, where alcoholic beverages are so widely used as social lubricants and so well-established as an essential ingredient in so many work and play situations.

In attempting to treat humanely persons who come to you for medical care and who, in addition, have alcohol problems, there are certain useful principles to keep in mind.

First, a physician must see relapses or recurrent drinking not as failures, but simply as the nature of the beast.

Second, do what you can without feeling guilty about what you can't do. Most physicians have a clear understanding of how to take care of alcohol-related medical problems, and should strive to do so while still being respectful of the patient as a human being.

Third, try to accept what the patients want for themselves with regard to the use of alcohol. An alcoholic who genuinely seeks treatment is generally not a problem. We are often angry at the person who has no interest in altering dependence on alcohol, and we become frustrated with a patient who is ambivalent about wanting treatment. With both of these, fasten onto the paradox with the patient: "It's ironic and sad, isn't it, that even though alcohol causes you so many problems, you're drawn to it again and again?" Allow yourself to share the irony and sadness with the patient without putting him or her on the defensive, or feeling that the burden for changing the situation falls upon yourself.

Fourth, when a patient does appear to be motivated to diminish a dependence on alcohol, recognize that partial attempts are seldom helpful. Like a change in diet or deprivation of cigarettes, abstinence from alcohol creates a psychological void which must be filled with something. Both you and the patient must understand this vital concept. If the patient cannot fill this need alone or with the help of friends and family (and many cannot), a self-help group is often a desirable alternative. Alcoholics Anonymous remains the principal referral resource for most alcoholic patients.

Fifth, avoid getting caught up as a partisan in family struggles concerning the patient's alcoholism. The patient's alcohol excess serves many intragroup functions in the family, and the dynamics are often complicated and difficult to understand without careful study. Either the alcoholic or the spouse or some other person may want you to play the role of rescuer or preacher or ally. Avoid these roles at all costs. Remain an empathetic and helpful resource. Say, "It's not going to do any of you any good for me to take sides. I know this is a difficult situation for all of you, and each of you is going to have to take responsibility for your own feelings and actions regardless of what I think is right or wrong."

The Cardiac Patient

There is something in sickness that breaks down the pride of manhood.
—Charles Dickens

My life is in the hands of any rascal who chooses to annoy and tease me.
—John Hunter

Cardiac disease is the Number One killer in this country; nearly half of all deaths are coronary related. Therefore, it is ridiculous to talk about a single personality type or a single set of emotional factors correlated with coronary disease.

Nonetheless, folklore and some research reports suggest that there is a certain personality who is particularly vulnerable to myocardial infarctions. The classic myocardial infarction (MI) patient, according to this view, is a man in his forties to fifties, hardworking, independent to the point of hating dependency on others, extremely time conscious, aggressive, and ambitious.

This discussion will focus on the so-called coronary-prone male personality, because it fits so many clinical stereotypes and is associated with certain characteristic doctor-patient relationship problems. I hope that much of this information will also be applicable to patients who don't precisely fit the stereotype.

It's important to understand that a heart attack is not only a source of stress, it is statistically most likely to occur at times of high life stress. What is the typical response to the chest pain that signals a heart attack? The average person with severe chest pain waits several hours before seeking medical help. He didn't want to disturb the physician, or thought it was gas pain; whatever the explanation the phenomenon remains the same.

Usually the patient tries to settle his stomach with antacids or alcohol or the like, perhaps even exercise. Since many coronary deaths occur during the first hour or so after the beginning of acute chest pain, this phenomenon is a significant source of mortality, and it is as prominent among physicians as laborers. The patient is often brought to the hospital against his expressed resistance, by a thoroughly frightened friend or spouse.

The reason I am stressing the delay aspect, which occurs before you even see the patient, is because the typical MI patient has a profound reluctance to admit the possibility of mortal illness. His reluctance (or fear, if you will) to see himself as sick, or have others see him as sick, will have significant impact on the kinds of treatment he will be willing to accept from you. Most of the common doctor-patient relationship problems occur after the acute episode is over.

On arrival in the emergency room, there is no question that the patient is taken seriously. The patient with typical cardiac pain is rushed to the front of the line, put in a "red room" or its equivalent, monitoring begun, IV started—all this may be even before you see the patient. He is given morphine and subjected to considerable attention, and the majority of patients find this reassuring. What you tell a patient in the emergency room is largely a matter of individual style. Most writers say, and my own experience is in agreement, that the most frequent error is telling patients too little rather than too much. Reflect for a moment on how many complaints you have heard from patients about being told too much information. I cannot recall any. If patients are told more than they wish to hear, they simply don't assimilate the information. But they don't complain about it. They do, however, complain about being told too little, about the manner of the person doing the telling (particularly brusqueness, insensitivity, et cetera) and about the excessive use of medical jargon.

Given your personal communication style, ideas to convey are that (1) the condition is serious enough to warrant admission, careful observation, and treatment; and (2) the condition is not so serious that the patient need abandon hope or confidence in his own ability to cope with what is ahead.

After leaving the emergency room, the patient is transferred to a hospital ward, probably an intensive care unit (ICU), and (increasingly) a cardiac care unit (CCU) in which only other cardiac patients reside. If conflicts are to develop between doctor and patient, they will usually do so here, though customarily not in the first few days.

The typical coronary-prone personality is a person who likes to be in charge of his own destiny. He may be willing to relinquish some of his independence, but customarily only to persons whom he regards with awe. He doesn't like being cared for by inexperienced professionals in training, and he doesn't like being dependent upon women for his bodily needs. He usually copes with anxiety by trying to take control of situations, and, in reflecting upon what has happened to him after he is no longer in pain and needful of morphine, he tends to become quite anxious indeed.

The typical coronary-prone patient is not only independent, he is competitive. He doesn't like being sick himself, and he doesn't like having other sick persons around him. The less he sees of sick people, the better he'll like it. If two patients with MIs arrive in the CCU on the same day, the one who improves less rapidly can often be expected to go into a bleak depression when the more fortunate fellow patient is discharged.

Other writers stress how few MI patients admit to being significantly stressed by watching a fatal arrest. The patients will talk about the mechanical efficiency of the crash-cart team, or they will complain that their visitors were required to leave the unit, or about how the noise prevented them from sleeping. But most will steadfastly refuse to identify with the stricken patient. Denial? Yes, but of an enormously adaptive sort. It also gives us another clear message that this is a patient who will flee from the patient role whenever he sees an opportunity.

Patients who have cardiac arrests may move in and out of consciousness and have flashes of understanding and recollection. Putting together the fragments may be very frightening indeed. Blessedly, most have amnesia for the event. Usually a return to conscious awareness is associated with bewilderment concerning all the people around and a dim sense that one's chest is sore. The nightmares may come later.

The best policy is to tell the patient exactly what has happened, frankly but simply. "Your heart stopped. The monitor alerted us instantly and we were able to restart your heart immediately. You are going to be okay now. Do you have any questions?" Most patients will simply react with stunned silence or shake their heads no. Most will not wish to face the full impact of what has happened to them, especially initially—some, never. Let them know that you will be available later to discuss the matter further with them, or they can ask questions of the CCU nurses. When the patient has had an opportunity to assimilate the bare facts of the event, someone should sit down with him, emphasize that survivors of cardiac arrest now number at least in the hundreds of thousands, and the fact of the event itself should not alter any basic expectations regarding positive outcome or the patient's ability to cope with having had an MI.

At first, patients who have had an MI are simply grateful for having survived. Then gradually they begin to think about their vulnerability, the recent dramatic evidence of their aging, and possible restrictions upon their future. In addition, the second and sometimes third weeks of hospitalization are usually boring, leaving the patient with great amounts of time for pondering. Depression often settles in a gloomy cloud. Typical sources of concern are decreased earning power, decreased competitiveness generally, decreased sexual ability, impaired physical prowess, and increased dependency. Depression is commonly dealt with by denial.

Early in the hospital course, describe to the patient what is ahead. Describe what an infarction is in anatomical terms. Tell the patient, "Your primary long-term problem will be in setting realistic goals and finding a happy medium between invalidism and reckless abandon."

Begin the patient on a carefully graduated exercise program, proceeding from passive to active exercises. Let the patient know that you will be regularly increasing his privileges in the hospital. Decrease in activity and excess caution not only are terrible punishments, but are a reflection of a rather narrow view that the only measure of the patient's health is his cardiac function.

Keep up with the newspapers, and be aware of community or national figures who return to full activity after infarction.

Expect anxiety. Most coronary-prone personalities do not like to admit that they are anxious, and will minimize their complaints in this regard. It is therefore useful to leave a standing order for minor tranquilizers, with the addendum that any given dosage can be omitted at the patient's request. That serves the double function of medicating the anxiety and giving the patient a sense of control over what actually happens.

Before discharge, warn the patient, "You will be depressed by your relatively restricted schedule until you are able to resume full activity, and you will feel weak because of inactivity and the stress that you have gone through. Often, that takes six weeks or more to subside."

Tell the post-MI patient that almost everyone who has an MI gets depressed, that this brush with his own mortality and limitations results in a perhaps necessary and certainly natural and understandable feeling of listlessness, sadness, and irritability. That will pass with time, and the patient can expect much or all of his normal vitality and zest to return. Most patients are reassured by such comments, though they tend to disbelieve them initially unless they know other post-MI patients who have done well.

Recognize that the patient was probably in stressful circumstances at the time of the infarction, which may well have played a role in precipitating it, and the patient will want to begin coping with those stresses. With this, as in all things, try to have the patient accept you as an advisor rather than an adversary.

Anticipate the patient's desire to be active, and try to see it as a blessing. Instead of preventing activity, counsel graduated activity. The most common doctor-patient conflicts occur when the patient attempts to be more active than his doctor thinks advisable.

Provide a specific conditioning program with specific, explicit steps to follow. Physical therapists can be an invaluable resource in this regard. A formal conditioning program builds confidence, provides structure, and gives the patient an increased sense of control and mastery. Tell the patient to start walking one block in the morning and one block in the evening, and gradually increase his activity until he is walking a mile to one and one-half miles twice a day.

Dietary counseling for the patient and the spouse is an excellent idea, because weight reduction is important for so many, yet so difficult to manage.

Whenever possible, include the spouse in all such counseling. Say in the presence of both, "Your relative inactivity over the next several weeks will make you hell to live with. You are going to mope around, be cranky and critical, and try to make everyone else feel as miserable as you. Being around the kids and the house all day will drive you nuts." The response to this is so stereotypic, I can predict it without any reluctance: both parties will grin and indicate their affirmation in some way.

Ironically, despite the trauma of having an acute MI, the recovery phase is far more exasperating for most coronary personalities and their families. They hate the weakness and being out of condition, and they should be forewarned that this is part of the natural course. Sleep disturbances are common, and the coronary personality is customarily reluctant to use sedatives and would prefer to tough it out. My rule of thumb is, as long as the patient is worried about sedative excess, I don't have to, and I customarily recommend a small supply of benzodiazepines for occasional use before bedtime.

With regard to sexual activity, authorities vary, but a good rule of thumb is that if a person can walk steadily up one flight of stairs, he can handle passive sexual play and intercourse that proceeds at a walk rather than a gallop. The more briskly he can walk up stairs, the more he can tolerate vigorous intercourse. Patients vary widely in their sexual desire and discomfort levels. I've had more than one patient tell me about adding nitroglycerin to the drawer in the bedside table, alongside such other accouterments of sexual activity as condoms, vaginal lubricants, and body oils—and resuming intercourse on the day of hospital discharge. The stereotypic coronary personality may wish to proceed as aggressively with sex as with everything else. Encourage your patients to experiment without fear, as long as they increase activities gradually, using shortness of breath and persistent angina as indications to moderate activities. You can tell your patients that intercourse-related coronary deaths, despite rumors to the contrary, occur very rarely, and—of these—mostly during or after extramarital rather than marital intercourse. Like so many other things, the act itself is less intrinsically stressful than the circumstances associated with it.

Bibliography

Baider L, Kaplan-DeNout A: Couples' reactions and adjustment to mastectomy. *Intl J Psychiatry in Med* 14:265–274, 1984

Bernstein NR: Medical tragedies in facial burn disfigurement. *Psychiatry Ann* 6:475–483, 1976

Bissell L, Haberman PW: *Alcoholism in the Professions*. New York, Oxford University Press, 1984

Boyd JH et al.: Different definitions of alcoholism, I. *Am J Psychiatry* 140:1309–1313, 1983

———: Different definitions of alcoholism, II. *Am J Psychiatry* 140:1314–1317, 1983

Burish TG, Bradley LA: *Coping with Chronic Diseases*. New York, Academic Press, 1983

Byrne DG: The stability of illness behavior after myocardial infarction. *Intl J Psychiatry in Med* 14:265–283, 1984

DerogAtis LR, Abeloff MD, Melisaratos, N: Psychological coping mechanisms and survival time in metastatic breast cancer. *JAMA* 242:1504–1508, 1979

Forester BM, Kornfeld DS, Fleiss J: Psychiatric aspects of radiotherapy. *Am J Psychiatry* 135:960–963, 1978

Goffman E: *Stigma—Notes on the Management of Spoiled Identity*. Englewood Cliffs, NJ, Prentice-Hall, 1963

Goodwin DS: *Alcoholism—The Facts*. New York, Oxford University Press, 1981

Greenberg GD, Ryan JJ, Boulier PF: Psychological and neuropsychological aspects of COPD. *Psychosomatics* 26:29–37, 1985

Kames LD: The chronic illness problem inventory. *Intl J Psychiatry in Med* 14:65–78, 1984

Lipp MR, Benson SG: Physician use of marijuana, alcohol and tobacco. *Am J Psychiatry* 129:612–616, 1972

Lipp MR, Malone ST: Group rehabilitation of vascular surgery amputees. *Arch Phys Med Rehabil* 57:180–183, 1976

Lipp M, Tinklenberg J, Benson S, et al: Medical student use of marijuana, alcohol and cigarettes—a study of four schools. *Int J Addict* 7:141–152, 1972

Madan R: Facial disfigurement in Garrett, JE, Levine, ES, (eds): *Psychological Practices with the Physically Disabled*. New York, Columbia University Press, 1962

Martin PJ, Friedmeyer MH, Moore JE: Pretty patient, healthy patient—a study of physical attractiveness and psychopathology. *J Clin Psychol* 33:990–994, 1977

Miller WR: Treating problem drinkers—what works? *Behav Ther* 5:15–18, 1982

Molinaro JR: The social fate of children disfigured by burns. *Am J Psychiatry,* 135:979–980, 1978

Pogrebin LC: Of beauty. *MS Magazine,* (December) 1983, pp 73–109

Schain WS, et al.: The sooner the better—breast reconstruction. *Am J Psychiatry* 142:40–46, 1985

Shontz FC: Severe chronic illness in Garrett, J. F. Levine, E. S. (eds): *Psychological Practices with the Physically Disabled*. New York, Columbia University Press, 1962

Silberfarb PM, Maurer, LH, Crouthamel, CS: Psychosocial aspects of neoplastic disease. *Am J Psychiatry* 137:450–455, 1980

Steinberg MD, Juliano MA, Lise L: Psychological outcome of lumpectomy vs mastectomy. *Am J Psychiatry* 142:34–39, 1985

Vaillant GE, Brighton JR, McArthur C: Physician use of mind-altering drugs—a twenty-year followup report. *N Engl J Med* 282:365–372, 1970

Wellisch DK, Jamison KR, Pasnan RO: Psychosocial aspects of mastectomy. *Am J Psychiatry* 135:543–546, 1978

7

Anxiety and Depression

Is it not marvelous how full people are—all people—of humor, tragedy, passionate human longings, hopes, fears—if only you can unloosen the floodgates!

—David Grayson

Two of the most common maladies you will encounter in medicine are anxiety and depression. They are so common that if you assume all of your hospitalized patients and a significant minority of your ambulatory patients are anxious and/or depressed to some degree, you will seldom be wrong. In fact, I'm going to argue that the absence of anxiety and depression may sometimes be more significant than their presence.

These are obviously strong statements.

First, you must understand that anxiety and depression are both spectrum disorders. There are very few people who can't stir up a little bit of anxiety or depression if you start asking them about their parents' health, their children's future, or the eventual likelihood of a nuclear "accident." What makes anxiety and depression significant is not their mere presence, but whether they are situation-appropriate, how long they last, how intense they are, how they affect an individual's coping style, and how much they interfere with what goes on around them. I find it useful to divide the spectrum of anxiety and depression into four categories.

Four-Stage Anxiety and Depression Scale

Stage One: Malaise. At this level a person exhibits some of the psychological or physiologic concomitants of anxiety and/or depression, but may or may not be aware of their presence or source. This is a low level of discomfort, with no significant interference with the person's functioning, and is almost universal in a new, potentially stressful situation such as hospitalization, a freshly diagnosed illness, or embarking on a major diagnostic work-up.

Stage Two: Coping Required. This is a slightly greater level of discomfort, and one which is also very, very common among patients with confirmed serious medical problems or hospitalization. At this level, the patient is usually aware of uncomfortable feelings, but may or may not be willing to acknowledge this discomfort verbally. This is a level of discomfort which all of us have faced, and most of us are reasonably good at handling ourselves. The following are typical comments, which represent familiar attempts by patients to cope with feelings of anxiety or depression: "I'll feel better if my spouse accompanies me." "I'll be okay as long as I have a book to read or television to watch." "I'm just going to think about the positive and not let my imagination run away with me." "I have a lot of confidence in my surgeon, so I'm really not *too* worried."

Stage Three: Coping Interfered With. At this level, feelings of discomfort are not manageable by ordinary and familiar coping techniques. There is danger of a vicious cycle or spiraling effect. For example, a patient feels anxious or depressed, tries to cope, feels inadequate, feels more anxious and depressed, requiring more of the already overwhelmed coping mechanisms. It is at this point that the patient's discomfort usually becomes apparent to health-care givers. The patient now begins to *look* anxious or depressed, or starts crying for help in whatever way he or she can, or starts drawing attention by unusual or noncompliant behavior. The patient is usually very much aware of having difficulty coping, and often tries to hide the fact from others. Very few people are comfortable telling others that their coping mechanisms are failing or that they feel themselves losing control, since in our society self-esteem is so intimately tied to coping.

Stage Four: Incapacitating. At this level the patient's coping mechanisms are frankly overwhelmed, and the patient becomes unable to be of assistance to himself or herself. Now there is no question that something is wrong with the patient, who may exhibit frank panic at one extreme or depressive withdrawal at the other. These conditions are usually very upsetting to people who know the patient, especially if they failed to observe earlier signs that these conditions were evolving.

The doctor's function, and indeed that of all health-care givers, is to help the patient move toward the more comfortable end of the spectrum. You can help prevent the more serious and extreme conditions by helping the patient at the earlier stages. If you ignore anxiety and depression at their minimal but most prevalent level, you can expect that a significant percentage of your patients will escalate to the more severe disorders. In short, giving prophylactic treatment to all of your patients will save both you and your patients grief in the long run.

Second, it's important to understand that anxiety and depression are not only symptoms, but also conditions in their own right. You will find many texts and teachers who insist on making a distinction between, for example, symptomatic depression and depression as a disease. I do not believe the distinction is clinically as useful as is often claimed. One must always assume that anxiety and depression are symptomatic of some underlying cause, then seek that cause and attempt to remedy it. However, at the same time, one must seek to treat the anxiety and/ or depression in its own right. Both conditions can assume lives of their own within a given patient, even to the extent of dominating all else that is going on.

Third, you will seldom find either anxiety or depression without the other. Most people who are anxious are unhappy about that anxiety, and therefore are likely to exhibit some evidence of unhappiness. Unhappiness, of course, is one of the forms of depression. Most people who are depressed anxiously seek ways of dealing with their depression. Certainly, it's a useful guideline to assume that anxiety and depression are present together. At the less serious levels, their treatment is very similar anyhow; and at the more serious levels, where the treatment may differ, the distinction between the two is more apparent.

Fourth, assume that the stress of illness and especially hospitalization will always produce an effect on the emotional life of the patient. It is in fact extraordinary that so many patients can assume without major difficulty the role of being a patient. Aside from more global concerns, all patients may have specific concerns about, for instance, injury to their bodily parts, and often with good reason. Many fear loss of control, not only of physiologic functions (such as bladder and bowels) but also of feelings. Many find it humiliating to be unclothed and exposed and essentially helpless in front of a succession of strangers. Many are frankly upset at having to leave their homes or their jobs or their social milieus, for your office or the clinic or hospital. Many are frightened of potential ridicule at the hands of people like ourselves, for whom illness and suffering and the apparatuses of treatment appear routine.

Fifth, anxiety and depression are among the most contagious of all disorders, for which not only the patients are at risk, but also people like you and me. Once a nidus of anxiety and depression is set up on a hospital ward or in a waiting room, you can expect it to spread. It will not only affect the other patients in the room, but also the nursing and medical staff who go into that room. Most persons, whether they understand the contagion theory of anxiety and depression or not, become instinctively uncomfortable; they tend to withdraw from and try to isolate the source of those uncomfortable feelings. You, yourself, often will feel an urge to avoid such patients on rounds, and to minimize the amount of time you spend with them during office appointments. If you have a number of patients who are anxious or depressed (e.g., in an oncology clinic), you are likely to catch a bout of patient-generated depression yourself. If you aren't careful, you will carry the contagion not only to your other patients, but also to your home as well. It will certainly affect your work, and it may affect your life in general. It's crucial that you learn effective ways of dealing with patient-generated anxiety and depression.

Assessment

I'm going to continue to talk about anxiety and depression together at this point, because customarily their evaluation involves similar approaches and techniques. I will take up notable differences between the two in a later section in this chapter.

Assessment of anxiety and depression is, by and large, fairly easy if you assume that anxiety and depression are already present, so that you only need to determine severity and extent, and not presence or absence.

There are a number of things you can do to help assure that your assessment of the patient will be comfortable and fruitful. They are the kinds of things that are useful in obtaining a history generally, honored and promoted in all textbooks on physical examinations, and accordingly difficult to practice in a busy hospital or practice setting. These include finding a time and place where you and the patient can communicate in a comfortable and relaxed manner. It's always advisable that you have enough time to be able to follow up clues, and to make sure that there will be no interruptions. Obviously excellent advice, but in practice very difficult to implement.

Learning to use time efficiently and effectively will certainly help. First, start off your interview sitting down. Even if you only have ten minutes for the patient's examination, spend the first minute or two sitting down while you take the patient's history. This serves the dual function of removing the rush-rush atmosphere from the examination, and ensuring that neither you nor the patient looks down at the other.

Next, make a point of establishing human contact, both by eye contact and by touching the patient. One simple yet effective tactic is to continue history-taking while you take the patient's pulse or feel for cervical adenopathy. Make sure that you keep the patient talking while you perform parts of the physical examination which do not require your complete attention. For example, keep the patient talking while you test his or her reflexes, evaluate straight-leg raising, or do rectal or pelvic exams. However, some doctors can bring off this kind of activity much better than others, and the "talking exam" is not without hazards. You want to be able to concentrate on what you are doing, and you don't want to give an impression of glibness when you are examining an area about which the patient has great concern. Focus on the matter at hand; let conversation be a part of that process as long as it seems comfortable for both of you.

Try to establish contact with the patient early in the exam by learning something about the patient as a human being, separate from his or her illness. The intent here is to establish a link between you which helps to establish the patient's individuality in your own mind, about which you and the patient can have some rapport, and something which you will not forget. Ideally, it may be something that you have in common. Good "links" include hobbies or likes and dislikes in food, activities, or places. Remember, you can't listen while *you're* talking, so focus on questions or comments which will get the *patient* talking.

The traditional vehicle for assessing the patient's psychological status is the mental status exam (which is discussed more fully in chapter 5, Confusional States). For the purposes of evaluating anxiety and depression, four questions (and their variations) will suffice. It's hard to believe that such pervasive disorders as anxiety and depression can almost all be evaluated with four simple questions, but this is substantially true.

Question no. 1: "What do *you* think is wrong with you?" Discover what the patient thinks is going on and how serious it is thought to be. Don't be content with a simple answer, e.g. "Psoriasis." What you're after, rather, is the patient's sense of whether this is going to get better or worse. Does the patient think it will turn into cancer? Does the patient fear it is something he or she will die from? It's useful to ask the patient these questions directly. Though you may feel like an idiot asking whether a condition may turn into cancer when you are evaluating a patient for a tonsillectomy, the question nonetheless has a couple of virtues. First, it will help expose the patient's often unrealistic fears about the condition (he or she may have read of someone who died during a tonsillectomy), and it will also help you become more comfortable in asking the question with patients who truly do have cancer or terminal illness. If you get in the habit of asking *all* your patients, "How serious is this?" "Do you think you're going to die from it?", you'll find that asking the same questions of a patient with an astrocytoma seems much more natural and comfortable.

A very common response to question no. 1 is, "That's what I came to you to find out, Doc." Do not dismay. Instead, respond: "I understand. But I'm wondering what you think is going on with you, because I often find that people have all kinds of fears and fantasies. For instance, have you worried at all that this might be cancer or some other

foul disease that you might die from?'' At this point, you will already
have a beginning feel for a potential major source of anxiety or depression in the patient, as well as an idea about possible ways to allay that
discomfort.

Many clinicians worry about asking question no. 1 for fear of "putting ideas into patients' heads." I have seldom found that to be a
problem. People who aren't worried about the issue before I raise it are
usually easily reassured after the subject is broached, if there is genuinely no reason for concern.

On the other hand, if in fact there is cause for concern, this is an
opportunity for the physician to start preparing the patient for the
inevitable diagnostic workup and to start building a collaborative relationship that will ensure the patient's cooperation: "Well, I think this is
worrisome enough so that you and I are going to have to work closely
together to get it evaluated quickly and thoroughly."

Question no. 2: "How much does this condition interfere with
your life or your future plans?" This question is particularly important
with any illness or condition that is potentially disfiguring or disabling,
or that in the patient's mind might cause extended hospitalization or
inactivity. Will it affect the patient's functioning on the job, or sexual
functioning, or ability to spend time with friends or in treasured activities? How much does this particular patient care about such things?
What other activities or sources of self-esteem does the patient have
available? How does the patient intend to cope with any incursions into
major sources of self-esteem or pleasure?

Try to understand the personal meaning of the disease to the patient.
Though it is truly difficult for most of us healthy types to accurately
empathize with our patients, try to do so. How would a cholecystec-
tomy affect me right now? What would happen to my professional
obligations and aspirations if I were out of commission for from 6 to 12
weeks? Is there someone to look after me as I convalesce? What if
there weren't? Would this mean that I would have to give up vacation
time for this year? (Next year too?) Would my income continue? What
if it didn't? What if my financial condition is marginal anyhow?

Any physical condition that is significant enough to put a patient into
a hospital is bound to have profound impact on his or her life outside
the hospital, and any condition worrisome enough to bring a patient to
a doctor's office can upset the psychic equilibrium of most folks. Be
very slow to say that any given patient's concerns are inappropriate.
You simply do not know what the situation looks like from inside his or
her skin.

However, *do* be suspicious if a patient expects no problems from
what is obviously a potentially very difficult medical condition. Do not
confront the patient's denial directly, but leave the door open: "Well,

some people have more problems with this condition than others. I expect you'll have some ups and downs too. I hope you'll feel free to talk with me if the going gets rough at all.''

Question no. 3: "How upsetting is this illness and/or hospitalization for you?" There are many, many ways of asking questions of this kind and you obviously have to find a manner that is comfortable for you personally. In addition, you have to find a way of phrasing the question so that the patient finds it easy to answer. If the patient at first demurs, you can respond by saying, "Many patients with this condition find it difficult to cope." Still, some patients don't like talking about being upset, being concerned that such a frank admission might diminish them in your (or their own) eyes. Such patients are much more likely to respond to a gambit such as, "You seem to be coping with all this much better than most people I've seen with this disorder. How do you do it?" That gives the patient an opportunity to focus on the coping rather than on any subjective feelings of distress. The question helps you to get some idea of the level of distress, as well as the resources the patient has at his or her command. At the same time, you are being very supportive. If the patient admits to being upset, get some idea of exactly how upset he or she has been. How much has being upset interfered with daily activities? How does it compare with levels of distress the patient has felt in the past? How has he or she coped with stresses other than illness (work, marital, military) in the past? Does he or she think it's going to get worse or better before the treatment is through? All these questions lead naturally enough to the fourth question.

Question no. 4: "How much has this gotten you down?" (Again, use language that is comfortable for you. "How low have you been feeling?" "How depressed have you been feeling?") Many patients who at first tend to scoff at such a question, will subsequently admit that in fact they have been feeling pretty discouraged. Again, if you think that the patient may well be depressed but tends to deny it, focus on coping. "How have you managed to keep your spirits up, when so many others are really worn down by this kind of disorder?" If the patient admits to depression, again inquire as to degree. "How has it affected your life?" "Have you gotten to the point where life isn't worth living?" If the answer is reluctant, or affirmative, ask "Have you had thoughts of suicide?" With this kind of progression, you are much more likely to get an honest and frank answer than if you were to ask out of the blue, in a rote review of systems, "Are you suicidal?"

With each of these questions your goal is to assess the levels of anxiety and depression, and balance them against the patient's coping abilities and resources. For clinical shorthand, you can rank these factors conveniently on the Four-Stage Anxiety and Depression Scale.

If you don't like that one, use your own, but find some framework that
makes sense to you and is useful clinically.

All four of the questions lend themselves to use with virtually all
patients that you are likely to encounter. They are questions that are
easy to ask once you have practice in doing so. However, many physicians feel uncomfortable discussing such matters with patients, especially when they save such questions only for patients who are obviously profoundly anxious or depressed. Before you try question no. 4
on a patient with fungating, metastatic breast cancer, practice on a few
patients with ingrown toenails; the experience will help prepare you for
the really tough ones.

Anxiety

*The reason why worry kills more people than work is that more people
worry than work.*

—Robert Frost

We've been talking about anxiety for some time now, and have not yet
bothered to define it. This has been intentional. Anxiety is a part of
normal everyday existence, something familiar to virtually everyone.
Like pornography and art, you may have difficulty defining it, but you
can identify it when you see it. It is not merely a symptom (i.e., something to complain about), but a condition which has true survival value.
It helps promote arousal, vigilance, and coping strategies. It helps
motivate us to adapt and change. It is a potential key source of energy
to your patients, and helping our patients to use anxiety effectively is a
continuing challenge.

The classic sources of anxiety are conditions of helplessness, separation, real or impending injury, social disapproval, and decreased self-
esteem. All of these are of course an integral part of the illness-patient
role. This is especially true in a culture such as ours where so much
emphasis is placed upon independence and self-sufficiency.

As a state of arousal, anxiety has many psychological and physiologic manifestations which are consistent with arousal generally. A
sense of dys-ease may lead to feelings of apprehension, dread, or even
panic. Under such circumstances, difficulty in concentrating and attending to tasks can be expected. As anxiety increases, one is likely to
become more irritable, perhaps even angry, restless, and active, both
verbally and physically.

Individuals often recognize anxiety in themselves by noting the
physical concomitants of anxiety. In this sense, any condition which
produces the physical manifestations of anxiety is a cause of anxiety
itself. This is an important point, because textbooks often emphasize

that the presentations of anxiety and various physiologic diseases are similar, and must therefore be subject to rigorous differential diagnosis. In fact, the subjective sensation is identical. A person *feels* anxious whether the source is hyperthyroidism or an impending breakup with one's spouse. In fact, most commonly, even when a person has a biologic disease that can explain the symptoms there will often be multiple psychological circumstances that also could explain the anxiety.

Common physiologic symptoms often associated with (and may be interpreted as) anxiety include the following: tachycardia, dyspnea, sweating, increased blood pressure, mydriasis, fatigue, sleeping and eating disturbances, palpitations, tremors, urinary frequency, changes in bowel habits, and headaches.

People differ in how sensitive they are to physical cues from their own bodies. Some people immediately experience the above symptoms as anxiety. Others will experience an obscure, omnipresent sense of threat, or danger. Some people will acknowledge this feeling when asked, and others are not comfortable in doing so.

There are many, many ways of responding to anxiety, and the whole panoply of Freudian "defenses" are postulated responses to anxiety. These include such traditional concepts as compartmentalization, rationalization, projection, denial, conversion, and many more. In terms of adaptation to illness, three are of special interest: regressive dependency, denial, and arousal to control the environment. All of these are potentially both useful and troublesome for the patient and care givers; the problems associated with each were discussed in chapter 1.

Depression

People can cry much easier than they can change.
—James Baldwin

Depression is an endemic disease in the United States this latter half of the twentieth century. Everyone knows what it is to be depressed, at least at a symptomatic level, and most people have had the experience of being weighted down by their depression. If you believe that depression, when present, should always be diagnosed, then depression is probably one of the most underdiagnosed phenomena in any medical practice. Almost *no one* is happy to be sick and consulting a physician, or in the hospital, and this simple level of reactive unhappiness is rapidly escalated by such factors as pain, severity or chronicity of illness, dependency, and being bedridden and among strangers, as well as other multiple simultaneous stresses.

Depression itself is a broad and ambiguous term. It may be used to refer to a mood state, a symptom, a condition, a disease process, or a subcategory of a disease. So much has been written about depression, it often seems that half the population is depressed and half is writing about it, with the two groups clearly *not* mutually exclusive.

Many authors emphasize the necessity of accurately diagnosing the specific type of depression at hand. I don't believe that it is worthwhile for a generalist to put much effort and time into carefully labeling a specific type of depression, but with a few exceptions. Assessing severity is important, and I think the framework given earlier in this chapter will suffice for most clinical situations. I believe that attention to differential diagnosis is crucial in two situations: (1) ascertaining possible organic contributions to depression, and (2) identifying lithium-treatable manic-depressive illness when present. If the patient has a psychotic depression, you will certainly want to treat the psychosis. Otherwise, the treatment of depression is entirely on a symptomatic basis, related to the clinical picture, severity, and contributing causes.

In fact, almost all depressions have multiple contributing causes. If the patient is hospitalized, you can usually expect that all of the following are likely to play a role with depression in any given patient: the fact of illness, conditions of treatment, loss of self-esteem, separation from loved ones, financial concerns, concurrent psychosocial factors, and fearfulness about the future.

Classic psychoanalytic thought emphasizes two specific sources of depression, which you may wish to see separately or as tied in with the more mundane sources listed above. The first theme describes depression as a response to object loss. That is, persons become depressed when they perceive an actual or threatened or even imaginary loss of some important person or thing. In fact, this is a useful concept for helping to understand depression in medically ill persons. Especially important here is the loss of a dream, or fantasy, or hope about one's future. A familiar example may be the teenaged football player who breaks his leg and then becomes depressed. In his mind's eye this broken leg is not simply a fracture with temporary disability, but rather a derailment of his life's dream: the big game, local and regional fame, scholarships, college athletics, national fame, professional athletics, wealth, and success. Many people have such scenarios in their minds for what is ahead of them, and illness often plays a key part in at least temporarily destroying such fantasies.

A second psychoanalytic concept often clinically useful in the general medical setting has to do with explaining depression as anger turned inward. The idea here is that anger is a difficult emotion for many people to express, and as a consequence the anger is internalized, resulting in depression. The useful aspect of this notion is to remind us to look for possible sources of anger in a patient who appears to be depressed. In particular, it's worthwhile wondering whether this patient has some anger which could profitably be expressed to us. Persons who begin to express their anger often rapidly get over their depression. It is then for us to decide whether we prefer the patient to be depressed or angry. Obviously, many patients will want to have some voice in the matter too. However, anger is often a transitional phase in the resolution of depression. We should not necessarily take the patient's anger as a personal attack.

Many psychiatrists have traditionally differentiated grief from other forms of depression. Grief is said to be a specific reaction to loss, appropriate in degree to the importance of the loss. However, it is often difficult to judge what is and what is not appropriate for another human being in terms of his or her own personal reactions to loss. We will discuss the treatment of grief as a separate entity in chapter 13 concerning the family.

Many psychiatrists place a good deal of emphasis also on differentiating neurotic or characterologic depressions from other kinds of depressions. The intent here is to identify persons for whom depression is not merely a reaction to specific events, but a life-style in itself. Such persons are unlikely to relinquish their lifelong habits simply to accommodate our omnipotent fantasies of curing them. To that extent, identifying these individuals can save each of us a lot of professional wear and tear. However, as we discussed earlier and shall reemphasize later on, the treatment goal in depression is generally to reduce it to a level manageable by the patient's own coping techniques, rather than to cure it entirely. In this respect, since this sort of depression fluctuates in intensity over time and in response to intercurrent events, the treatment of characterologic depression is little different from any other kind.

I have specifically avoided up to this point defining and describing depression in detail. I have tried rather to present depression as a phenomenon common to all human experience, which you will intuitively understand. However, for the sake of reference, I think it useful to describe briefly some of the common manifestations of depression. *Psychological manifestations* include depressed mood, sadness, lack of enjoyment from ordinary sources of pleasure, narrowing of interests, a sense of worthlessness, decreased concentration and attention, apathy, pessimism, indecisiveness, a sense of helplessness and/or hopelessness, obsessive worrying, decreased emotional responsiveness, and guilt. *Physiologic manifestations* of depression include psychomotor retardation, easy fatigability, lassitude, insomnia, and early morning awakening, changes in diet and/or weight, decreased libido, and an infinite variety of somatic complaints (usually worse in the morning). As with anxiety, any physiologic condition which reproduces these symptoms and signs (e.g., anemia, myasthenia, diabetes mellitus) may be interpreted by the physician (or experienced by the patient) as depression.

Treatment of Anxiety and Depression

Treating anxiety and depression to the medical-surgical patient, as opposed to the primarily psychiatric patient, can become one of the most gratifying things you have ever done. It's gratifying because it is simple, and because your treatment will almost always be successful in alleviating severity, if not in total cure. Almost all anxieties and depressions are self-limited and will improve no matter what you do. However, you can certainly make these conditions improve more rapidly than they would on their own, and, in the process, make your patients' course of illness much more pleasant and improve your rapport with them at the same time.

The best way to approach treatment in such cases is to have an outline in your mind of what you want to do. I suggest the following set of approaches, symbolized by the acronym SLANT (Sit–Listen–Accept–Nostrums–Therapy), as a basic model upon which you can build your own treatment of most patients.

SIT

No matter how much or how little time you have with a patient, sit down. Even if you are in the room for only two-and-one-half minutes, make sure that this time really belongs to the patient, and that you will not be distracted by outside pressing concerns. While you're sitting, look directly at the patient. Impress the details of his or her face in your mind. Look for attributes of character which you can respect. A strong jaw, gnarled hands, a twinkle in the eye, an interesting tattoo, a wrinkled brow—anything. But search for something that will help establish that patient as a unique person in your eyes, and let the respect you feel show on your face. Before you depart, give the patient some warning, so that your departure won't come as a rude surprise. One convenient technique (e.g., in a three-minute visit with one minute remaining) is to stand up, walk to the patient's side, and touch the patient reassuringly. An easy way to do this is simply to take the patient's pulse, holding the wrist for a full minute. Leaving even an upset patient needn't be difficult as long as the patient knows what to expect in advance. Most patients are keenly aware of how busy you are, and are grateful for whatever time you can spend with them.

LISTEN

Duke's Dictum:
Don't analyze,
Listen.

—Edward Kennedy (Duke) Ellington

The first rule of listening is to come in terms with our own anxiety in sitting silently with a patient. Our words in this situation have only one function: to help get the patient started talking. Except for that one function, we will do best if we keep our mouths shut. It's difficult to both talk and listen at the same time, and our function with the patient is to listen. Listen not so much for details as for broad themes. Recognize the obvious. If a patient looks scared to death say, "You look scared to death." If the patient starts crying while you are conversing with him or her, say, "You're feeling pretty upset aren't you?" Avoiding the obvious gives the patient the message that you are uncomfortable with the patient's feelings and that the patient should be too. This serves to put the lid on the patient's feelings while, at the same time, undermining your relationship.

Listen for things about this patient that you personally can relate to and respect. Listen for broad areas of concern, especially about the patients' illnesses and how those illnesses will affect their lives. Listen for how the patients have coped with similar stresses in the past. Good questions for getting the patients started talking include the following: "How are your spirits doing?" "How is your family taking all this?" "How is this illness going to affect the way you live your life in the days ahead?" "How have you coped with rough times like this in the past?" The specific content, while potentially useful, is less important than the process whereby the patients have an opportunity to ventilate their concerns to a willing and interested listener, who also happens to have responsibility for the patients' health care.

ACCEPT

The therapeutic effect of the patient's talking and your listening will be undermined if you sit there with a look of disdain or boredom on your face. You have to convey the impression that their concerns and sadness meet with acceptance in you. You don't necessarily have to agree, but you have to show some understanding that the patients' feelings are real to them and make sense within their framework. Do *not* attempt to reassure the patient directly. Instead, allow the patient to be reassured indirectly by your manner and your acceptance. Help the patient to understand that this emotional state is natural in context. "If you're worried about losing your job, it's no wonder that you're upset." "Having teenagers in trouble puts a lot of stress on a family." "I can understand how frustrating all this is for you." Do *not* deprive patients of the validity of their feelings by saying, "Don't be upset," or, "There, there now, it will all be better by and by."

In order to be truly accepting, you have to be willing to acknowledge that you cannot sit in judgment of someone else's feelings. That is easier said than done, especially when that person's feelings become an obstacle to you in something you must do or feel you must do. Take the following example from a familiar medical school setting:

The patient is a 22-year-old woman with an acute surgical abdomen, most likely from a ruptured ectopic pregnancy. You are a senior medical student who has been told by the department chief, Dr. Scalpel, to get the surgery permit signed, and then get up to the operating room and start scrubbing. You are going to be first assistant (a real coup on your part) and you have dreams of being offered a coveted residency slot. You go in to see the patient and, though she is in obvious discomfort, she is terrified of surgery and refuses to sign the surgery permit. What do you say now?

A representative though perhaps extreme range of choices includes the following:

1. "You stupid girl! You're going to die if you don't have this operation, and it would serve you right!"
2. "Look I really need for you to sign this. Dr. Scalpel is letting me be First Assistant and my whole career hangs in the balance."
3. "Try not to be frightened. There's really nothing to be afraid of. It's silly to be so scared."
4. "Well, we certainly can't force you. We'll give you a while to think it over and the nurse will be in from time to time to see if you have changed your mind."
5. "It must be terrible to be so uncomfortable and yet so frightened of the remedy. How can I help you?"

There is no certainty that any of the above would lead to an absolutely predictable response, but the odds are clearly in the following direction:

Alternative 1

Everybody loses. While the feelings are perhaps understandable, the action and words are ill-chosen. The patient's fear is transmuted into fury. She complains to her family, Dr. Scalpel, and the hospital administrator, and demands to be transferred to another hospital. Enroute, she expires from hypovolemic shock. The family sues, and the hospital settles out of court. If you are lucky, you are allowed to graduate with your class, but the evaluation in your student records folder says "arrogant to patients and loses composure under stress."

Alternative 2

You get high marks for honesty, but low marks for everything else. You neglected to maintain the primacy of the patient's needs above all else, and have therein confirmed the patient's fear that no one truly cares about her and her welfare. She continues to refuse surgery. If you are lucky, she won't tell anyone what you said. If you are unlucky, the scenario could resemble alternative 1.

Alternative 3

You get high marks for intentions, low marks for technique and zero for acceptance. Clearly, you mean well, but the patient isn't frightened because she wants to be. If she knew how to be otherwise, she probably would. You have lost credibility by saying there is nothing to be frightened of. There *is* something frightening her, even if neither of you knows what it is. You probably have also harmed your relationship by telling her she is being silly, which many patients would see as a put-down, reflective of lack of empathy. The deciding factors here will probably be the clarity with which your good intentions show through—and how much time the patient has to make the decision before she bleeds out.

Alternative 4

This is a tricky one. If you choose this course as part of a gruff, let-nature-take-its-course philosophy, then you aren't giving yourself credit for a large enough repertoire of responses. The patient, alone in a room with only her fears and falling hematocrit, is unlikely to see safety and salvation where before she saw only terror. But you never know. However, if you choose this course because you know that the nurse on duty is a warm, empathetic listener who is much more likely than you to persuade this woman, then you may have chosen well. A recognition of one's own limitations can be the most fruitful course, even if humbling.

Alternative 5

Excellent! You have fastened onto the paradox in this woman. You accept her fear, yet you refuse to let it become a barrier between you. As a matter of fact, you are using it as the basis for your relationship. Keep up this line of gentle probing and you will have your surgery permit, the patient will have the operation, and you will have a grateful patient, too. Before that is achieved, expect some tears and a gush of information: a relative has died under anesthesia, there is fear of abdominal scarring, she had an illicit sexual experience for which this condition is seen as punishment, she fears what she might verbally reveal during anesthesia induction, etc. Once you have properly set the stage, patients will often reveal many intimate concerns, and you can then begin to help them with their fears. But most of them first demand that you demonstrate—in your manner and in your words—that you give a damn about them as they are, and will accept them on those terms.

NOSTRUMS

Nostrums provide evidence to patients that you and the other people who are looking after their health care actually care about them. Nostrums are evidence of caring. They are designed to help increase the patients' confidence in their treatment. You can also use them to help patients feel that they have more control over and participation in their own treatment. Often as not, nostrums involve gestures which represent compromises in textbook treatment of the patient's disorder in favor of reducing the patient's subjective discomfort, minimizing dependency, maximizing independence, and enhancing self-image. For example, while letting the patient know that you are doing these things because you want to help him or her feel better: offer a mint from your pocket; call the patient's family to ask, "How do you think he's doing?"; give ice chips to a patient who is officially NPO; remove an intravenous tube with 250 cc left to go because you know it is uncomfortable for the patient; ask the person on weekend call to stop in specifically to see the patient and say, "Hello from Dr. X"; ask the patient to choose between two different acceptable medications, after explaining the differences between them; allow a patient to discontinue bedrest prematurely for "the sake of his spirits"; and change the patient's medication regimen along the lines that the patient wishes, even though it isn't quite what your consultant would have preferred.

The secrets in nostrums lie in the treatment of the whole patient, not just his or her physiologic or even specific psychological problems. The intent is to make the patient feel special and useful, someone who merits the esteem of others. Some hospitals—and some hospital staffs—are very good at this, putting a flower on each meal tray, serving wine or beer with dinner, handing out suggestion-box cards to patients, making sure that each patient personally meets the Chief of Nursing or an assistant hospital administrator.

You, however, can do your own bit independently of whatever your hospital or medical group does or does not do. You can integrate into your own treatment any of the suggestions outlined above. You can help a depressed patient feel useful (perhaps the greatest gift of all) by asking him or her to read to a blind patient or to talk to a new patient who is facing a procedure which the depressed patient has already survived. You can ask your patients to evaluate the services they receive—including those you provide. You can ask your patients to teach you, to help you be a better doctor, to correct you when you screw up, and to pat you on the back when you do well. In short, you can let your patients know you really care.

As a consequence, your patients will be partially immunized against the disease which afflicts most patients, but you yourself will be more susceptible to feelings of responsibility when anxiety and depression do occur. Whether the achievement is worth the price is something that each of us has to decide for ourselves. However, we have more to offer our patients than sitting and listening and acceptance and nostrums—and it's hoped you will have a clearer idea about these alternatives as we go along.

THERAPY

The most important therapy you can give an anxious or depressed patient is measured doses of yourself. If a patient has confidence and respect in the treating physician, and feels that the views are reciprocated, the restorative effect for the patient can be enormous. These kinds of feelings develop best with regular investments of time on the part of the health-care givers. Even a few minutes at a time, if they come regularly enough and the patient knows that he or she can count on them, will be sufficient.

Familiarize yourself with the techniques described in the Appendix. I doubt that all of them will seem comfortable to you, but each embodies principles which may be useful to your patients and yourself. Each can be used in any stage of anxiety and depression, often with good effect. The patients' acceptance of the various techniques will depend not only on their social and cultural background, but also on your manner in bringing the technique to their attention. If you fervently believe in meditation, at your insistence even a doubting patient may be willing to give it a respectful try. Be careful to be respectful in return; don't shove a technique at patients if they are clearly uncomfortable with it and regard it as a gimmick. For more complicated cases, you will want to consult the recommendations and discussion in chapter 8, Psychotherapy and Counseling, or consider requesting a consultation or referral.

Drug Therapy of Anxiety and Depression

I have specifically kept chemotherapy till almost last, because it is
what most people think of first in treating anxiety and depression. The
emphasis in this chapter clearly is on nondrug therapy of these disorders. However, as long as you include nondrug approaches to anxiety
and depression as a matter of course, don't be afraid to use chemotherapy liberally. Of course, drugs can be useful adjuvants in your treatment of patients and their problems. There are, however, a few cautions which should be kept in mind.

Know the specific target symptom you are attempting to influence.
Is it the patient's subjective complaint of anxiety? Is it rapid pulse or
diaphoresis? Be very cautious about obscuring manifestations of related physiologic problems. Is it a specific behavior on the patient's
part? If so, make certain that what you are trying to reduce or eliminate
is truly maladaptive for the patient and not representative of his or her
own attempts to cope. Is it complaints by hospital staff about the
patient's behavior? If so, perhaps your efforts will be better spent
helping the staff to become more forgiving with the patient, rather than
changing the patient's behavior per se.

Recognize when the use of drugs is your own response to frustration
with the patient and his or her complaints. Always be wary of to what
degree you are treating the sufferer, and to what degree you are treating your own needs to have a compliant, noncomplaining patient. Be
particularly cautious when you are prescribing multiple central nervous system depressant drugs (narcotic and nonnarcotic analgesics,
sedatives, tranquilizers, and other drugs with central nervous system
depressant effects). Be certain that any given psychoactive medication
is not dangerous or contraindicated in this particular patient with this
particular condition, when coupled with the particular medications that
he or she happens to be taking.

Anxiety and Anxiety-Related Problems

With all the preceding cautions, I recommend the following medications. Dosages may need to be higher for those patients who are large
in size or have established drug tolerance, and lower for patients who
are very thin or elderly.

For sleep

Treat insomnia freely with medication in any short-term situation,
especially hospitalization. Sleeping in a strange bed is difficult for
many people, especially in a frightening and noisy place like a hospital.
Feel free to repeat the dosage at least one time, as long as there are not
medical contraindications.

1. Flurazepam (DALMANE) from 15 to 30 mg
2. Diphenhydramine (BENADRYL) from 25 to 50 mg

In long-term hospitalizations and for outpatient treatment, a different approach is necessary. Routine bedtime sedation leads to drug tolerance and possible addiction. In order for you to have their cooperation, patients must understand this consideration. Once they do, they are far more likely to accept your reluctance to prescribe sedatives on an every night basis, and you can either help them find other ways of inducing sleep (see Appendix) or encourage them to make productive use of episodes of sleeplessness by using the time for other activities.

Anxiety

The dosage requirements of the two agents below vary considerably from one individual to another and are recommended for stages one, two, and three, i.e., less than incapacitating. You can use both of them over a fairly flexible dosage range. Given at bedtime, each is likely to have some residual antianxiety effects the following morning.

1. Diazepam (VALIUM) from 2 to 10 mg, usually two to four times a day
2. Chlordiazepoxide (LIBRIUM) from 5 to 25 mg, usually two to four times a day

Antianxiety agents sometimes relieve coexistent depression and sometimes increase depression. Watch each patient for changes in depression levels as you treat anxiety.

Incapacitating anxiety

Be certain to ask the patient if he or she has had similar episodes in the past. A surprising number will have had such episodes, and will know which drug at which dose will be most helpful for them. Remind yourself of the side effects of all the following agents, and watch for them carefully.

1. THORAZINE from 15 to 100 mg intramuscularly (or orally by elixir), may be repeated hourly in the absence of significant hypotension and central nervous system depression.
2. VALIUM from 2 to 10 mg intravenously (slowly), may be repeated hourly in the absence of hypotension and/or central nervous system depression. (*Note:* Intravenous use of central nervous system depressant agents requires the ready availability of resuscitation equipment for respiratory or cardiac arrest.)

Depression

Drug therapy for depression tends to be generally controversial, with most of the evidence suggesting that we should not expect too much from antidepressant drugs, even though most clinicians can point to occasional dramatic successes, seemingly attributable to tricyclics. Even though there is good statistical evidence that these agents are useful in some patients, it is still unlikely that the introduction of such drugs accounts for more than a small percentage of the variance from non-drug-treated patients.

When I was a psychiatrist with an active psychotherapy practice, I prescribed my share of antidepressant medications. Now, as an emergency medicine doctor, I loathe them, primarily because they are a major factor in many serious and sometimes fatal overdoses.

If you do prescribe antidepressants, you are obliged to prescribe them in small amounts, with a total amount which represents a sublethal dose (usually less than a one-week supply). You need to see the patient frequently, usually on a weekly basis, to titrate the level of depression, monitor the many side effects and potential drug interactions, and adjust dosages. All antidepressant medications tend to have a delayed onset of clinical improvement, varying from two to three weeks, so patience is required for both patient and physician. Because of toxicity and delayed clinical improvement, antidepressant medications require an *absolutely reliable* patient who will take medications *exactly* as directed, and for whom there is no danger of an overdose.

If you have a patient who qualifies for antidepressant medication, consider using a tricyclic antidepressant such as amitriptyline (ELAVIL) or imipramine (TOFRANIL). A convenient schedule would be to begin either medication at 25 mg every eight hours. Increase the nighttime dose by 25 mg each day until a total dosage of 150 mg per day is reached. Keep it at this level for from three to four weeks before evaluating the therapeutic effect. If there is no therapeutic effect visible at that time, many psychiatrists recommend increasing the dosage to up to 350 mg per day (Some would say more and some would say less, though I would taper the drug if no effect had been seen by this time.) If no effect has been seen after maximum dose has been maintained for from three to four weeks, taper the drug. If a positive therapeutic effect is reached, maintain the drug at that level for from three to six weeks longer (some would say more), then gradually taper the drug.

The newer "second generation" antidepressants (the tetracyclics, triazolopyridines, and dibenzoxazepines) constitute a large, diverse group which has not as yet been demonstrated to offer any significant clinical advantages over the conventional tricyclics or even the potentially very toxic monoamine oxidase (MAO) inhibitors. Therefore, use them (if at all) only with reliable back-up. If you arrive at such a point, consider psychiatric consultation and/or referral.

Consultation and Referral

How often you utilize mental health consultation and referral depends (among other things) upon your own skills, the kinds and numbers of patients you have, and the talents and availability of mental health personnel. In general, you should be able to manage and treat prophylactically any patient with Stage One or Stage Two anxiety and depression; but you should routinely request help with patients in Stage Four.

Patients with Stage Three problems fit neatly into neither of the above categories. In short, whether to manage the problems with or without specialist input requires some judgment. If you feel you can ameliorate the problem by comfortably using the SLANT technique and by mobilizing other talented persons, give it a try. If in doubt, call a consultant and ask for advice.

One good approach is to call up the mental health consultant and say something like this: "I'm taking care of a gentleman who is quite depressed and is having trouble coping effectively with the circumstances of his illness. He is not suicidal. I believe I can manage the situation on my own now, but I just wanted you to be aware of what is transpiring, in case I need you to see him. Here are the details and here is what I plan to do. Do you have any suggestions?"

Most consultants in such a circumstance would be pleased by your interest and gratified that you wish to tackle the problem yourself but want their guidance. They would also appreciate having had advance warning if the situation should happen to deteriorate.

Bibliography
Aneshewsel CS, Frerichs RR, Huba GJ: Depression and physical illness. *J Health Soc Behavior* 25:350–371, 1984

Baldessarini RJ: *Biomedical Aspects of Depression and Its Treatment.* Washington, D.C., American Psychiatric Press, 1983

Bird B: *Talking With Patients.* Philadelphia, Lippincott, 1955

Blazer DG: Impact of late-night depression on the social network. *Am J Psychiatry* 140:162–166, 1983

Clayton PJ, Barrett JE (eds): *Treatment of Depression—Old Controversies and New Approaches.* New York, Raven Press, 1983

Gray JA: Anxiety as a paradigm case of emotion. *Brit Med J* 37:193–197, 1981

Hollister LE: Mental disorders—antianxiety and antidepressant drugs. *N Engl J Med* 286:1195–1198, 1972

———: Second-generation antidepressants. *Ration Drug Ther* (December) 1982, 16(12):1–5

Jenner FA: Advances in antidepressant treatment? *Practitioner* 225:1378–1385, 1981

Kashani JH, Priesmeyer M: Differences in depressive symptoms and depression among college students. *Am J Psychiatry* 140:1081–1082, 1983

Kreuger DW: The depressed patient. *J Fam Pract* 8:363–370, 1979

Leckman JF: Anxiety disorders and depression. *Am J Psychiatry* 140:880–882, 1983

Perry JC: Depression in borderline personality disorder. *Am J Psychiatry* 142:15–21, 1985

Priest RG: The treatment of anxiety and depression in general practice. *Practitioner* 226:549–556, 1982

Rippere V: Depression, common sense and psychosocial evolution. *Brit J Med Psychol* 54:379–387, 1981

Schiffer RB: Depressive episodes in patients with multiple sclerosis. *Am J Psychiatry* 140:1498–1500, 1983

Shader RL, Greenblatt DJ: Antidepressants—the second harvest and DSM III. *J Clin Psychopharm* 1(2):51–52, 1981

Walker JI: The anxious patient. *J Fam Pract* 12:733–738, 1981

———: Drugs for psychiatric disorders. *The Medical Letter* 25(635):45–52, 1983

Winokur G: *Depression—The Facts.* New York, Oxford University Press, 1981

8

Psychotherapy and Counseling

Attempts to enhance a person's feeling of well-being are usually labeled treatment. . . .

—Jerome Frank

If little else, the brain is an educational toy. While it may be a frustrating plaything—one whose finer points recede just when you think you are mastering them—it is nonetheless perpetually fascinating, frequently surprising, occasionally rewarding, and it comes already assembled; you don't have to put it together on Christmas morning.

The problem with possessing such an engaging toy is that other people want to play with it, too. Sometimes they would rather play with yours than theirs.

—Tom Robbins

If you can get a half dozen psychotherapists together in one room and arrive at a single, specific definition of psychotherapy, let me know. I'd be delighted to join the ensuing celebration. Even the terms psychiatrist and mental illness are distressingly elusive to persons wishing to define them. An American Psychiatric Association task force spent several years trying to define the latter terms, and the best they could do is roughly approximated by the following: "A psychiatrist is someone who treats mental illness, and mental illness is whatever psychiatrists treat." A symmetric set of definitions, but hardly enlightening.

Psychotherapy is variously described as (1) helping people function more comfortably at whatever level they choose to, (2) helping people make sense out of apparently meaningless suffering, (3) assisting individuals in their search for insight and self-identity, or (4) anything which a psychiatrist does and can get paid for. There are numerous wordier descriptions as well.

The point is that the *concept* of psychotherapy is so diffuse as to be practically meaningless. Mind you, I am referring to labels and concepts which relegate one person's helping another to the province of a scientific technique; I am not referring to the process itself. I believe firmly in one person's ability to help another see things in new ways, to offer consolation and guidance. I myself have been helped so often by friends, relatives, and even strangers that I am amazed that I still remain so helpable.

Further, some people are more skilled at the process than others, and even the very skilled can become better with additional learning and experience. In that sense there certainly are experts in human guidance, but demonstrating that this expertise correlates with any specific academic degree or certification may be difficult.

The terminology surrounding psychotherapy depends on theoretical constructs, and the latter are heavily dependent upon currently dominant cultural explanations for natural phenomena and contemporary standards of well-being. If your perspective is medical-psychiatric, you will talk about therapy; if sociologic, the term will be counseling; if theologic, then ministering; if educational, then tutoring or teaching.

When mental illness was regarded as infestation by the devil, the logical treatment was prayer, isolation, exorcism, neglect, and occasionally physical abuse. With this treatment, some individuals got better, some got worse, and some stayed the same. Now that bedevilment is seen as mental illness, the spectrum of results stays the same. The only quarrel is whether the treatments and the percentages of those improved and those deteriorated are significantly different—and of course what one means by "improvement."

With that lengthy and obviously opinionated introduction, let me clarify the intent of this chapter. I would like to provide a useful perspective for the nonpsychiatrist which will make it easier for you to be a helpful person to those patients whose human problems are complicating their medical problems and vice versa. That is, when you decide that you want to "psychotherapize" a patient, this chapter may give you some sense of how to go about doing it.

Psychotherapy is a tool that you can learn to use in some situations, even though you make no pretense at using it expertly. No matter how good you get at this process, there will always be persons around who are better at it than you, who work at it more, and who have had more experience and training. The latter group will most prominently include psychiatrists, and referral to them needn't depend upon a conviction that there is anything extraordinarily technical or mystical about what a professional psychotherapist (counselor, minister) does with the person you refer.

Levels and Types of Psychotherapy

Rather than play Ping-Pong with words, I will continue to use the term *psychotherapy* to refer to the purposeful efforts of one person to help another with ordinary human problems, based upon the shared understanding that the attempt at "talking it out" will be worth the time spent.

Psychotherapy deals with problems of various degrees of intimacy. At the most superficial level, the individual (in this instance, the patient) talks with the therapist about problems which might be discussed with almost any other friend or acquaintance. Generally, these are easily recognizable problems of daily living common to general experience: the kids are unmanageable, the tension at work is terrible, the aging parents are burdensome. At a secondary level, psychotherapy deals with problems sufficiently personal that they may be discussed with only a few treasured intimates, if the patient has such intimates available. These issues commonly concern embarrassing and secret personal traits or feelings: "I hate one of my children," or "Though everyone thinks I do well at my work, I've never gotten any pleasure from it and feel listless and bored," or "I wish my parents would die." The third level involves concerns so intimate and emotionally charged that the individual may not think about them even in solitude, and they remain mostly in the unconscious.

This chapter deals only with the first two levels; the third is beyond the scope of this book. However, it is important to know that such a level exists. Even though neither you nor the patient knows what goes on in the unconscious, the latter still influences thoughts, feelings, and behavior.

Whatever level of problem you are dealing with, there are dozens of different sets of ideas about what techniques and theoretical perspectives you should use as you proceed. Despite the number and types of these schools of psychotherapy, the approaches have more in common than they have differences. Most of the ideas are conveniently lumped into four groups.

PSYCHOANALYTICALLY ORIENTED THERAPY

This approach attempts to understand and treat human problems by probing a person's innermost thoughts and feelings, derived largely from previous early experience, bringing unconscious "neurotic" conflict to the level of consciousness. All approaches which do not use this approach are generally regarded as symptomatic and lacking in class. A typical psychoanalytic strategy is to analyze the relationship the patient has with the therapist, because the latter is presumed to provide clues to the patient's personality and unresolved childhood conflicts on which the personality is based.

BEHAVIORISTIC THERAPY

This approach is derived heavily from laboratory studies of learning processes. Thoughts and feelings are conceived as existing only insofar as they lead to behavioral manifestations: e.g., anxiety does not exist unless it leads to specific physiologic correlates such as muscle tension or increased gastric acidity. If you can't perceive the physiologic manifestations of anxiety in your body, the behaviorists ask, how do you know you are anxious? The aim of treatment therefore is to change behavior: its frequency, its stimulus–response link, its intensity. Strategies vary, but therapy is seen largely as a relearning process, achieved by means of conditioning, training, modeling, desensitization, and so forth.

HUMANISTIC THERAPY

This approach emphasizes "self-actualization" and realizing your own potential largely by means of personal understanding, heightened awareness, and, especially, getting in touch with your own feelings. Common maxims include "Know what you are, feel what you are, do what you are" and "The only reality is one's own emotional experience." Typically, humanists tend to regard psychoanalysis as too aridly intellectual and behaviorists as mechanistic computer programmers.

TRANSCENDENTAL THERAPY

This approach emphasizes a number of humanistic goals, but further seeks integration of the awareness of one's self with one's place in the universe. Common catchwords include "higher consciousness," "spiritual integration," and "religious experience." Realizing one's own potential is predicated upon spiritual and mystical and psychical considerations.

Enormous time, effort, and money has been expended to demonstrate that any one or a variety of psychotherapeutic methods are significantly more successful for any particular problem than simply allowing a patient's difficulty to run its natural course. Scrutinizing the reports of such studies leads me to the conclusion that the evidence does not yet convincingly support the unique effectiveness of any particular psychotherapeutic style.

Most comparative studies suggest insignificant differences in proportions of patients who improve by the end of treatment, regardless of the various treatments used, the degree of experience of the practitioners, and so forth. When patients improve in psychotherapy (and there is a slight preponderance of studies which favor psychotherapy over no treatment at all) there is no consistent feature of the treatment except that some sort of relationship was developed with an identified helper.

The difficulties of assessing outcome in long-term psychotherapy apply equally to any long-term educational process. Measures of maturation and success are so nebulous, and intercurrent variables so numerous, that meaningful cost-effectiveness studies may well be impossible.

The end result is therefore that if and when you decide that you are in a good position to psychotherapize a patient and you decide you want to do so, you needn't feel obliged to first become immersed in Freudian or Jungian theory. Your intent is to form a purposefully helping relationship, to provide the patient with a bit of perspective or insight which will lead to new values or new ways of feeling or behaving. You will also wish to avoid putting your foot in your mouth and avoid looking or feeling like an ass in the process.

Perspectives for the Would-Be Psychotherapist

Suffering ceases to be suffering in some way at the moment it finds a meaning.

—Viktor Frankl

How to avoid putting one's foot in one's own mouth is a recurring problem for most of us. It takes a particular knack in doing psychotherapy, because you are dealing with intensely personal issues and you're playing on another person's turf. No matter how open the patient may be, there is always information that the patient has that you don't. It is therefore helpful if you approach the task with some humility, recognizing at the onset your own limitations and the limitations of the situation. A lucky person gets reasonably good at running his or her own life; being an expert at running somebody else's life seems to me to be a contradiction in terms. An expert is supposed to know all the relevant facts, and it's difficult enough to know all the facts about one's own life.

The information which follows is separate from the specifics of goals and tactics in psychotherapy which we will discuss a bit later on. My intent is to provide perspective, based upon some arbitrary observations of human behavior, which will get you into a proper mental framework for doing psychotherapy.

Your potency as a therapist depends not only on your attentiveness and genuine caring for, and empathy with, your patient, but also on your ability to convey these qualities in a nonintrusive fashion. Generally, the process requires considerable emotional energy on the part of the therapist. Truly helping someone with an intensely human problem, and watching them grow as a consequence of that help, is one of the most rewarding things I can imagine. In order to do it well, I have to be confident that I have the energy to spare and that I am not robbing my energy storehouse of supplies that properly belong to myself, my friends, and my family. Some psychiatrists manage to do 40 to 60 hours of psychotherapy a week. When I was doing psychotherapy, and when things were going very well for me personally, I could do up to 20 hours a week; when they were not going so well, I was lucky to be able to do a decent job of psychotherapy five hours a week. Sometimes, as one friend said, I would pay people not to tell me about their problems at all. The point is simply that each of us has to be aware of our own limitations, that these limits vary from one to another of us, and vary within each of us over time.

The most common error in psychotherapy is not that it is done poorly, but that it isn't done at all. Remember our working definition of psychotherapy: the purposeful efforts of one person to help another with ordinary human problems, based on the shared understanding that the attempt at talking it out will be worth the time spent. There is nothing in that definition that says you have to meet with the patient an hour at a crack, or any number of times a week, or even that you have to meet more than once. The only requirement is that two persons think enough of one another to spend some time together focusing on one person's problems. That in itself is likely to have some palliative effects.

Many physicians are uncomfortable with their own potential for influencing patients. Our democratic and scientific traditions interact to emphasize objective and rational doctor-patient relationships, with the two relating as coparticipants in the treatment process. Certainly, treating the patient with respect for his or her right to self-determination has gotten heavy emphasis in this book. Yet we would also be amiss if we didn't recognize that our role as physicians still gives us enormous potential for influencing our patients. Grappling with the terminology on the subjects is like chasing soap bubbles in the air— whenever you trap them, they seem to go "pop" and lose their substance. But the terms are identifiable: charisma, power of personality, certain "presence," making people think that one "really cares," "bringing energy to the situation," and so forth. Whatever it is, the effect is related to confidence in one's own way of viewing and doing things. Healing correlates not only with the patient's faith that the treatment process will be successful, but also with the physician's faith and optimism too. The latter is good stuff to have around whenever you can harness it for the mutual benefit of yourself and the patient. Things can get sticky, however, if you've got a lot of this mystical quality but your best interests diverge from those of the patient. Be very alert to the patient's welfare when you are feeling particularly charismatic; if in doubt, call for consultation before things get messy, rather than afterwards.

Remember that some amount of mental conflict is a fact of life for most of us. You needn't feel obliged to charge in and start therapizing everyone who is doing some struggling. I hesitate to describe suffering as healthy or unhealthy, because I'm not convinced that placing suffering on a health spectrum makes more sense than placing it on an existential or spiritual spectrum. Nonetheless, suffering has potential usefulness. Telling some patients to "tough it out" can therefore sometimes make sense if you're confident that the patient can do so, that the patient perceives that you are empathetic and not just sadistic, and that the patient agrees that suffering intelligently makes more sense than other available options. If suffering is a fact of life for a given person at a given time, ask in your own words: "Given that you are suffering so much, what value can you get out of this for yourself?" Does the patient's distress, for instance, become more manageable by expressing it openly? Will it in the long run add to the patient's sense of self-worth as a person who can survive such suffering? Is it a necessary step in this patient's long-term adjustment to life changes which are underway?

Remember that every behavior is multiply determined. There is more than a single contributing cause to virtually everything. If you seek simple answers, you will find them—at the expense of missing or ignoring other equally simple answers. The question of causality can be as complex as you wish it to be. For instance, if you blame a patient's anxiety on the fact that his wife left him, you will later find out that her departure occurred when she found out that he had a homosexual lover, which was related to some peculiar circumstances at work which were related to yet some other event; the anxiety turns out to be an intermittently appearing thread which appears again and again throughout the entire fabric. Or, if you blame a patient's apparent neurodermatitis on what you regard as her neurotic life-style, you will inevitably later find out that she also has a nickel sensitivity. Therefore, never say: "That" (meaning any one thing) "is or is not *the* cause." Instead, say, "Yes, that could be contributory," or "Yes, I think that is a very significant contributing factor."

There are easy questions and easy answers; the difficult task is fitting the two together correctly. When a patient asks you a question of fact, he or she frequently seeks an answer separate from the specific content of the question. For example, when a patient asks you about the side effect of a certain medication, there may be less concern with the specific answer (which the patient may well be aware of already) than with assessing your knowledge and ascertaining evidence that you have thoughtfully weighed the relevant considerations before prescribing the medication. That doesn't mean that you should refuse to answer direct questions from patients or always look at them skeptically and inquire, "I wonder why you ask that?" It does mean that you should always be alert to the question behind the question and deal with that, too, as the occasion dictates: "I'm glad you asked about side effects; I've been thinking about that issue myself and weighing the potential benefits versus possible harm."

In a related and common circumstance, a patient presents you with ambivalent feelings about a situation, and asks for your advice; e.g., "I'm trying to decide whether to return to work or to file for disability. Which do you recommend?" No matter what you advise, the patient will follow the contrary path 50% of the time. A good general rule is never to side with one-half of the patient's ambivalence. How you respond depends on how much time you have, and how psychotherapeutic you wish to be. The most superficial (but honest) response is: "I'm sorry, that's a decision I can't make for you." To add another layer of depth, say, "That depends on how much you value your work, what your pain tolerance is, a few other physical variables I can tell you about, and probably some personal considerations I'm not aware of." If you have more time and more interest, say, "Tell me more; what are the circumstances as you understand them?"

In the same way that I recommend you not side with one-half of patient's ambivalence, I recommend that you not side with one person of a couple or of a family, at the expense of any others. A good rule, certainly for adults, is: couples deserve one another—or, more generally, individuals tend to deserve the people with whom they have continuing relationships. Whenever you are tempted to say: "He's great, but she's a bitch" (or vice versa), two conditions probably apply. The first is you aren't owning up to the role your own values play in the situation. What you really mean is, "I like his particular idiosyncrasies, but not hers" (or vice versa). Of course, your taste in people has no more relevance to whom your patient chooses to have a relationship with than does your taste in ice cream flavors.

The second factor is that you are not fully informed about the details of the couple's relationship, the kinds of complementary functions they serve for one another, and how illness or other intercurrent events have altered the psychological balance sheet they have implicitly set up between them. I remember one very sick male patient, courageous and stoic, who nonetheless was bitterly disappointed that his family never visited him or showed their concern in any way. The ward staff were furious at the family for their neglect of this fine patient. While the staff correctly perceived that the patient behaved bravely and honorably in the hospital, they were not aware that his behavior on the outside was, to put it charitably, far more complicated—and included contemptuous philandering in front of his wife, incestuous physical abuse of his two eldest daughters, and selfish squandering of limited family funds. The wife had for a long time provided most of the glue which held the family together. Before your sympathies career from him to her, you should know that she had both virtues and unsavory qualities as well. Often, this kind of information just never comes out unless you maintain an awareness that people who choose one another tend to deserve one another; getting the details involves giving people an opportunity to talk, expressing your interest, and providing a nonjudgmental response.

Goals for Psychotherapy

Words of comfort, skillfully administered, are the oldest therapy known to man.
—Louis Nizer

One ceases to be a child when one realizes that telling one's troubles does not make it any better.
—Cesare Pavese

While words have the potential to heal, merely babbling is rarely very helpful. You are much more likely to get somewhere through talking if you have some sense of what you wish your destination to be. The next step in doing psychotherapy is therefore setting goals. Not as simple as it sounds. Many individuals have difficulty articulating what they want, and persons in turmoil—the ones who are most likely to seek psychotherapy—have even more difficulty.

However, just because the patient isn't able to articulate a goal doesn't mean that you as the therapist shouldn't have a goal in mind. How else will you know when to stop therapy, to change your tactics, or to refer the patient? I think a reasonable goal for a nonpsychiatrist doing psychotherapy is simply to help the patient to cope more effectively and comfortably with current life stresses. For most, that will involve fortifying old coping techniques; for some, that will mean learning new ones. While therapists often like to view therapy as a growth process, most people's unarticulated goal is to remain the same or "to return to the way I was," but feel better. We'll talk more about the specifics of enhanced coping after considering some other types of goals.

Seeking the meaning of life in psychotherapy is like seeking it in college or in a job. You may find some meaning—that's certainly a laudable intent—but then again you may not. Meaning in life doesn't come from words or even experience alone; it comes from inside. People have been seeking personal meaning, happiness, and self-esteem in the external world for thousands of years, and the goal has remained elusive. If a patient identifies "the meaning of life" or "personal meaningfulness" as a goal of psychotherapy, avoid the trap of saying you can help. If you have found *the* meaning in life for yourself, say, "I know what that is for myself, but I can't guarantee it will fit for you." Most of us would respond more accurately by saying: "I've been looking for that too; if you find it first, let me know." What you can offer in psychotherapy is likely to involve goals far more limited and concrete.

Other potential goals include decreasing the incidence or severity of certain symptoms or improving interpersonal relations. In each case, make certain that the goal is truly the patient's and not one imposed on the patient by yourself. Most symptoms and interpersonal struggles serve some adaptive function for the individual involved. Just as not everyone wants to give up smoking or lose weight, not everyone wants to have more socially acceptable ways of (e.g.) expressing anger.

Some persons, both therapists and patients, are interested in psychotherapy not because they have any specific goals, but because they like the process. It can be enormously satisfying for some individuals to talk endlessly about themselves to someone with a seemingly endless capacity to listen and accept. Therapy ad infinitum. Chronic patient and chronic therapist. It's obviously important to be aware of your own motivation for providing therapy. There's nothing wrong with getting pleasure from the process yourself; I believe that it's impossible to do the job conscientiously and well unless you do enjoy it, but beware of your own loneliness and need to be needed if they play a more important role in the decision to initiate or perpetuate treatment than do the patient's needs.

Coping

How is it that so many people manage to cope with stress without breaking down? God knows there is enough stress and strain in this world and especially during illness and hospitalization. Most people are amazingly resourceful most of the time, and everybody's resourceful some of the time.

Few individuals in our culture come anywhere near exhausting their inner resources at any given time. Those who survive best are those who can gain greatest nurturance from resources—either internal or external.

The physician's task is to recognize the patient's coping style and help the patient to use it effectively. If the patient wants to change coping styles, or if the coping style proves persistently unsuccessful, usually that's a job for an experienced professional counselor or therapist. When you are trying to gauge the level of the patient's coping effectiveness, you will necessarily do so in a subjective fashion. The four-stage anxiety and depression scale (see chapter 7, Anxiety and Depression) provides a rough index to quantitate your assessment: malaise, coping required, coping interfered with, and incapaciting.

Coping styles refer to characteristic ways of perceiving, thinking, and acting in dealing with the demands of living. In perceiving, individuals may practice selective inattention to stressful stimuli, or hypervigilance, or anything in between. In thinking, some individuals may ruminate and some may utilize varying degrees of denial, and each individual attaches varying levels of conscious importance and emotional impact to potentially stressful stimuli. In acting, some individuals habitually avoid dealing directly with stressful events, some habitually capitulate to them, and some actively strive for mastery over external stresses. Each style has its potential advantages and disadvantages, depending upon the nature of the stresses and the environment. Some styles work better when you have an argument with an automobile mechanic, and other styles are more likely to be adaptive for a prisoner in a penitentiary. No one style is adaptive across the whole range of human experience.

In broad outline, coping behavior serves to (1) keep the level of distress manageable, (2) maintain or restore a sense of self-worth, (3) enhance problem solving, and (4) maintain or restore social identity and relationships.

Given the broad outlines of style, there are dozens of specific techniques which an individual can use to implement one's own coping style. Most behavioral characteristics have some usefulness to the persons employing them: e.g., intellectualization, religiosity, a sense of humor, alcohol ingestion, somatization, sociability.

Coping styles are seldom either adaptive or maladaptive without further qualification. Most styles have adaptive and maladaptive aspects, the balance of which changes depending upon the setting. For example, most physicians use a lot of obsessive-compulsive techniques for organizing time and marshaling energies. The approach generally works quite well in a professional setting, but becomes a pain in the neck in a leisure setting: the motor won't switch to idle simply because you try to relax on the beach. It makes no sense to abandon all our

obessive-compulsive traits entirely—they're just too damned useful—
but it helps to be able to save them for when they are most useful, and
use other techniques, too, as appropriate.

Most of us need reminding about this from time to time with specific
patients. Their weaknesses when seen from another perspective may
be their strengths too. Be very wary about trying to therapize a trait
which for the patient, consciously or not, is a coping technique. We've
already talked in other sections about such behavior styles as denial,
alcoholism, and clinging dependency. Rather than tackling any of these
head-on in psychotherapy sessions, you will do far better to diminish
the anxiety which is likely to bring these behaviors to the fore, or to
help the patient mobilize other internal or external resources.

Remember, failure of coping occurs when stresses overwhelm resources. You can therefore help the patient cope by decreasing the
number or intensity of stresses, by altering the patient's perceptions so
that events previously perceived as stressful are no longer perceived in
that fashion, or by augmenting internal and/or external resources. In
the latter category, whatever you do to augment the patient's physical
health will be a useful adjunctive measure in promoting psychological
coping.

Tactics for Enhancing Coping

Given that you have decided that you are interested in trying your hand
at psychotherapy, and that the most common applicable goal is enhancing coping abilities, the next question is one of tactics. Whom do
you choose to do psychotherapy with, how much time do you devote
to the process, where do you do it, and how do you proceed?

Usually, for a nonpsychiatrist physician, choosing a patient with
whom to do psychotherapy is more a matter of exclusion than selection. You have contact with potentially needy patients every day, so
the key ingredients are time and interest. You have to have enough
time available so that you won't feel that your energies are being mis-
spent, and you have to be sufficiently interested in the patient so that
you won't resent the time you spend together. You can't empathize
with everyone, so I would suggest that you automatically exclude from
psychotherapy any patient that you don't like. Exclude, too, patients
who are actively psychotic and high-risk patients (e.g., imminently
suicidal) about whom, if worse comes to worst, you will feel guilty for
not having referred in the first place. Include anyone you would enjoy
helping, if the patient feels he or she would benefit by talking to you.

The amount of time you devote to psychotherapy, the frequency
with which you meet with patients, and the duration for which you see
them depends upon you, how much time you have available, and the

total number of patients you are seeing in psychotherapy. Many generalists who see patients for counseling about personal problems tend to see such individuals at the end of their working day, but for some, the idea of having to sit and listen to somebody's personal problems at the end of a long working day tends to get burdensome. Some see patients as a change of pace in the middle of the afternoon, or over the lunch hour. There are no hard and fast rules. In general, let the patient know what to expect with regard to how much time you feel you can devote to psychotherapy and at what frequency. It's fair to say to a hospitalized patient, "I'll stop by after rounds for the next several days to talk with you, and then we can decide together whether to continue. I'll try to be here about 5:30, but I may be later if things get hectic." Almost no patient will object to such a loosely scheduled therapy meeting, as long as you do keep your word and eventually show up.

Finding a private place in which to talk with patients is no problem when you have your own office and an ambulatory patient, but may be extremely difficult in a busy hospital setting. Often, the patient is confined to a multibed room, and you have to do the best you can by lowering your voices, closing the drapes, and occasionally asking understanding roommates to leave the room for a while. You can turn on a radio or TV to drown out your conversation for others, but you and your patient may also find that distracting. Examining rooms, nurses' lounges, chaplains' offices, even linen rooms, may sometimes provide a substitute for you with the ambulatory hospital patient, but all of these may be subject to heavy traffic in a busy hospital. You simply have to do the best you can to provide the patient with a reasonably private setting for uninterrupted conversation.

The principal benefits you will wish to provide for your patient during the course of psychotherapy are (1) a helping relationship with you, and, (2) if possible, a conceptual framework for making sense out of suffering. Patients want to be treated by a person, not a machine. They want to relate to someone who is interested, seems to feel positively towards them, and is respectful of patients as worthwhile human beings. At the time of physical illness, the patient's relationship with you may be the most important and powerful relationship. Illness often provides a time apart, a private time, a lonely time. That time can be available for a variety of intrapsychic endeavors: introspection, meditation, reading, writing, creativity. The nature of the illness experience and your key role as the patient's physician gives you extraordinary leverage in being psychotherapeutic. If both you and the patient are lucky, you can help the patient find one way of understanding life's sufferings. That will be enough. You do not have to provide the patient with promises to cure, with definitive answers to all of life's riddles, with advice or criticism or even praise.

PHASES OF THE PSYCHOTHERAPEUTIC PROCESS

Almost every kind of treatment you can think of involves an evolution
of the various components. Even the suturing of a simple laceration
usually follows a prescribed pattern: cleanse the area, inject anes-
thetic, glove, drape, debride, suture, apply dressing. The point is simply that in doing psychotherapy you must allow the process to unfold in
a natural manner. Don't go rushing in to give advice when your understanding of the problem remains superficial. Patience is a key virtue,
both for you, so that you don't go tripping over your own premature
pronouncements, but also as a trait to demonstrate to the patient. Time
will work to your advantage more often than not, and patience is a
device for helping time to do its work.

Making contact

The first step in developing a psychotherapeutic relationship is to
make contact with the patient. As the patient's physician, looking after
physical health, you already have such contact. One of the purposes of
your initial history and physical exam, in addition to getting information about the patient, is to provide the patient with a favorable predisposition toward *you*. You have already spent time sitting with the
patient, listening, demonstrating your thoroughness and general competence, showing some of your acceptance of the human being. That's
an enormous advantage which the average psychotherapist does not
have when setting out to do psychotherapy on someone just met. You
do not have to define the patient as a psychiatric patient in order to do
psychotherapy. You are simply caring for the patient as a whole.

Making a contract

In order to proceed, both you and the patient should have some idea
about what you're trying to do, and have reasonable agreement in the
matter. Arriving at a "contract" with the patient simply means that
you make it a point to establish such agreement. The contract may be
implicit, as when you and the patient start discussing some of the
patient's personal problems without making a conscious decision to do
so, and then you say: "Why don't we continue this discussion tomorrow?" Sometimes, one or both parties will feel better if the contract is
explicit: "I believe it might be helpful for you to discuss some of those
personal problems with me, and, if you are agreeable, why don't we
meet several times to talk about it?"

Problem definition

The next phase is to arrive at some preliminary statement of what
the patient's problem is, so that the two of you will know what it is
you're trying to work on. I say "preliminary statement" because usu-

ally the problem definition evolves as you discuss it further. It is not necessary that your statement of the problem and the patient's statement of the problem be identical; they merely have to be compatible. For instance, the patient may describe the problem as "my wife hates me," whereas your statement may be: "You and your wife are in a marriage which has some hate in it." In general, where there is more than one person involved, try to define the problem in terms of the relationship, rather than in terms of one individual. Avoid blameful or negativistic statements wherever possible. Don't feel obliged to make a problem statement which differs from the patient's, unless you are certain that your understanding is great enough to do so.

Discussion of problem(s)

Discussion of any psychological problems should proceed in a manner similar to discussion of any physical problems. Ideally, you will let the patient speak freely, without interrupting for questions. You only use questions to get information which you need to know but which doesn't come spontaneously. Usually, one question is enough to start the patient on a line of discussion which will cover other, unasked questions as well. The information you need to know is as follows: How does the patient know there is a problem? What is the effect of the problem on the patient? On others? On such areas of vital functioning as family, friends, job, and finances? What makes it worse, and what makes it better? What self-treatment has been tried?

What you want is a clear understanding of the problem as it exists in vivo for the patient. Once you have that, you can begin to ask about the past, in the same manner you would in taking any history of a present illness. When did the problem begin? How did it evolve? Has the patient ever had a similar problem before, and, if so, how did he or she cope with it? What treatment was received and where? Was it helpful or not? Ask if anyone else in the family has had the same or similar problems. When you know about the present and the past, ask about the future in the same way. What are the patient's expectations? How is this expected to affect life over the future? Will it get better or worse or stay the same if nothing is done?

Formulation

Formulation provides a useful way of organizing your approach to the patient's problem. It's a personal statement; you must recognize that another therapist might conceptualize the problem in an entirely different way, using a different theoretic or cultural perspective. Provide one reasonable framework for discussion and thinking, and that usually will be enough.

The statement should be brief, no more than a sentence or two, and should include some of the patient's own wording: for example, "Your depression seems to me to result from guilt—what you call your 'unpaid debt' to your parents—and the fact that you believe your illness will prevent you from achieving your goals and discharging what you call your obligations." Avoid elaborate formulations and dogmatic statements.

An additional value of a stated formulation is that it allows the patient to see what you are thinking and give *you* feedback at the same time you are providing feedback to the patient. If the patient's response is "that doesn't make any sense to me," you must either rethink your formulation or try expressing your thoughts differently. Don't automatically chalk the patient's response up to denial or resistance. Effective communication requires that both the broadcaster and receiver be using the same wavelength. If in doubt, remain quiet and spend some time listening again, or comment on the process: "It's frustrating, isn't it, when we're both trying so hard and have difficulty finding a mutually meaningful way of understanding what is happening?" Remember that your formulation needn't be static; it will usually evolve over time along with your understanding of the patient.

Discussion of alternatives

Once you have a clear formulation of the patient's problem, solid enough to serve as a basis for discussion, you can begin to think about alternate means of palliating or resolving the problem. Do not assume that you must make choices for the patient. Only the patient can take responsibility for life-molding decisions. Alternatives can cover the entire range of coping behaviors. In general, physicians tend to err in the direction of nudging the patient toward active problem-solving behavior. Many individuals needn't *do* anything in this active sense: they will feel better simply after talking a bit or crying or even sulking. In this sense, you can usefully foster enhanced coping by commenting, "One of the ways of dealing effectively with problems is simply what you are doing now with me." Help the patient consider alternatives as each of you become aware of them, but avoid foisting your own preferences on the patient.

Ending therapy and providing follow-up

When you and your patient enter into an agreement to do psychotherapy, you make an estimate, at least in rough terms, of how long you expect to be engaged in the process. As you near the end of therapy (when your estimated time is from 70 to 80% completed), it's useful to assess what has gone on in the time that you have spent together and what will happen with the patient when therapy with you is completed. Have you accomplished what you intended? What has been beneficial, and what has not been beneficial? Asking these questions is to your advantage in improving your own skills. Does the patient need continued therapy? Do you have the time and energy available to continue as therapist? Should you renew your original therapeutic contract with the patient or develop a new one? What other alternatives are available? In any event, you will want some follow-up. If you will be seeing the patient for care of general medical problems, you can keep track of the patient's personal problems at the same time. If there is no medical reason to continue your relationship, say, "Give me a call in a month or so and let me know how things are going: I'm interested, I care, and I'll be curious to see how things turn out."

THE BASIC VERBAL PROCEDURES

We are proceeding on the assumption that your goal is to enhance patients' coping abilities. Your task is to help patients find the skills and strength *within themselves* to do the job. You assume that you don't have to put anything into the patient; instead, you help the patient to mobilize resources which are already there. Everything you do will therefore be directed toward helping the patient find skills and strengths heretofore unperceived, for some reason not mobilized.

The three basic verbal procedures you have are making an observation, asking a question, and offering an interpretation. The usefulness of each depends upon focusing the patient's attention on subject matter which you deem important to the task at hand: early in treatment that will be clarifying the problem; later it will involve identifying alternatives and making choices.

You should recognize that these three verbal procedures—observation, question, interpretation—get progressively more intrusive as you proceed from the first to the third. Generally, you do best to start with the least intrusive, observation, and proceed to question and interpretation only as you decide that they are clearly more likely to be helpful than harmful. If you jump directly to interpretations, you will often simply be ventilating your own prejudices and premature conclusions, and they will seldom be as helpful as you intend them to be.

Making an observation

What you choose to make an observation about is a matter of judgment, but the observation itself should be free of your opinions. At the simplest level it may simply be a restatement of what the patient has just said: "You say you are upset with your family." Or it could be a description of behavior: "The nurse says you haven't had any visits from your family," or "You look like you have been crying," or "You started to cry when you mentioned your father." Often an observation is sufficient to focus a patient's attention, to promote further thought and discussion. If not, it's reasonable to make an observation on the process: "You haven't picked up on any of my comments," or "You don't seem very talkative today." Don't prod the patient with your observations, however; sit patiently and quietly and give the patient time to mull over whatever is going through his or her mind. There may be something the patient wants to say, but he or she may not be sure whether you can be trusted to listen quietly and nonjudgmentally. If in doubt, be quiet and sit patiently.

Asking a question

You, of course, have been asking questions all your life and may be reluctant to see a question as a big-deal psychotherapeutic technique. Fair enough, but questions involve some subtleties which you can usefully keep in mind. Questions tend to be more intrusive than observations because they imply that you expect an answer, and the person being questioned is expected to know the answer. They also tend to imply a bit more of a value judgment than does observation. For instance, "you are crying" may simply be a statement of fact, whereas "Why are you crying?" implies that the act requires some sort of explanation. Also, a question suggests ignorance on the part of the questioner in a way which may be disproportionate to reality. For example, if you told a young nulliparous woman yesterday that she has a uterine mass and the treatment of choice is hysterectomy, you can reasonably assume that her tears today are related to the information she received so recently and how that will affect her childbearing potential, her sense of femininity, and her fantasies for the future. Asking "Why are you crying?" doesn't adequately reflect your understanding. You would do far better to restate the question: "I know this is a rough time for you; I'd really like to know what's going on in your head. Can you tell me what the tears are about?"

Offering an interpretation

An interpretation is an explanation of a circumstance in a way which suggests causal relationships or motives that are not readily apparent or which relate specific events to general principles. Everyone loves to make interpretations; it's a wonderful way to demonstrate erudition. However, any interpretation is subject to considerable cultural and personal bias. Dramatically different interpretations of any given sequence of human behavior could be expected from a fundamentalist minister, a Marxist neurobiologist, a Freudian analyst, and a Hindu mystic. That doesn't mean that any one of the interpretations would necessarily be more or less valuable per se than any of the others. It depends on the manner in which it is given, and whether the patient is receptive to a given cultural perspective.

An interpretation may be helpful to a patient so long as the process is not coercive, either implicitly or explicitly. Do not imply that your interpretations are the only correct way of viewing things. You will do best to present an interpretation as a thought or possibility or as the way that *you* conceptualize things, rather than as a representation of natural law. For the purposes of enhancing coping, your interpretations will be most useful if they help the patient find self-esteem in circumstances where little or none was found before, and assist the patient in seeing unwelcome events as part of a natural and dynamic evolution. For example, "I know you don't like crying in front of strangers, but in my opinion if the tears are in there, it's best to get them out." Or, "The guilt feels lousy, but in my experience it's an extremely common part of the grieving process that many people seem to have to go through." However, be careful to avoid Pollyanna-ish platitudes such as "It's good to cry." Many individuals will rebel at such simplifications, and your therapeutic effectiveness will be undermined.

After an interpretation, inquire, "Does that make sense to you?" If not, where does the problem seem to lie? Perhaps your interpretation was premature. Perhaps you have been looking at things too narrowly from your own perspective, and not listening carefully enough to the patient. If it fits your style, feel free to say "I guess I missed the target with that one; maybe I'd better shut up and listen for a while." As long as you don't overdo it, you'll seldom get in trouble by expressing a little humility. You may even catch the patient off guard; humility isn't a trait the general public attributes to physicians as a rule.

Alternatives to Psychotherapy

The number and kinds of alternatives you can offer instead of psychotherapy depend on what you perceive the function of psychotherapy to be in the first place. If you believe it is to enhance individual coping, then anything you do to reduce stress or to augment the patient's internal or external resources will be of value. If you believe that counseling is a human skill rather than a superspecialist's procedure, then the number of potential counselors extends far beyond available physicians or even other health professionals. If in doubt, feel free to request a consultation from a psychotherapist or pastoral counselor.

Consider the methods listed in the Appendix; use them if they seem comfortable to you and your patient.

Don't forget that patients can be of help to one another even without professional supervision. Numerous self-help and cooperative-assistance organizations are available to help your patients, but your patients may never learn about them unless you or someone else takes responsibility for telling them.

Patients may or may not help one another on an informal basis. If you make it a habit to nudge patients toward self-help groups, that will take a lot of responsibility off your shoulders for support and patient instruction. Remember, however, that the quality of any specific group in your area depends on the people involved, how much knowledge and energy they have, and whether they will take the initiative in contacting your patient. Typical groups include Alcoholics Anonymous, TOPS (Take Off Pounds Sensibly—for people who are overweight), Ostomy Societies (for patients with ileostomies, colostomies, and ureterostomies), Reach for Recovery (operated by the American Cancer Society for women with mastectomies), and the Multiple Sclerosis Society.

The value of medically supervised group support for patients with disabling or disfiguring or chronic illnesses has been a part of medical folklore for decades. Joseph Pratt, a Boston internist, began organizing group meetings for tuberculosis patients in the early 1900's, using the meetings both for teaching patients about their disease, and to allow them to express feelings about their shared experiences.

Since that time, the popularity of group meetings for persons with physical ailments has run an erratic course. However, if they suit your taste they can be useful to both you and your patients, and fun as well. You can set aside a certain amount of time each week or each month, say an hour at the end of the working day, for a gathering of patients who share a common problem such as hypertension, asthma, amputation, or myocardial infarction. You will do best to keep the atmosphere primarily social, but make it a point to weave in rehabilitation issues and whatever educational material you think is relevant. Try to avoid giving a formal lecture, unless it is a brief one. The emphasis should be on shared experiences, with one patient teaching another. That gives the patients an opportunity to feel helpful, as well as helpable. Encourage people to talk about problems and unpleasant experiences, but don't be surprised if they would rather talk about their successes. Remember to keep the enhancing of coping ability as your priority, both individual coping and various members of the group helping one another.

Bibliography

Adler G: Special problems for the therapist. *Intl J Psychiatry in Med* 14:91–98, 1984

Andrews G, et al.: General practitioner as psychotherapist. *Med J Aust* 2(12):655–659, 1980

Anstett R, et al.: Selecting patients for brief office counseling. *J Fam Pract* 13:195–199, 1981

Browne GB, et al.: Psychotherapeutic intervention and health service utilization. *J Fam Pract* 14:593–600, 1982

Chard PS: Psychosocial problem assessment—to counsel or not to counsel. *Family Medicine* 17:21–23, 1985

Cristol AH: Studies of outcome of psychotherapy. *Compr Psychiatry* 13:189–200, 1972

Eysenck HJ: The effects of psychotherapy—an evaluation. *J Consult Psychol* 16:319–324, 1952

Ficken RP, et al.: Management of mental disorders by family practice residents. *Family Medicine* 16:170–174, 1984

Forester B, Kornfeld DS, Fleiss JL: Psychotherapy during radiotherapy. *Am J Psychiatry* 142:22–27, 1985

Frank JD: *Persuasion and Healing.* Baltimore, Johns Hopkins Press, 1961

Frankl VE: *Man's Search For Meaning.* Boston, Beacon Press, 1959

Ginsberg G, Marks I, Waters H: Cost-benefit analysis of a controlled trial of nurse therapy for neuroses in primary care. *Psychological Med* 14:683–690, 1984

Kutz I, Borysenko JZ, Benson H: Meditation and psychotherapy. *Am J Psychiatry* 142:1–8, 1985

Lipp MR, Malone ST: Group rehabilitation of vascular surgery patients. *Arch Phys Med Rehabil* 57:180–183, 1976

Luborsky L, Singer B, Luborsky L: Comparative studies of psychotherapy—is it true that "everyone has won and all must have prizes?" *Arch Gen Psychiatry* 32:995–1008, 1975

Malan DH: The outcome problem in psychotherapy research. *Arch Gen Psychiatry* 29:719–729, 1973

Orleans CT, et al.: How primary care physicians treat psychiatric disorders. *Am J Psychiatry* 142:52–57, 1985

Rodin G: Expressive psychotherapy in the medically ill. *Intl J Psychiatry in Med* 14:98–105, 1984

Sanderson P: Pastoral counseling and dimensions of healing. *RI Med J* 64:33–35, 1981

Schwartz AN: Counseling—listening with the third ear. *Geriatrics* 35:95–102, 1980

Skuse D, Williams P: Screening for psychiatric disorder in general practice. *Psychological Med* 14:365–377, 1984

Walker JI: Office psychotherapy—supportive techniques and indications for referral. *Postgrad Med* 70(4):34–43, 1981

9

Pain and Addiction

Physical discomfort is only important when the mood is wrong.
—Robert Persig

Those who do not feel pain seldom think it is felt.
—Samuel Johnson

We must all die. But that I can save him from days of torture, that is what I feel is my great and ever new privilege. Pain is a more terrible lot of mankind than even death itself.
—Albert Schweitzer

The most common and compelling symptom in all of clinical medicine is pain. Therefore the ability to interpret and treat pain is crucial to one's functioning as a clinician. These tasks can also be extremely complex and filled with emotional overtones for the patient, the physician, and other medical personnel.

In many ways, the treatment of pain is the fundamental transaction in medicine. We as physicians have a near-sacred responsibility to relieve suffering. As a consequence, analgesics, in addition to their specific chemical effect, can assume almost sacramental properties. Abuse of the sacrament amounts to sacrilege when the physician withholds analgesics unnecessarily, or the patient takes analgesics like candy for pleasure or trivial reasons.

Pain defies definition. The sensation itself is difficult to describe even for the most articulate, since the experience is a uniquely subjective phenomenon.

In order to understand what pain is like for a given patient, the physician must depend upon teachings of others, or what the patient communicates, or personal experience.

There is no test for clinical pain. Researchers have endeavored to measure pain and its concomitants, but the effort has produced little that is clinically useful. Most laboratory studies have singled out pain threshold ("I can feel it") and tolerance ("That's all I can take"), but their relevance to clinical pain remains dubious. Somehow, experimental and clinical pain remain mysteriously different.

Pain must be envisioned as both a psychological and a neurophysiologic event. Such variables as attention, distraction, anxiety, trust in care givers, motivation, and even a patient's ethnicity affect the perception of, and reaction to, pain. The pain experience is also highly situation-specific; soldiers and athletes with high-morale, can sometimes tolerate appalling injuries with apparently minimal distress.

Once pain has been expressed by the patient, either verbally or nonverbally, it also becomes a psychological issue for those caring for that patient. There is probably no more uncomfortable situation for the physician than hearing a patient cry out in agony. How the physician responds to pain behavior in patients depends upon the physician's emotional ability to relate generally to a patient in pain, the relationship with that particular patient, and the physician's personal feelings about stoicism versus immediate gratification.

Treatment decisions are based upon this chain of events: (1) perception of pain by the patient; (2) the patient's threshold for expressing pain; (3) the patient's manner of expressing pain; (4) the perception by the physician of the patient's problem; (5) acceptance by the physician that the complaint is genuine and appropriate; and (6) a treatment decision.

Acute Pain

While treating acute-onset pain is a routine experience for most physicians, the experience of acute-onset pain is almost always exceptional and unique for the patient.

Very few individuals enjoy pain, and almost all seek to escape severe pain in whatever way they can. While there is considerable variation from one individual to another, many patients can be expected to become cranky, childlike, and impatient in requesting relief. Pain, and the complaints which it precipitates, are often worse at night when the environment is quietest, when there are the fewest distractions. Thus, pain is most likely to become intolerable when the patient's personal physician is least available—and the patient therefore may seek attention from an on-call physician or an unfamiliar emergency medicine doctor. To many patients, the way a doctor responds to a pain complaint is the most important single criterion by which the patient can judge the physician's ability and caring.

Each of us must learn how to use ourselves effectively with a patient in pain, both in terms of using analgesic medications and in terms of using ourselves and our own personalities to help minimize the need for analgesic medications.

Aside from diagnosing and treating the source of pain, the single most important decision a physician must make in treating pain is to define the goal of symptomatic treatment, and it is crucial that both doctor and patient are in substantial accord. The only way to achieve this is to describe your goal to the patient and make sure that you have the patient's agreement. When this does not occur, the chances for friction between doctor and patient and others become increasingly great.

Generally there are two choices—(1) freedom from pain, and (2) tolerable discomfort. If the goal is a pain-free existence, narcotic analgesics are the quickest and surest way to achieve it. The customary treatment is increasing doses until either relief or toxicity is achieved. While many doctors believe that their patients should have minimal pain, for instance, in the postoperative period, most patients nonetheless remain in moderate-to-severe distress.

If the agreed upon goal is tolerable discomfort, we must have a clear idea of what we mean by tolerable, and to whom. Usually the physician can tolerate a good deal more pain in the patient than the patient can tolerate in himself or herself. However, this is not always the case, and some of us insist upon treating pain aggressively even when the patient finds the level of discomfort acceptable.

Pure chemical control of pain and pain complaints is a rather narrow way of approaching the problem. Since sensitivity to, and tolerance for, pain varies so much with mood and environment stimuli, there are many things a physician can do besides medicate to help the patient become more comfortable. The doctor must recognize that he or she is not only treating the patient, but also the patient's family and, in the hospital or emergency department, the staff. If the patient is in pain, or appears to be in pain, the doctor will hear many requests to "please do something." Managing these aspects of pain control remains a continuing obligation.

Because of this there is a tendency in all of us to either undertreat or overtreat. Indeed, it is difficult to say just what represents the optimum level of pain amelioration, especially if there are multiple factors involved. A frequent postoperative problem consists of balancing palliation of pain with concerns about respiratory tidal volume, ability and desire to cough, and so on.

Reasons for undertreatment of pain can range from lack of knowledge to a variety of psychological considerations. Few of us know with great precision exactly how the effective doses of many analgesic medications vary with pathophysiology, activity, and drug interactions.

Undertreatment may also be related to stoicism and denial, either on the part of the patient, the physician, or the person who is administering p.r.n. medications. Some physicians may be reluctant to admit that their treatment, or the withholding of it, may result in significant pain for the patient. Undertreatment can also be related to undue weighting of other factors, such as concern about respiratory or central nervous system depression, the addiction potential of the patient, or the physician's own fear about addiction generally.

There are some specific reasons for overtreating pain patients. Physicians who are reluctant to become involved, or even those who become heavily involved with a given patient, for example a terminal patient, may medicate that patient to a semistuporous state. Physicians with their own fears regarding personal suffering may do likewise. Sometimes overtreatment stems from an attempt to mollify persons around the patient who are uncomfortable in dealing with patient complaints. And often overtreatment with analgesics stems from the physician's lack of appreciation of how pain sensitivity is related to psychosocial factors.

We now have abundant evidence that patients who are carefully instructed and encouraged, and who trust their physicians and nurses, feel less pain and need less pain medications than other patients. On the other hand, it is important that you not take the patient's pain as evidence that you have not done your job properly. All the patient instruction and encouragement in the world will not totally eliminate pain for all patients. Simply ask, "Have I done what I can to make this patient comfortable, aside from medications?" Remember to ask, as well, if there are other people (nurses, physical therapists, family social workers) who can help too.

Chronic Pain

Chronic pain must be viewed as an entirely different phenomenon. Acute pain is a psychological and biological event; chronic pain must be viewed as a matter of life-style and identity.

Anyone who has had much contact with patients who have chronic pain know that many such patients are extraordinarily difficult to treat. The patient with chronic low back pain, refractory to treatment, is a familiar example. Such patients have usually had considerable experience with a variety of physicians, their trust of physicians is low, and they have already experienced many treatment failures. While such patients seem to be seeking relief from pain, physicians often get the impression that such patients are resistant to change and, at some level, are reluctant to give up their discomfort. Some view chronic pain as a sign that the patient is seeking the sick role.

Chronic pain patients customarily reject any psychological explanations, as do all somaticizing patients. What to tell patients, and how to relate to them, then becomes a continuing major concern for physicians and other health personnel.

The pain is frequently undiagnosible, in that its extent and persistence cannot usually be explained on the basis of apparent organic disease. By definition, the suffering is unrelievable for any extent of time, and as such poses an enormous challenge to the physician. As a consequence, the physician often feels compelled to use increasingly more invasive diagnostic measures, and increasingly more drastic therapeutic measures.

Chronic pain carries with it a high addiction liability which is usually of far more concern to the doctor and other medical personnel than it is to the patients. This factor in itself frequently becomes a source of concern to those around the patient.

EVALUATION

Evaluating the chronic pain patient is a difficult and complicated task. Nonetheless, there is much that a physician can do to help a patient who is "addicted" to a life of pain and pain medication.

The following suggestions are directed to the physician who sees such a patient within the context of general medical or general surgical responsibilities. You simply have to do the best you can. However, we should understand that if you have a formal pain clinic available to you as a referral disposition, they can sometimes do a more thorough and effective (and expensive) job than an individual physician working unaided.

Evaluation should consist of five sets of questions.

1. *Standard Information.* This is the kind of material that you elicit from all patients with almost any presenting complaint. Ask about onset, duration of symptom, time pattern, what makes it worse, and what makes it better. Ask how it is affected by activity, medication, eating, sleeping, and position.

2. *Pain Behaviors.* Ask, "When you are in pain, how would I know it?" How do the spouse and other family members know it? How do those individuals respond to the patient in pain? What do they say, how do they show their feelings, and what do they do?

3. *Functional Impairment.* How often does pain interfere with activity? How often must the patient rest because of the pain? What doesn't the patient do because of pain? What would the patient be doing if he or she did not have any pain? Would he or she be working full-time or part-time? Does the patient's response seem realistic? How

would the patient's social and psychological life be different? How would it change his or her sexual life, involvement with children, etc.?

4. *Current Coping.* Ask the patient how he or she has managed to cope, given all the pain apparently being endured? How does he or she manage to keep spirits up? Can he or she have fun and pleasure from ordinary activities? If sitting is so very uncomfortable, how does he or she manage to go to the bathroom? What personal resources are used to manage social occasions? How are financial problems managed? How much disability compensation is being paid? Is there litigation pending? What would happen to disability payments and pending litigation if the patient were to return to work?

5. *Expectations.* What does the patient want from you and from treatment, with regard to changing pain and medication dependence? What are the expectations and how realistic are they? How much does he or she think will have to be done alone, and how much does he or she think will be done by others?

Pain behaviors by the patient technically fall under the category of operants, a term derived from Pavlovian behavioral psychology. Operants are behaviors which elicit certain responses. Pain behaviors include any method the patient has for communicating the experience of pain: a grimace, words, screams, guarded or splinted movement, or social withdrawal. Operants can be controlled by their consequences. If an operant is systematically followed by a favorable response, it is likely that the operant will occur again in response to similar stimuli. If the operant is not systematically followed by a positive response, the behavior will tend to disappear. If the operant is followed by punishment (aversive consequences), you can expect a temporary decrease in activity, and avoidance behavior. In other words, the patient will shop for medical care elsewhere, whenever he or she has the opportunity.

CONCEPTUAL BASIS OF TREATMENT

Chronic pain disproportionate to the pathologic process can be viewed as a habit disorder, a maladaptive life-style to which the patient is seemingly inextricably bound. As with other habit disorders, you have *no chance* of changing the patient's behavior unless you and the patient work together as allies. Attempts to force the patient to do something against his or her wishes will result in frustration for both of you.

The first step, therefore, is to arrive at a treatment contract. Ask the patient, "Do you wish to live more comfortably with pain and decrease your dependence on medications at the same time?" Unless you get a firm and believable, positive response to this question, there is no sense to proceed further.

The second question is, "Are you willing to work hard to achieve that end?'' An alternative, if both you and the patient agree, is to maintain medication dependence, increasing doses as tolerance develops.

Prior to arriving at the contract with the patient, it is fair to emphasize that the patient has bona fide organic and psychological reasons for having pain, but that in addition the pain has come to play an enormous role in the patient's life, and altering life patterns is always difficult. Emphasize that while mutual trust and cooperation between yourself and the patient will make the task easier, getting over the pain habit will nonetheless require an enormous amount of hard work and courage on the patient's part.

The task in treating chronic pain is like getting Pavlov's dog to stop salivating. Pain must be viewed as a complex learned behavior, in which the patients are systematically rewarded for pain behaviors. The patient perceives discomfort, complains, elicits a response (administration of narcotics), and the discomfort is replaced by mild euphoria. Though pain behaviors may originally have been associated with specific pathologic, painful stimuli, chronic pain behaviors may bear little or no relationship to the original stimuli.

I personally doubt the usefulness of labeling chronic pain patients with any psychological diagnosis. My bias is that anyone can learn a pain habit or behavior if the conditions are right. Labeling the pain and the patient as being functional, psychiatric, or supratentorial only serves to stigmatize and alienate the patient.

The optimal conditions for developing a pain "habit" are shown in the familiar example of a laborer with a meniscus injury. Going to work (well behavior) leads to pain. Refraining from work (sick behavior) results in rest and relief. Work itself is only marginally rewarded, with little recognition, minimal chance for a career advancement, and marginal financial rewards. Disability may result in nontaxable financial rewards, the net value of which may differ little from ordinary salary. In such a situation, it is simplistic to talk about this patient's pain as being "psychogenic." It is a complex consequence of true organic injury, social values, and psychological and economic reinforcement.

Other rewards for pain behavior may include attention, assistance with mundane daily burdens, and certain avoidance behaviors, the exact nature of which may be obscure to the clinician who has only marginal contact with the patient and family. An example may be the person whose chronic back pain helps to minimize the frequency of sexual intercourse with his or her spouse, in a relationship in which there is considerable unexpressed anger.

BASIC TECHNIQUES OF CHRONIC PAIN MANAGEMENT

The focus of this section is to help make the unbearable bearable for the patient, with minimum reliance on medication. Most of the approaches mentioned here work best within the context of a formal pain clinic in which multidisciplinary input and structured organizational control are an integrated part of the treatment process. However, such formal programs are expensive and rarely available as a resource to the average patient or most physicians, and therefore one must do the best one can with what is available. It is crucial for each of the approaches mentioned that you be working *with* the patient, rather than *on* the patient. Patient motivation and a good working relationship between doctor and patient are the key ingredients to success.

Surgical techniques

In their attempts to cure chronic pain, competent surgeons in good faith have at various times attempted to sever virtually every nervous connection from the periphery to the sensory cortex. Both diseased and healthy tissue has been ablated. No matter what technique is used, recurrence of pain after surgery remains distressingly common. A customary pattern for such patients is a series of surgical procedures, gradually escalating in invasiveness and proximity to the sensory cortex.

Placebos

Since a collaborative working relationship between doctor and patient is so important in the treatment of chronic pain, placebos (with only one exception) should never be used. Placebos represent an attempt by the physician to trick patients into believing they are receiving chemically active medication when in fact they are not. If the fact of the attempted trickery becomes known to the patients, any hope for a collaborative working relationship is usually destroyed. Therefore, the single circumstance in which the use of placebos is justified is when you tell the patients in advance that placebos may be included in treatment. The patients should of course consent to this treatment approach before it is instituted. In practice, most patients will readily submit to a treatment regimen which includes intermittent use of placebos along with chemically active agents, as long as the advantages for doing so are carefully explained to them in advance. It is clearly to the patient's benefit to be treated with the least toxic medication possible and placebos provide this advantage.

Acupuncture

Nobody knows why acupuncture works, but there can be no doubt that it does work when used by skilled practitioners with carefully selected patients. The traditional Chinese explanation for acupuncture's effectiveness depends upon correcting an imbalance of bodily humours via implantations on a series of body meridians. Others believe that acupuncture is nothing more than a hypnotic technique. Still others emphasize "counterirritation" phenomena, relegating acupuncture to the level of a highly sophisticated mustard plaster. Whatever the explanation, the effective use of this technique requires instruction beyond the scope of this book.

Hypnosis

Hypnotism as a general technique is discussed more fully in the appendix. Its use in pain reduction is well accepted, and the evidence is now overwhelming that hypnotism can be useful for pain related to parturition, dental extractions, some surgical procedures, and even painful burns and terminal cancer.

Behavior techniques

Pain clinics that have been most successful at treating chronic pain patients utilize a variety of methods derived from operant conditioning theory. The following approach is ideally implemented on a hospital ward devoted to treating chronic pain patients, but I have used it successfully on general medical-surgical wards as well. Making it work with outpatients requires a highly motivated patient, a cooperative and involved family, and an amenable pharmacist.

1. Gradual decrease and elimination of pain medications. First, establish a baseline by allowing a patient to take p.r.n. medications for several days. Make certain that the patient does not have a supply of medications stored up for surreptitious use. Rather than searching the patient, or having the nurse do so, explain to the patient the importance of total honesty between you. Say that many patients bring pain medications into the hospital with them, that you expect such behavior as a matter of course, but that the treatment requires that all pain medications be carefully measured and recorded. If the patient lies to you, he or she is the loser, not you. This is easy to say, but if you are very involved with the patient, your heart will be on the line, too.

After establishing a baseline, figure the total amount of analgesics consumed during an average day, then divide the total into a set number of standard doses. Give the standard dose at fixed time intervals, which is slightly shorter than the p.r.n. time interval. For example, if the patient has been taking DEMEROL every four hours, plan on giving the medication every three hours. This makes the giving of the medication contingent upon time, not upon pain behaviors by the patient. Whenever possible, mask the dosage given by diluting oral medication in some strong-tasting beverage, such as fruit punch. Advise the patient that you will be gradually decreasing the dosage on an irregular basis over an agreed-upon time interval. Usually, if the patient is on high doses of narcotic analgesics to start with, a minimum of ten days to two weeks is required to get significant decrease in medications.

Reduce the total dosage of medication by approximately 10% a day, but do not decrease all doses uniformly. For example, on a given day, you may reduce every other dose, while keeping the alternating doses the same as the previous day. Your task will be considerably easier if you can get a pharmacist to rise to the challenge and prepare the appropriate unit dosage containers in advance.

2. Working to quota. Most pain patients work to tolerance: that is, they pursue a given activity until pain interferes, and then they stop. In order to work to quota, one must first establish baselines for daily activities. During the first several days on the program, have the patient keep track of how much activity he or she performs. Depending upon how active the patient is, activity may be defined as time sitting up or time out of bed or time walking. When you have obtained an average daily activity time, divide the number by 2 and require the patient to be up and active for specific periods of time on both the day and the evening shift. Then increase this activity time by 10% each day while the patient is in the hospital. The patient is not allowed to discontinue activity because of pain. Emphasize that the quota has been derived from the patient's own daily activities and is therefore fair. Keep the patient working to quota.

3. Identification and reduction of positive reinforcers. Try and figure out as best you can how the patient has been systematically rewarded for pain. Does his wife say, "You poor dear!"? If so, point out to the patient and spouse that this activity may in fact reinforce pain and you will therefore request her to remain silent while the patient is up and about. If she is unable to remain silent, request that for her good and for the patient's good that she not be present during the patient's activity periods. Identifying such reinforcers can be simple and rewarding for both you and the patient. However, elimination of all positive reinforcement may be impossible. This is especially true if the reinforcement is financial, and the patient's continued disability payments are dependent upon continued pain behavior.

Addiction and Addicts

Reality is just a crutch for people who can't deal with drugs.
—Lily Tomlin

Cocaine is God's way of saying you're making too much money.
—Robin Williams

While illicit drug use is a frequent focus of comedians, addicts themselves are seldom regarded as amusing by medical staff. Often they are viewed with negative emotions ranging from fear to frank hostility and even loathing. Our attitudes toward addicts are seldom well concealed, and addicts in turn tend to stay away from health care facilities unless they have acute medical problems—or unless they cannot conveniently get drugs in any other way. It's worthwhile to keep in mind that much addiction begins with the assistance of physicians' lax prescribing habits with people in pain, which is one reason addiction is being discussed in the chapter on pain.

The irony is that physicians who approach addicts with friendliness and trust tend to have much more satisfactory relations with them, than do those who are suspicious and standoffish. However, if you expect that trust to be always well placed, you will be disappointed— addicts sometimes seem destined to abuse trust in the same way they abuse drugs. Thus, the temptation to be a rescuer to an especially appealing person with a "drug addiction problem" is primarily a phenomenon of the young health professional whose supply of compassion still flows unhindered by a history of having been and having felt ripped-off.

A further irony is that while addiction constitutes a medical diagnosis, physicians in general are not allowed to treat addiction per se, unless that treatment is provided under the aegis of a certified treatment program. Instead, we treat associated medical conditions and their concomitant pain.

Indeed, it is usually in terms of pain and requests for its treatment that an addict comes to our attention. The familiar triad is: (1) severe distress associated with (2) conditions with few objective physical findings (e.g., migraine, sickle-cell disease, low back pain) in (3) a patient who has very specific ideas about medications ("The only thing that ever works for me is DEMEROL").

Successful outpatient treatment of such patients, once they are recognized, relies on a consistent institutional response and good communication among care givers. One doctor in a clinic or group practice must take responsibility for determining the nature and extent of the patient's organic illness, deciding what appropriate treatment should be, and then communicating the specifics about reasonable drugs and dosages to the other doctors who will see the patient while on call or in the emergency department. In the absence of such a policy, each successive doctor who sees the patient will prescribe (or not) according to personal prejudices, and the addict will soon learn which prescribers are least demanding of stoicism in their patients.

Another challenge in caring for the addict is finding some way to look after the patient's health without sacrificing the doctor's integrity. Do you, for instance, give instruction in sterile technique to an addict who comes in repeatedly with cellulitis at injection sites? How do you respond to obviously illegal behavior when it goes on right under your

Table 9.1 Management of Drug Addicts Admitted to General Hospitals for Medical–Surgical Conditions

Common Features	Treatment Alternatives
1. Impending withdrawal	1. Support the habit *vs.* Ignore the problem *vs.* Withdrawal regimen
2. "Antisocial" behavior on the ward	2. Limit-setting *vs.* Permissiveness
3. Illicit drug use on the ward	3. Urine drug screen, search visitors, etc., *vs.* Benign neglect
4. Poor reliability and compliance	4. Limit-setting *vs.* Acceptance
5. "Disproportionate" pain complaints	5. Hard-line approach *vs.* Meeting all requests
6. Threat to leave "against medical advice"	6. Court order to stay *vs.* Good riddance
7. Staff dissension and turmoil, feelings of being manipulated	7. Patient care as priority *vs.* Staff care
8. Patient's clinical condition obscured by psychosocial problems	8. Problem-limited treatment *vs.* Attempts at comprehensive care

nose? The questions have particular salience when you are caring for a hospitalized addict.

Narcotic addicts get seriously ill just like anyone else, and when they enter the hospital a sequence of fairly predictable problems develops concerning their treatment and behavior. Addicts can have any disease which any nonaddict might have, but they also have an especially high incidence of hepatitis, AIDS, bacterial infections (endocarditis, thrombophlebitis, cellulitis at injection sites), and pulmonary emboli.

Characteristically, the addict views hospital staff with suspicion and fear, expecting them to be unsympathetic and punitive, fearing that they will report the addiction to police, and that the patient's dependence upon drugs will be manipulated by the hospital staff in order to force acquiescence in areas where the addict would otherwise not yield control.

In return, the staff usually regards the typical addict as hostile, belligerent, untrustworthy, and uncommunicative in any meaningful way. The staff expects that when addicts are around, both hospital property and belongings of other patients are likely to disappear mysteriously. Staff view all of the addict's visitors with suspicion, assuming that they are the source of illicit drugs on the ward.

Table 9.1 lists a number of common features of the addict hospitalized for medical disorders, together with the treatment alternatives that each feature presents. The table is designed to stimulate your thinking about the kinds of choices you will have to make in treating the addict. There are no right and wrong answers, but I have my own preferences that I regard as a reasonable compromise approach to these complicated problems.

As with outpatients, when you are taking care of a hospitalized addict, I suggest that you have only one person write all medication orders and take primary responsibility for coordinating the patient's care. This includes anticipating potential nighttime problems, and writing clear notes in the chart to guide physicians on call who may have to care for the patient's sudden and perhaps dramatic demands. The same individual should take full responsibility for discussing all gripes with the patient, explaining the rationale behind all treatments, and providing support for nursing staff who are barraged with the patient's demands and complaints.

Avoid an authoritarian stance in which you put yourself in the position of telling the patient what you will and will not allow him to do. Instead, in your conversations with the patient, put the limits on yourself. For example, instead of saying, "No, you can't do this, and I won't let you do that," say, "I'm sorry, but I cannot in good conscience prescribe that much medication, or do what you ask." Express sympathy that your limitations make things difficult for the patient, but say, "These are the realities and my limitations, and let's see how we can work best within them."

On short hospital stays, I suggest you ignore any illicit drug use in the addict. Unauthorized intravenous drug use upsets most of us but should be expected, since in many cases we have provided the patient with an intravenous line. Confrontations over such issues during short hospitalizations usually result in far more turmoil than they are worth. However, you will have to provide support for the staff and other patients who may be upset by this. Help to mollify them by pointing out that the patient will soon be leaving the hospital and life will be more comfortable for all concerned, including the addict. With longer hospital stays, your hospital staff and the other patients may well not be able to tolerate continued illicit drug use. In that case, explain "our limitations" to the patient, describe what compromises are and are not possible, and determine what policing procedures are necessary. Explain to the patient that breaking laws are police matters, and continued lawbreaking in the hospital will result in the police being called in. *Do not* require that either you or the nursing staff be police surrogates; chances are you will do the job poorly, you will feel uncomfortable in the role, and your other hospitalized patients will be frightened by your aggressive and punitive approach to the addict.

Anticipate that any addict may decide to leave the hospital precipitously, "against medical advice." Early in the patient's hospitalization, perhaps even during your initial history and physical, tell your patients something like this: "I know that you are hurting. I will try to help you as much as I can, but I have my limitations and there may be some aspects of your treatment with which you will be uncomfortable. I am sorry, but those are the realities. For your part, you must guard against running out when the going gets rough. You will sometimes feel like leaving the hospital on impulse, but I hope you will fight that impulse when it occurs. We want to give you the best treatment we can, and we don't want you to leave the hospital prematurely."

The decision to arrange withdrawal or maintenance of a drug should be made dependent upon the wishes of the patient, his or her probable length of stay, and hospital policy. Food and Drug Administration regulations allow you to maintain a patient on methadone when he or she is a bona fide heroin addict hospitalized for the treatement of a medical condition. As long as the patient is hospitalized for the treatment of the medical condition per se rather than for treatment of the addiction, the administration of methadone need not take place within a Food and Drug Administration-approved methadone program. Two different kinds of addicts are candidates for methadone maintenance during a medical-surgical hospitalization.

First, are the addicts who are already enrolled in a methadone-maintenance program and who should be continued on methadone while hospitalized. However, you must be aware that addicts have a tendency to exaggerate their methadone needs, and you must contact the methadone maintenance program physician to confirm the fact of the patient's enrollment and identify the proper dose of methadone. After confirming the dose, do not change it and do not attempt to detoxify the patient. Give the dose orally on a once-a-day basis. If the patient is NPO, you should give the methadone parenterally, but lower the dosage by one-half. For example, if the patient was receiving 100 mg of methadone by mouth daily, give him only 50 mg parenterally, but in a divided dose twice a day; that is, 25 mg twice a day or every 12 hrs intramuscularly.

Try to maintain contact with the patient's methadone-maintenance program, both to facilitate discharge planning, and as a resource for yourself in the management of the patient's hospital behavior. Experienced drug counselors can provide a good deal of support to the patient, and at the same time assist you in communicating with the patient and helping to minimize impulsive or antisocial behavior.

The second kind of addict, the "street addict," presents a somewhat different problem. If street addicts are genuinely addicted, you should continue to support their addiction until the acute phase of the illness is over. Attempting to withdraw them from drugs during an acute medical or surgical crisis will only make the management of their medical condition more difficult and is unlikely to achieve any long-term change in their addiction.

However, it is crucial that the giving of methadone to street addicts be made contingent upon the appearance of physical signs of abstinence or withdrawal syndrome, either spontaneously or subsequent to administering narcotic antagonists. There are many addicts who use narcotics intermittently ("chipping and dipping") and cannot be said to have bona fide dependence on opiates.

Never base the administration of methadone solely on subjective complaints. Some individuals believe that the only valid sign of opiate withdrawal that cannot be feigned is gooseflesh. Other signs, in order of increasing severity of withdrawal reaction, include lacrimation, rhinorrhea, diaphoresis, dilated pupils, tachycardia, fever, diarrhea, vomiting, and clinical dehydration.

Do not expect that withdrawl symptoms will disappear promptly after the administration of methadone. Significant effects are only seen from three to four hours after oral administration and from 30 to 60 minutes after parenteral administration. Some physicians use short-acting narcotics for initial treatment of withdrawal until methadone takes effect. Others prefer sticking to the administration of methadone alone, and they encourage the addict to be patient while awaiting the effect of the methadone.

Most street addicts can be maintained on a total daily dosage of approximately 40 mg of methadone in divided doses, so long as they do not know the dosage being given. If the addict does know, you can expect that he or she will ask for a higher dose. If the addict insists upon knowing the dosage, respond: "I know it's frustrating for you to not know the dosage. I can understand your being upset. Nonetheless, my experience has been that if you will trust me, I can be of most help to you with you not knowing the dosage. If you have objective signs of withdrawal, I will increase the dosage as necessary."

If you have clear evidence that the patient is an addict, currently on drugs (as evidenced in urine tests), undergoing withdrawal (as evidenced by the physical signs previously mentioned), and wishes to be withdrawn from opiates with the assistance of a methadone-withdrawal program, then I suggest the following regimen: give methadone 10 mg PO every six hours for four doses; then decrease the dosage 10 mg per day. Many addict patients will criticize such a schedule, but it is widely used and fair. *Do not* reorder the methadone if the patient spills it, vomits, and so forth, and make it clear to the patient in advance that this is your plan. You may also give an antiemetic before the methadone dosage to help prevent emesis, if that is a problem.

With the addict undergoing withdrawal, with multiple physical complaints and often dramatic behavior, you must always be alert to the danger of overlooking medical conditions unrelated to the withdrawal itself. Since the addict customarily has limited pain or frustration tolerance, he or she can be expected to mask discomfort from organic pathology with increasingly higher doses of drugs. Such conditions may therefore go unnoticed until the onset of the withdrawal.

Patients on withdrawal regimens should receive nighttime sedation and tranquilizer supplements in the same manner that you would provide to any other patient. Addicts customarily require higher dosages of both kinds of medications than the average patient. Frequently, addicts have sleeping patterns that differ markedly from those of most patients. Do not use narcotics or barbiturates for nighttime sedation.

Patients who are being maintained on methadone may nonetheless require analgesia for other medical problems. Management of such patients is subject to all the problems discussed earlier in this chapter concerning chronic pain. Nonetheless, if you see the patient having pain, you will probably wish to use analgesia. Remember not to neglect the other psychological and social techniques of raising the pain threshold and tolerance to pain. You may use opiates for the treatment of pain in addicts, as you would for any other patient. However, because of the addict's tolerance to narcotics, he or she will demand higher doses more frequently than the average patient. There is some evidence that pentazocine (TALWIN) acts as a narcotic antagonist and therefore may precipitate a withdrawal reaction in a patient dependent on opiate.

Methadone itself should not be used for pain associated with surgical procedures or intercurrent medical problems, because of the time required to build an effective blood level and because of its long-acting nature.

A patient with barbiturate addiction requires careful attention, since withdrawal syndromes can occasionally result in fatality. The progression of symptoms includes anxiety, muscle twitches (sometimes becoming massive and uncontrollable), nausea, vomiting, delirium, seizures, perhaps progressing to status epilepticus. Any patient who takes more than a gram or two per day of barbiturates should be considered a potential candidate for seizures, but it is often difficult to know how much credence to place in the patient's history recital.

Therefore, for any patient whom you suspect of being a barbiturate addict, I suggest the following assessment procedure: Give 200 mg of secobarbital or pentobarbital intramuscularly. If the patient is put to sleep by this dose, you may conclude that his or her previous intake has been negligible and no withdrawal program is necessary. If no toxic symptoms appear in 30 minutes (somnolence, slurred speech, ataxia), give another 100 mg orally. Repeat the oral dosage every hour until toxic symptoms occur. For maintenance purposes, you can consider that the amount necessary to produce toxicity equals the patient's daily needs. Withdrawal or maintenance is then dependent upon substituting a long-acting barbiturate (such as phenobarbital) for the short-acting preparation in a manner similar to methadone being substituted for heroin. The dosage equivalency is 30 mg of the long-acting preparation (phenobarbital) to 100 mg of the short-acting preparation. For instance, if the patient required 900 mg of secobarbital to reach toxicity, his or her daily requirement is 270 mg of phenobarbital. This total daily dosage can be given in divided doses, usually every six hours. Maintain the patient at full dosage for several days to stabilize, then gradually reduce the phenobarbital by 30 mg per day. If the patient at any time sleeps through a scheduled dose of barbiturate, that dosage can be omitted on the assumption that it is not necessary to prevent withdrawal symptoms. Barbiturate addicts rarely need additional medication for sedation or tranquilization.

Bibliography

Bickford J: Outlaws, bandits and renegades—treatment of alcoholics and drug addicts. *Hosp Community Psychiatry* 34:362–363, 1983

Biener L: Perceptions of patients by emergency room staff—substance abusers versus non-substance abusers. *J Health Soc Behavior* 24:264–275, 1983

Drossman DA: Patients with psychogenic abdominal pain. *Am J Psychiatry* 139:1549–1557, 1982

Fordyce W: An operant conditioning method for managing chronic pain. *Postgrad Med* 53:123–128, 1973

Fultz JM, Senay EC: Guidelines for the management of hospitalized narcotic addicts. *Ann Intern Med* 82:815–818, 1975

Gaston-Johansson F: Pain assessment. *Pain* 20:69–76, 1984

Keefe FJ, Wilkins RH, Cook WA: Direct observation of pain behavior in low back pain patients during physical examination. *Pain* 20:59–68, 1984

Lief TP, Allen HD, Bloom WA: Drug abuse and the private practice of medicine. *Intl J Addictions* 16:731–739, 1981

Lipner J, Harris B, Katz S, et al.: Hospital management of heroin addicts undergoing cardiac surgery. *Brit J Addict* 68:341–344, 1973

Marks RM, Sachar EJ: Undertreatment of medical inpatients with narcotic analgesics. *Ann Intern Med* 78:173–181, 1973

Margolis RB, et al.: Internists and the chronic pain patient. *Pain* 20:151–156, 1984

Maruta T: Substance abuse by patients with chronic pain. *Curr Psychiatr Ther* 21:155–160, 1982

Mendelson G: Compensation, pain complaints and psychological disturbance. *Pain* 20:169–177, 1984

Reich J, Tupin JP, Abramowitz SI: Psychiatric diagnosis of chronic pain patients. *Am J Psychiatry* 140:1495–1498, 1983

Robinson GM, Sellers EM, Janacek E: Barbiturate and hypno-sedative withdrawal by a multiple oral phenobarbital loading technique. *Clin Pharmacol Ther* 30:71–76, 1981

Roy R: Pain-prone patient. *Psychother Psychosom* 37:202–213, 1982

Scott LE, Clum GA: Examining the interaction effects of coping style and brief interventions in the treatment of postsurgical pain. *Pain* 20:279–291, 1984

Serban G (ed.): *Social and Medical Aspects of Drug Abuse*. New York, SP Medical and Scientific Books, 1984

Smith CM, Barnes GM: Alcohol and drug problems in medical patients. *NY State Med J* 82:947–951, 1982

Ward CF, Ward GC, Saidman LJ: Drug abuse in anesthesia training programs. *JAMA* 250:922–925, 1983

Washton AM, Resnick RB: Recent advances in opiate detoxification. *Natl Inst Drug Abuse Res Monograph* 43:44–50, 1983

White AG: Medical disorders in drug addicts. *JAMA* 223:1469–1471, 1973

10

Psychosocial Conditions Disguised as Physical Illness

Neurosis has an absolute genius for malingering. There is no illness which it cannot counterfeit perfectly. It will produce lifelike imitations of the dilatations of dyspepsia, the sickness of pregnancy, the broken rhythm of the cardiac, the feverishness of the consumptive. If it is capable of deceiving the doctor, how should it fail to deceive the patient?
—Marcel Proust

Psychosocial factors play a role in almost all illness, either in the initiation or perpetuation of a disorder, or in the way a given complaint or problem is communicated to you as the patient's physician. Most of our grandparents accepted as common sense the notion that personal burdens and social trauma predisposed individuals to physical illness, and recent life-stress research has given this notion a solid statistical confirmation. Persons who go through divorce and job hassles and personal tragedies are more likely to become physically ill than those who don't. Since virtually everyone goes through personal tragedy at some stage in life, it is really more correct to say that any given individual is at greatest risk for physical illness at times of significant psychological and social stress.

At the same time, we are learning through biofeedback that the conscious mind has enormous potential for altering physiologic functions that heretofore have been regarded as immune from voluntary control. Many people can be taught to lower their blood pressure, slow their heart rate, decrease gastric motility, and even reduce perspiration at will.

Under the circumstances, it makes no sense to talk about functional conditions and organic conditions as being two totally separate entities. We know better. Mind and body are intertwined in a manner which we do not understand, but which nonetheless is indisputable.

We must therefore view illness not only as a consequence of specific etiologic agents, but also as a consequence of the patient's natural defenses failing to ward off disease. These defenses include the strength of the patient's spirit, as well as antibody levels and the friskiness of leukocytes. In order to treat disease, one must therefore attempt to restore and maximize psychic host-resistance and recruit the patient's energy and spirit into the treatment process. To be able to use such resources effectively, the physician must have some understanding of the patient as a person, as well as the circumstances of his or her life situation before, during, and after treatment.

Alas, in many high-volume impersonal medical clinics or busy private practices, you will have only fragmentary access to such information, and you will often have to proceed on bits and pieces of knowledge plus your own intuition.

Despite the fact that psychological and social factors play a role in the clinical presentations of *all* patients you will see, psychological factors play a much greater role with some patients than with others. You can't call all patients who are under psychological stress "crocks," but most physicians find it difficult to organize their thinking about "functional" patients without using labels which end up having derogatory connotations. It is helpful to have some sort of conceptual framework in which to organize your thinking. Traditionally, the labels clinicians use to identify such patients reflect the clinician's assessment of three sets of variables concerning—

1. The degree of organic basis to the symptoms;
2. The degree to which the illness behavior is consciously or unconsciously motivated; and
3. The degree to which the patient's behavior is "justified."

For example, if we find no organic basis for the patient's complaint and we regard the illness behavior as unconsciously motivated, we label the patient as having a conversion reaction. If there is no organic basis for the complaint and we believe the patient's illness behavior is consciously motivated, we call that person a malingerer. If we believe that the malingerer has no morally justifiable reason for such behavior, we additionally call him or her a sociopath.

This schema suffers from some flaws.

First, there is simply no reliable way to determine whether a person's behavior is consciously or unconsciously motivated. Usually, in fact, it is a mixture of both, but one never knows for sure. Interrater reliability on this subject is terrible. The best you can do is ask the patient, but there is something a bit ludicrous about asking a person's conscious mind to assess the unconscious, when the latter is by definition out of reach of the former. The brain is governed by principles which it cannot understand, and we rarely do much better with someone else's mind than we do with our own.

Second, determining the degree to which a patient's illness behavior is "justified" is fraught with problems. It's impossible to put ourselves in another person's skin, to truly understand what a stress or illness experience is like for that person. Most of us find value judgments easy enough to make, but we must recognize them as uniquely personal, reflecting moral standards and training which are more a matter of class and ethnicity than fundamental spiritual truth. The challenge in clinical medicine is to maintain the integrity of our own beliefs without letting judgmentalism prevent us from being of assistance to our patients. My own bias is that very few of the judgmental, pseudodiagnostic labels we attach to patients are helpful either to us or the patients.

Much of the rest of this chapter will be devoted to scrutinizing many of the labels used to designate various portions of the functional-organic spectrum. Most of them are the subject of endless attempts at clarification in the literature, the results of efforts by both clinicians and theoreticians to resolve some vexing theoretical problems. All the terms are widely used and misused and, to some extent, all reflect the physician's frustrated endeavors to diagnose and cure organic illness in patients whose problems are more complex than "just organic." You will notice considerable overlap from one term to another.

As we go through each of the terms, I encourage you to ask, Is this a meaningful term or does it simply represent a diagnostic wastebasket? If the latter, is such a diagnostic wastebasket necessary? For what? Does each term help the patient? How? Does it simply serve to label patients in a derogatory fashion, distancing them from us, serving to limit our responsibility in their care?

Psychophysiologic Disorders

The first thing you need to know about psychophysiologic disorders is that they officially no longer exist. They were removed from the nomenclature when the third edition of the *Diagnostic and Statistical Manual* was published in 1980. Since I was very much a part of the haggling and negotiation which led up to that change, and take great pleasure in and some responsibility for those developments, I feel justified in saying that you need to know what psychophysiologic disorders *were,* even though they no longer *are.*

The term *psychophysiologic* traditionally identified a distinctive group of diseases, rather than the patients who had those diseases. The terms *psychophysiologic* and *psychosomatic* often were used interchangeably for those disorders characterized by physical symptoms, caused by emotional factors, involving a single organ system, usually under autonomic nervous system innervation. The coding system in this nomenclature required that the affected organ be specified, such as *psychophysiologic cardiovascular disorder*. This classification derived from the idea that there was a core group of uniquely psychosomatic diseases, usually known as the "holy seven"—thyrotoxicosis, neurodermatitis, peptic ulcer, rheumatoid arthritis, essential hypertension, bronchial asthma, and ulcerative colitis.

There are numerous problems with this diagnostic approach, which when taken together help to explain why the diagnosis itself was seldom used. In general, the most likely reason for a patient being given a psychophysiologic diagnosis instead of some other appropriate alternative, was that the patient had been evaluated and diagnosed by a psychiatrist. For example, if the patient saw a psychiatrist he or she might have been given a diagnosis of psychophysiologic gastrointestinal reaction, while if the same person with the same disorder saw an internist, the diagnosis might have been pylorospasm.

In addition, this diagnostic approach unfortunately tended to imply that psychological factors were important in a limited number, but not in the vast majority, of diseases. By extension, the system perpetuated a dualistic conception of the mind and body. A patient who had a psychophysiologic disorder had a problem that was "in the mind," and the patient who had gastritis had a problem that was in the gut. One patient therefore became the province of a psychiatrist and another became the province of an internist or generalist. In both cases, effective collaborative efforts to treat multiple contributing factors in the development of the disease did not occur.

And finally, the concept of autonomic versus voluntary nervous system control continues to undergo reassessment. As biofeedback teaches us that many heretofore involuntary functions can be brought under some measure of voluntary control, it is clear that arbitrarily dividing diseases in terms of voluntary and involuntary organ systems is less clinically useful than we have previously thought.

The new nomenclature should be an improvement. The official psychiatric nomenclature resides in a document called the Diagnostic and Statistical Manual (DSM). Code numbers for diagnoses contained within the DSM are designed to mesh with those in the International Classification of Diseases (ICD), although the criteria for parallel diagnostic categories are not necessarily identical. Both the ICD and DSM are evolving documents. The DSM was first adopted in 1952 (DSM I), underwent substantial change in 1968 (DSM II), and evolves even more dramatically in the subsequent document (DSM III). This enormous flux is variously viewed as a tribute to the vitality and flexibility of psychiatry, or as evidence of the multiple, fundamental disagreements which permeate the field.

The relevant section in the new classification is titled "Psychological Factors Affecting Physical Conditions," but, for convenience, we shall refer to it here as Section 316 (which is the code number attached to this diagnosis in DSM III). This label includes—

1. The traditional psychosomatic disorders;
2. Anything that would have been diagnosed as a psychophysiologic disorder under the criteria of DSM II; and
3. Any physical condition in which psychological factors are significant in initiation, exacerbation, or perpetuation of the disorder.

The section is unique in that it is to be used only in conjunction with another diagnosis; that is, any clinician using Section 316 must always diagnose the physical disorder. This feature will ideally encourage attention to both the physical and psychological aspects of the disease, rather than narrowing the clinician's focus to one at the expense of the other.

If the initials and numbers and professional jargon seem burdensome, please bear with me. The classification system will be discussed in more detail later in this chapter, at which time I hope it will seem not only natural and simple, but also a welcome alternative to anything else available.

Conversion and Hysteria

Like many of the other terms discussed in this chapter, the concepts of conversion and hysteria are blurry around the edges. The term *hysteria* is sometimes used to designate—

1. A specific symptom, as an hysterical conversion symptom;
2. A disease state which predisposes to the development of conversion symptoms;
3. A pathologic personality type, as an hysterical character or an hysterical personality; and
4. A nonprofessional, pejorative description of a highly emotional, dramatic style of behavior seen most frequently in females.

The term *conversion reaction,* in classic psychoanalytic theory, refers to the substitution of physical symptoms for repressed instinctual impulses, with the specific symptoms having symbolic relationship to the underlying conflict. The symptoms resolve the unconscious conflict in a way so that the patient with a conversion reaction is no longer anxious. There are reams of material discussing the psychodynamic origins of conversion reaction in early childhood development. However, weighty discussions of pregenital versus phallic-oedipal etiologies have relatively little clinical relevance for the nonpsychiatrist.

There is considerable overlap between the concepts of conversion reaction and psychophysiologic disorders. The former is said to affect only the voluntary nervous system and the latter the autonomic nervous system. The former is said to be a purely psychological phenomenon with no tissue changes, and the latter were sometimes said to always have tissue changes. I personally don't find these distinctions very useful. The disuse atrophy of conversion paralysis is no less significant a tissue change than the short-lived inflammation associated with peptic ulcer disease.

Many more recent and less psychoanalytically inclined authors have emphasized the communication value of conversion. These writers emphasize conversion as a means of seeking the sick role, a way of nonverbally communicating distress within the context of the doctor-patient relationship, and the usefulness of conversion in achieving secondary gain.

The term hysterical personality arose at a time when dramatic exhibitionistic activity, crowned by florid and patently psychogenic symptoms (e.g., swoons and faints), was culturally the province of females. It came to be used to describe the type of person who was most apt to develop conversion symptoms: essentially, women who could play a certain kind of turn-of-the-century feminine role to the hilt. In general, the term has been very loosely used, especially by men, to designate a woman with some or all of the following characteristics: attractiveness, youth, overt seductiveness, histrionic affect, dramatic language with verbal excess, and demanding or dependent behavior as a way of controlling interpersonal situations.

In the last half of the twentieth century the relationship between "hysterical character structure" and actual conversion remains uncertain.

One clear historical message is that any patient labeled as a conversion reaction or hysterical character may nonetheless also have physical disease. In fact, it has been striking for me to see how many individuals who have classic psychoanalytic conversion reactions ultimately are found to have organic disease.

However, the term is likely to haunt us and patients for a long time to come. Whenever you see the diagnosis used, demand that the criteria for its use be explicit and precise, and that the patient's condition fully satisfies these criteria. Also, make provisions for further physical assessment of the patient at appropriate intervals, so that occult organic disease will not be missed.

Hypochondriasis

People who are always taking care of their health are like misers, who are hoarding a treasure which they have never spirit enough to enjoy.
—Laurence Sterne

The term *hypochondriac* is used sometimes as a specific diagnostic term and sometimes as a generic, to encompass all patients who could be less delicately called bellyachers, chronic complainers, doctor-shoppers, neurasthenics, organ-recital patients, and chronic neurotics.

Hypochondriasis may be defined narrowly as a worried preoccupation with body processes, such that essentially normal biologic functioning is recurrently interpreted as disease. However, elaborate variations to this conceptualization abound.

There are many tortuous theoretic explanations about what goes on in people's minds to make them become so worried about essentially normal bodily functioning. Some writers differentiate a primary hypochondriasis (in which the conviction of illness is central to a person's life-style and interactions with others) versus secondary hypochondriasis (in which fear of illness becomes a reaction to, or a defense against, some other terrible circumstance or problem). Among the factors implicated by such writers are repressed hostility, castration fears, lack of self-esteem, oral envy, guilt, masked depressions, destructive parenting, and poor interpersonal relations. In each case, the hypochondriacal symptoms are seen as providing a partial solution for neurotic conflict.

I personally don't find such theoretic explanations of much assistance. If I look hard enough for repressed hostility or castration fear in any given patient, I can usually find some evidence whether the patient is a hypochondriac or not.

The situation is complicated a bit by the fact that many "ordinary" patients will have hypochondriac interludes. An active man who has a myocardial infarction in his thirties will often become intensely aware and fearful of normal variations in bodily function. Similar phenomena can be expected with the friends and relatives of a 25-year-old woman who dies suddenly from a ruptured berry aneurysm, leaving all who knew her with extraordinary concern for their own biologic processes.

Whatever the precise pattern, patients who refuse to be reassured that they are indeed healthy present a vexing and difficult challenge to the physician. If we say that "nothing is wrong," we know in advance that the patient will probably seek care elsewhere. However, in a complex medical center, usually some abnormality can be found, however trivial. The bind for the physician then is: Do I reinforce the conviction of illness by emphasizing the abnormal finding, or do I push the patient towards a conviction of health that he or she seems unwilling to accept? The fear for most of us is that, if we reinforce the conviction of illness, we are helping to create a "crock" who will come back to haunt us and other physicians in the future.

The hypochondriac views hypochondriasis somewhat differently than does the physician. The patient is convinced of illness, and concerned that the expert care he or she has been seeking is not achieving the desired results. Explanations are wanted, not simply negative workups. He or she is likely to believe that the doctor is not bright or aggressive enough, or—more commonly—that the doctor is not sufficiently caring or does not really take the patient seriously. The patient tends to develop some cynicism about medical care generally, and yet feels desperately in need of medical care. Such people will consequently often attempt to diagnose their own conditions, reading widely, developing an extraordinarily detailed layman's knowledge of certain diseases, and treating themselves with various remedies.

Treatment of the hypochondriac (which will be discussed in more detail at the end of this chapter) relies upon minimizing disparity between the goals of the patient and the goals of the doctor.

The Disability-Compensation Patient

Patients in this category often have a variety of other labels appended to them (professional cripple, the actively dependent) or their condition (accident neurosis, traumatic neurosis, compensation neurosis, and litigation neurosis). By whatever label, the illness behavior and lives of these patients are dominated by the desire for financial remuneration and other forms of compensation our society gives to persons we consider disabled. To the extent that the various factors can be sorted out, compensation factors appear to be more important to these patients than the technical and physical limitations imposed by their physical disabilities.

This group is to be differentiated from the truly disabled for whom the physical limitations dominate the clinical picture. Where one draws the line between the two groups depends upon the personality of the patient involved, the nature of the social reinforcement system, and the values and biases of the clinical staff.

Why is it that some individuals become disabled when stricken with injuries or illnesses that impose few or no limitations on the activities of others? Again, beware of oversimplification.

Most psychological explanations emphasize that individuals who utilize illness and accidents for their own gain are the ones most likely to have accidents in the first place. Various personality types which have been singled out by one author or another include the following:

1. The passive, dependent, immature individual, who seeks to avoid competition either for fear of failure or because even the possibility of success is frightening;
2. The intrapunitive individual who emphasizes inner flaws as a means of self-punishment, to atone for feelings of guilt;
3. The angry person, for whom disability is a weapon with which to punish others—those who are specifically important, or even society at large (by requiring society to pay financial penance);
4. The self-dramatizing individual, for whom crises and unexpected events are a way of life and a means of relating to other people; and
5. The aging worker who has been dedicated to a job for years, who no longer feels the same satisfaction from that work or who can't tolerate it any longer, but who has no financially secure alternative other than disability.

Whatever the explanation, it is apparent that for many people there is much to gain and little to lose in seeking compensation for physical disability.

There are a number of paradoxes at work here. While there is a proud tradition of working in this country, and while most of adolescence is spent preparing to find a satisfying job or occupation, the prime ambition of many is nonetheless to retire early on a guaranteed income. Total disability may be some individuals' sole access to that goal. Partial disability offers only restricted benefit; it is difficult for the partially disabled to obtain employment, and benefits are often reduced or eliminated with employment.

These paradoxes are translated into reality by the multiple individuals who are concerned with the patient's disability. Each of these—the attorney, the physician, the insurance agent, the employer, the union representative—has his or her own narrow goals, and all may be working at cross purposes.

Given, then, the disability, it becomes natural enough to want whatever compensation is possible in a less-than-ideal situation. There is no punishment for trying. Quite the opposite. There is a broad current in present societal attitudes that fosters disability: "You might as well try and get what's coming to you; that's what you paid your taxes for."

The courts are often generous, and the trend has been to require a less direct connection between disability and working conditions and/or military service. (For example, one 56-year-old man was awarded workmen's compensation when he suffered a stroke while sleeping, because his physician attributed the stroke to overwork.)

Any patient who has filed for compensation, but who is uncomfortable with the disability, is necessarily afflicted with ambivalence: should he or she seek a doctor who will effect a cure, or simply one who will attest to the degree of disability?

If the chosen physician is reluctant to attest to disability, or tries to "cure" the patient before the validity of the disability is confirmed, the patient may adopt an attitude of "the doctor is trying to cheat me out of what is mine." Reciprocal hostility is usually the hallmark of the relationship.

It's easy to see how treatment is doomed to failure in the narrow sense. Cures are impossible without the patient's wholehearted cooperation, and the best we can hope for from such patients is ambivalence.

Since many of us get our satisfaction from curing, we have to find alternate sources of reward. Otherwise the relationship will deteriorate, we will get no enjoyment from our task, and our dissatisfaction with one patient may affect our work with other patients as well.

To proceed comfortably with such patients, you must make a set of assumptions:

1. The degree of impairment is not a medical question; it is a legal or administrative decision that depends in part on medical documents;
2. The degree of disability can rarely be accurately determined in a clinical setting; it can be determined only by how the patient functions in a natural setting; and
3. The physician's duty is merely to describe accurately apparent defects in the patient's ability to perform specific functions within the clinical setting.

With such a narrow definition of responsibility vis–a–vis the patient, you can proceed to do your job reasonably well and find satisfaction in a job well done. However, if the patient shows any inclination, I suggest attempting more.

Ask: When did this patient's disability career begin? Is it juvenile–onset disability or maturity–onset disability? Why has this patient opted out of conventional means of support? To what degree have the health-care system and physicians fostered the disability role in this patient by encouraging passivity, dependency, and avoidance of risks?

Try to help the patient ask, disabled for what? Physically fit, for what? What kinds of abilities can the patient salvage and nurture, without necessarily interfering with the compensation process?

Achievement of adequate treatment and relative satisfaction for the participants depends on a series of principles:

1. Keep potential doctor-patient hostility at a minimum. Avoid getting into an adversary position. Don't attempt to be a policeman, and don't act as if your patient were a criminal. Put limits on yourself rather than on the patient. Acknowledge the awkwardness of the situa-

tion. For example, do not say, "You are not nearly as disabled as you pretend—I can't let you get away with that." Instead, say, "This is an awkward situation for both of us—I would like to heal you, and you would like to get whatever financial assistance you feel is coming to you. I will do my best, and I will try to describe honestly your disability as it appears to me."

2. You can't expect significant improvement in the patient's condition until all compensation issues are settled, if then. There is little hope for improvement if the person has no desire to return to unhappy work or sees no reasonable alternative. Don't try to cure the uncurable; that will only result in frustration for both of you. Ultimately, "cure" depends upon getting rid of reverse incentives which initiate and perpetuate disability. This is a matter of social policy over which clinicians are likely to have little control.

3. Help prevent disability and compensation from becoming a major factor by getting your patient mobilized as soon as possible. Keep the patient functioning in family, community, and job—the longer away from any one of the three, the more uncomfortable he or she is likely to feel in resuming normal role functions. Acknowledge that our natural desire to hospitalize the patient for extended testing or observation or to insure maximum healing may unwittingly help to create a disability-compensation patient.

4. Help your patient and the family to set realistic hopes and goals for themselves. Often that will depend upon devaluing physique and physical accomplishments, and focusing on other kinds of attributes and accomplishments. They will need your help in setting realistic performance levels. If you cannot do that accurately, be honest about it, and ask for consultation with other competent people. Don't mislead the patient with false projections about what can be expected. Find out if there are any organized groups of patients who share the same disease or disability who can help your patient know what to anticipate and how to cope effectively.

Invalidism

Invalidism is continued disability disproportionate to the physical findings following an acute illness or injury. The disability is presumably the result of psychological factors, especially fear. The classic example is myocardial infarction, after which the patient is almost totally immobilized by the fear that any activity will precipitate another infarction and death. In such a case, the patient is often labeled as having a "cardiac neurosis."

Most individuals suffering from invalidism see themselves as extremely fragile, having only a tenuous hold on life. They tend to overinterpret symptoms, seeing normal aches and pains as concrete evidence of serious problems. The relationship with hypochondriasis is obvious, though it is customary to view hypochondriasis and invalidism as distinct conditions.

Multiple factors have been implicated in etiology. Some individuals have suffered from hypochondriasis all their lives, whereas no such history is evident in others. Other patients appear to adopt invalidism at the behest of their families: the patient's neediness and dependence serve an important function in terms of gratifying the caretaking role of other members of the family. Therefore the pressure is for the patient to persist in a weakened and debilitated position.

One aspect of the etiology of invalidism deserves special emphasis for us: the iatrogenic. Physicians often do two things that tend to promote invalidism. First, there is a strong tradition in medicine to opt for the conservative course whenever the patient's status is doubtful. For instance, whenever a cardiac patient complains of chest discomfort, there is a strong tendency to encourage the patient to abandon activity. Bedrest seems safest in terms of the patient's cardiac status, and we are less likely to consider how cessation of all activity will affect the patient's morale and long-term adjustment. In taking this approach, we reinforce the idea that, in the event of doubtful stimuli, the patient should interpret them as threatening.

A second way in which physicians reinforce invalidism is the use of scare techniques. Physicians will sometimes emphasize the frightening aspects of illness to cow the patient into obedience to the recommended treatment program. The reasoning usually goes as follows: if the patient gets well, he or she will be grateful for the marvelous job we did in healing; if the patient doesn't get well or runs into problems, we will have warned him or her from the beginning that the situation was a perilous one.

Treatment of invalidism depends upon recognition of the fundamental paradox: with regard to recommending activity or inactivity, you're potentially damned if you do and damned if you don't. The aggressive risk-taking approach may aggravate the patient's condition, but conservatism may foster invalidism.

It's not a decision which you as a physician have to carry all by yourself. The patient and family can reasonably participate in the decision if you tell them what you know, express your concerns about what you don't know, and relay the information empathically. Emphasize that it's difficult for you and for the patient and family to live with this kind of uncertainty, but the decision about activity depends upon philosophy as much as the medical facts of the case. Does the patient wish to see himself or herself as a cautious person, fearful, shrinking from the slightest sign of overexertion, or does he or she wish to appear as courageous, a risk-taker? Which approach will lead to greater enjoyment in life, and which will lead to an enhanced self-image for the patient? These are questions which only the patient can decide.

It's important in presenting these alternatives that you do not browbeat the patient. Pushing may have the opposite effect of what you intend. Patients must understand that you respect their concerns. The trick is to focus not on the symptoms in isolation, but upon the patient as a human being. Teach patients how their feelings affect the problem. For example, anxiety will not only increase the patient's perception of pain and lower tolerance to it, it may also help to promote the conditions in which pain is likely to occur.

Finally, help the hospitalized patient prepare for an active life outside by aiding him or her to experience graded increases of activity while in the hospital.

Malingering, Factitious Illness, and Munchausen's Syndrome

The term *malingering* describes a condition in which the patient deliberately feigns the symptoms of the illness or disability in order to gain advantage or evade responsibility. The term *factitious illness* describes a condition in which the patient deliberately creates or produces signs of illness or disorder in order to seek some advantage. *Munchausen's syndrome* is variously described as chronic factitious illness or chronic malingering.

Though each of the terms is often used as an epithet, the label is justified only by concrete evidence, essentially by patients' giving themselves away.

The appropriateness of the label depends upon what aspect of causation we or the patients choose to emphasize: the secondary gain, psychologic and characterologic predispositions, or the consciousness of the act that brings the patient to medical attention. For most individuals, these terms are not truly diagnoses, but describe ways of responding to stress or conflict by adoption of the sick role.

In practice, it may be difficult to separate these conditions from others described in this chapter—for example, hysteria. The malingering group of conditions is largely regarded as being conscious, whereas hysteria is commonly thought of as being unconsciously determined. In actuality, hysteria has many volitional components, and the terms described here are often influenced by unconscious factors. In any case, very little human behavior can be understood wholly in terms of conscious versus unconscious behavior. Many authors believe that the syndromes described here are indicative of severe psychiatric disorder, a perspective that I will not emphasize here.

The whole issue of conscious versus unconscious evolution of symptoms doesn't deal with the question of whether the patient feels justified in his or her complaints. Consciousness is a multilevel phenomenon; it may include or exclude awareness of symptoms, the extent of fabrication, the reasons behind the fabrication, or the ability to control the degree of distress and complaining.

Whatever the degree of conscious participation in the fabrication of symptoms, emotional factors underlying the phenomenon can be complex. In theory, a malingerer or a person with a factitious illness has a clearcut goal. When that goal is achieved, the symptoms tend to disappear. In practice, things are seldom so simple.

MALINGERING

Just as self-made billionaires keep on driving even when they have all the money they can spend, malingerers may adopt their behavior as a way of life. They may use it to alter a balance in social relations, get themselves off the treadmill of their normal occupations or family settings, seek revenge on the social system, or outwit and demonstrate their superiority over you, the physician. The latter quality seldom endears malingerers to their physicians. Malingerers can also be inspired by a desire for free board and lodging or the seeking of sanctuary, possibly from police.

It is difficult to discuss any of these patients and remain free of prejudice or moral judgments. While it's easy enough to list the various factors that may predispose a given individual to malinger, in practice most physicians find malingerers difficult to understand, to empathize with, and to treat.

For example, the apparent secondary gain may be small relative to the pain and suffering the patients put themselves through in the process of undergoing diagnosis and treatment. In the doctor's compulsive need to rule out any elusive organic contributing factors, such patients are often subjected to incredible and heroic diagnostic and therapeutic measures. The paradox, of course, is that hospitalization and diagnostic workups tend to reinforce the validity of the patients' complaints, often enough producing genuine iatrogenic illnesses as well.

FACTITIOUS ILLNESS

This is usually regarded as a subgroup of malingering, wherein the patient produces lesions or symptoms of disease with the intent to deceive others. This is to be differentiated from self-mutilation in which there is no attempt to deceive. Examples of factitious illness include the patient who injected albumin into his bladder in order to simulate nephrotic syndrome, or patients who produce cutaneous ulcers "of unknown cause" by applying acid or burning themselves with cigarettes. The literature repeatedly mentions that one of the difficulties in diagnosing such patients is a reluctance on the part of the physician to believe that the patient is capable of the act. Often it's difficult to reconcile the etiology of the lesion with the character of the patient. This is especially true when the phenomenon occurs in people with whom we can readily identify, most commonly middle-class individuals of education, apparent stable social situations, and personal attractiveness.

MUNCHAUSEN'S SYNDROME

Chronic factitious illness, or Munchausen's syndrome, is also known by a variety of less regal but more colorful descriptions (hospital hobos, hospital addicts) and diagnoses (polysurgical addiction, hemorrhagica histrionica, and laparatomiphilia migrans). The syndrome is named after Baron Hieronymus Karl Friedrich von Munchausen (1720–1791), a peripatetic fellow who wandered from one city to another telling tales.

Identification of these individuals relies upon a triad of characteristics exemplified by—

1. Pathologic lying, malingering, and impostureship;
2. Rootless and wandering lives;
3. A masochistic perpetuation of self-injury, and a seeking out of painful, often dangerous diagnostic and therapeutic procedures.

The lengths to which such patients will go in order to gain admission to a hospital can be awesome. For example, one case cited by Blackwell included a history of cardiac arrest, laryngeal stridor, hematuria, renal stones, abdominal pain, bleeding, anemia, neurodermatitis, and fever. Though the history was by no means readily available from the patient, careful medical detective work revealed that the patient had had 178 hospital admissions in 83 different hospitals over a period of 9 years. While such a dramatic achievement on the part of a Munchausen patient is probably exceptional, Munchausen patients are nevertheless now common enough so that every medical student can expect to see several during training years. In fact, Munchausen patients seem drawn to complicated and turbulent medical centers, where they can expect to have a different physician on every admission.

A somewhat chilling variant of the Munchausen patient is the Munchausen parent. One can see such parents taking their essentially well children from one medical center to another in a continuing search for organic illness. Most who search long and hard enough ultimately find that some diagnosis can be tacked on to their children—perhaps scoliosis, or some interesting variant in the child's immune system. In any event, the imprinting of health-care-seeking behavior in the children of such parents gives us an idea of how Munchausen's patients may develop.

MANAGING MALINGERING AND ITS VARIATIONS

Assessment of these patients is extremely difficult, because the better you diagnose, the less the patient likes it. It is one situation where the patient knows more about the diagnosis than you do. The physician must constantly attempt not to overinvestigate or overtreat; yet, unfortunately, it is precisely these patients who are most likely to be overinvestigated and overtreated.

Physicians in general are lousy at discovering dishonest behavior on the part of their patients. It would speak poorly for us if we didn't trust our patients; the patients would almost certainly sense our attitude, and an adversary relationship would ensue. In that sense, the malingerer represents a breach of trust in the doctor-patient relationship. Nonetheless, the malingerer's behavior usually makes good sense to the malingerer, otherwise he or she wouldn't perform that way. The physician may simply be caught in the middle because of the authority given by society to document illness. For most of us, because of the complexities of the problem, the malingerer's behavior is best seen as an unusual but understandable product of joyless work, interpersonal frustrations, and dreary lives.

When faced with someone who may be a malingerer, physicians often resort to a series of tricks or ruses (usually called "gomer tricks") designed to make such patients unwittingly reveal their true abilities. However, the most comfortable role for most physicians is that of helper and healer, not detective and adversary. Pitting ourselves against the patient rarely does much to enhance our own esteem as physicians or our pleasure in our work. It should be enough to identify the facts in the case, share them with the patient, and not take upon ourselves the burden of prosecuting and punishing the patient for his or her fraudulence.

We can observe discrepancies, inconsistencies, and our own uncertainties about our findings, and say so in the medical record: e.g., "These findings (or lack of them) should be interpreted in the light of other objective information not available to us regarding how the patient functions outside the clinical setting." In some ways, malingering is inevitable with our society's compensation system and the concomitant dependence upon medical authority for exempting individuals from ordinary responsibilities.

It is useful to remind ourselves that deciding the morality of our patient's complaints is rarely seen as one of the physician's functions, whether the problem relates to an abortion, venereal disease, or enuresis. The same is true for malingering. It is crucial that you retain your cool in dealing with the patient. You will want to proceed doing your best even if the patient is clearly not doing his best.

You must continually ask, Where does my primary loyalty lie? Traditionally, the answer has been "With the patient." To risk changing this answer may mean a fundamental change in how you deal with many of your patients.

With a suspected malingerer, the question always arises, Should I confront him or her with this malingering? You should, as with all patients, tell your patient what you have or have not found; the question is, How? Most important, maintain a composed, nonjudgmental, nonaccusatory, nonresentful manner. Then give the patient an opportunity to respond to your factual description. If no further comments or questions are forthcoming, keep your counsel to yourself and let the patient go. Speculate to yourself and your colleagues as you wish about the patient's motivation, but write up the report as factually as you can. If the patient wishes to contest your findings, you could say: "We have examined you very carefully. I have told you what we have found and what we haven't found. I think it might be useful to reassess the matter in three months, but I think we are being a bit nearsighted in focusing only on the physical complaints at the expense of the rest of your life. How much do you think your, for example, job and marital turmoil are affecting your health?" If the patient expresses interest in this line of reasoning you can follow up in the manner described at the end of this chapter. If no interest is expressed, say: "We would really like to help you. Our interest is in your welfare. We don't believe it would be in your benefit to subject you to more tests or more procedures at this time, neither are any additional consultations indicated. We would be glad to reassess your condition at an appropriate interval. You, however, must do what you think best with the information which we have given you. You are free to seek information or care elsewhere if you choose, though we cannot in good conscience recommend that at this time."

Angry and direct confrontations with malingerers, even with considerable evidence of the factitious nature of the complaints, rarely produce positive results. In most cases, the outcome is a breach in the relationship. In addition, if the confrontation takes place in a setting where other patients can overhear, they will have been treated to a scene wherein a doctor angrily denounces and humiliates another patient. While they may understand and even justify your behavior, very few of them will trust you more as a consequence.

THE CROCK

The crock is also known by a variety of other names—professional patient, illness addict, psychoceramic patient, the incurable patient, the rotating patient, the thick-chart syndrome, and the neurasthenic. Definitions range from the philosophic ("when illness is a way of life") to the comedic ("when the medical record outweighs the patient").

However they are labeled, these patients usually are characterized by multiple major and minor complaints, often with a history containing many operations, visits to many different clinics with notes from dozens of different doctors. The patient seems to drift from one complaint to another, some seemingly having a physical basis while others do not. If the patient has been seen by a psychiatrist, the report will probably emphasize that the patient is chronically depressed and masochistic, with massive dependency needs which are only gratified when the patient is physically ill and taken care of by others.

These patients see themselves somewhat differently, often as conscientious persons who have worked hard to look after themselves and others for many years. They find satisfaction in doing for others, and would do more if only they weren't plagued by all those physical problems. They see themselves as having made many personal sacrifices, often unappreciated, and having had many personal disappointments which they largely attribute to illness.

The disparity between the patients' self-image and that perceived by others suggests some compromise perspectives. The patients have not always been illness addicts; how did they become that way? A harsh assessment is that the illness life-style was adopted as a crutch; he or she couldn't make it in the normal competitive struggle of life and therefore opted for sickness as a way out. A more sanguine view is that the process of adjusting to illness has become a major achievement for these individuals, which they are now unwilling to relinquish. Coping with life in spite of illness gives life a special flair, which makes them feel particularly worthwhile. In fact, their primary source of self-esteem comes from viewing themselves as persons who cope in spite of the adversity of illness.

This latter view is particularly useful in that it is respectful of the patients and suggests several approaches to comfortable coexistence with them.

Successful treatment of the "crock" depends upon approaching the patient respectfully. If you radiate disdain or contempt, your contacts will be grossly unsatisfactory for both of you. You must understand that the patient's strength is in illness, and you must be able to give credit for the ability to function despite what he or she sees as limitations. It's a tricky line to walk. You must not deprive the patient of illness, and yet at the same time communicate the following: "My interest is in you, not in your illness. Don't tell me about your symptoms, tell me about you."

Once you have recognized the "crock," undertreat all somatic conditions. Focus on functioning despite the problems. If you successfully treat one symptom, the patient will simply develop another one. Recognize that your role with such patients is that of validator of physical illness, and a source of approval for the patients as they cope despite illness. Accept the symptoms as being genuine to the patient; accept the patient as someone who is worthy to you. Applaud strength of character in the face of perceived adversity. (Never say: "This illness is not so bad." Instead ask, "How do you manage to cope as well as you do?")

Most of us tend to respond in ways that are good medical practice but that not only result in no improvement for the patient, but in fact conspire to perpetuate the original problem. These patients are worrisome in that we are always concerned that there may be something organic going on that we have missed. We are aware that being a crock does not give a patient immunity to organic disease, and we therefore tend to perform diagnostic studies whenever we can't put our finger on what is wrong.

Recognize that these patients need their symptoms. Say, "We won't be able to cure you, but we'll try to help you. However, your principal task is learning to cope despite your physical problems." The most effective thing you can do for such patients is to offer a bit of yourself and whatever respectful attention you can give.

There is an irony here related to the changing nature of medical care. "Crocks" used to be the treasure of the young doctor just opening an office, the patient who would reliably be in the waiting room week after week, helping to pay the office rent, perhaps bringing in some fresh-baked bread in the bargain. Now crocks are an anachromism: there's no room for them in a busy ambulatory clinic and no one to finance their hospitalization for "tune-ups" or brief social admissions.

Some patients who fit this category welcome psychiatric referral, but most do not. Most will see such referrals as a rejection on your part, an attempt to deny the validity of their complaints. Psychiatric referral therefore should be dependent upon the fulfillment of two criteria: 1) the patient is interested in psychiatric referral, and 2) the psychiatrist to whom you will refer the patient is interested in taking care of patients of this type. Otherwise the outcome of the referral will be unsatisfactory to the patient, to you, and to the psychiatrist.

I want to emphasize here that if you *are* able to treat an "illness addict" in the manner suggested, you will be extremely gratified by the results. There is no more devoted and appreciative group of patients than "thick-chart patients" who are appropriately treated. They are so used to rejection and condescension at every hand that simply according them some human dignity will be rewarded many times over.

Treating Patients with Psychiatrically Based Medical Complaints

The first major treatment decision is how far to pursue the diagnostic work-up without perpetuating the vicious cycle in which increasingly vigorous and intrusive diagnostic measures result in iatrogenic problems. In general, it is best to assume that both organic and psychosocial factors are playing a role. Take physical complaints seriously, but perform invasive diagnostic procedures only on clear indications. If in doubt, temporize or defer; the patient can always be reinvestigated at a later time, and leads followed up when the indications are clearer.

Distinguish in your mind between contributory factors, sufficient factors, and necessary factors. Psychosocial factors may often be contributory, but be wary of assigning them responsibility for total causation. If you are a persuasive person, it's easy to talk people out of their symptoms whether the cause is psychological or organic.

When all else fails, do an adequate history and physical. Items of special interest in the history (where possible, to be confirmed by persons other than the patient) include current psychosocial stress, clear information about how the patient has handled stress in the past (has he or she resorted to sickness?), how much work and school time has been lost due to physical illness, and evidence of modeling of illness behavior by parents or other significant people in the patient's past. Ask about finances: is there litigation or claim pending? Observe the patient's relationships with those who come to visit: do they enjoy keeping him or her in a dependent and sickly role?

I have expended considerable effort in this chapter to discredit what I regard as misleading and pejorative labels. The question then naturally follows, How can one describe psychosocial factors which play a role in the initiation, exacerbation, or perpetuation of physical disease?

I suggest you follow the model used in DSM III for psychologic factors in physical disease, the 316 category described earlier. First, adequately describe or identify the patient's physical condition or complaint; e.g., angina pectoris, whiplash injury, chest-wall pain. The presence of this information on the chart will remind you that the patient's physical condition will need your continued attention. Then, follow that entry with a 316 notation, indicating that emotional factors play a prominent—or probable but clinically unverified—role in this condition; say, e.g., "Stress contributory." The 316 entry will remind you that you will have to pay special attention to psychosocial factors but will not make you think that the psychosocial part represents everything, or mislead you into believing that you have a detailed understanding of the patient's psychodynamics or the degree of conscious premeditation involved in the patient's complaints.

When you have difficulty sorting out how much is organic and how much stems from psychosocial factors, explain your diagnostic bind to the patient and ask for guidance. Say, "We want to get to the bottom of your symptoms, but we don't want to subject you to unnecessary tests or procedures. We need your help in sorting out possible contributory factors. How much do you think stress is contributing to what's going on with you?" Most patients respond very positively to this kind of approach. However, if your patient becomes defensive and protests, "You're saying it's all in my head," say, "No, we do not think it's all in your head. You are obviously in distress. We are simply wondering whether emotional stress is making your condition worse than it would be otherwise." Give examples of how stress can produce headaches, final-examination diarrhea or businessmen's ulcers. If you haven't already done so, ask how things are going in the five crucial areas that encompass the vast majority of human problems: relationships with loved ones, personal finances, trouble with the law, sexual satisfaction, and sense of fulfillment on the job.

Discussing psychosocial etiologies of physical symptoms needn't be the ordeal that it is often made out to be. Your first priority should be to get a clear understanding of what aspects of psychogenicity you and the patient feel the most and least comfort with. Does the idea of "psychiatric disease" make you uncomfortable? Do you feel that people who use illness to solve personal problems are greedy or inadequate? Do you dislike working with or helping people who have character foibles? Does the idea of the patient's secondary gain make you envious? Do you get upset when a patient struggles to hold onto an illness, when your primary source of satisfaction is in curing illness? Whatever your own particular stumbling block, try to put it in perspective and strive to approach the patient as one human being to another. Then follow this simple outline:

1. What we have found is this. (List both positive and negative findings, paying more attention to items readily understandable to a lay person and less to esoteric laboratory tests. For example, "Your cardiogram and chest x-ray were essentially normal, but you are a bit overweight and your family's history of heart disease must certainly trouble you.")

2. What you have is this. (Give the patient a name to attach to the physical aspect of his or her problem. The label needn't be either fancy

or esoteric; e.g., "Your pain is in the chest wall itself, and is sometimes called pleurodynia or chest-wall syndrome.")

3. The customary explanations are this. (Try to make his or her symptoms understandable to the patient. As you describe the bodily mechanics that play a role in the symptoms, include a reminder that "stress and tension, of course, lower your threshold for feeling pain and make you worry about it more once you feel it.")

4. What you can expect is this. (Give the patient some notion of what represents a reasonable prognosis. Feel free to describe a range of prognoses, especially when you feel that the patient needs to hold onto symptoms. In that event, emphasize that for some individuals, this condition can be chronic or recurring, but with courage and determination the patient should be able to continue with most daily activities.)

5. What we can do is this. (Explain to the patient that you do not want to cause more troubles with the treatment than he or she already has with the illness. Emphasize that all medications and all treatments have side effects. Note that doctors disagree on exactly how the patient's condition should be treated, but you believe in taking the safest course possible. Then prescribe nontoxic symptomatic treatment, including changes in activity or habits, as necessary.)

6. The way we will follow up is this. (*Always* emphasize that if the condition persists or recurs or becomes worse, the patient should seek reevaluation in a reasonable length of time. Then put a clear note in the chart, documenting your thinking, so the next doctor who sees this patient will have the benefit of your insight and will not feel the need for putting the patient through a diagnostic wringer. In general, follow-up is best arranged through the format of multiple, brief structured visits. See the patient yourself if at all possible. Use consultants as necessary, but try not to refer the patient elsewhere. Continuity is important, and your patient may see referral as rejection. It is unlikely that other clinics or other doctors will be any more enthusiastic about or any better at treating such patients than you are.)

Maintain a respectful cheerfulness with your patient. Avoid showing resentment. Don't burden the patient because your need to cure has been frustrated. Reward healthy behavior and don't reward sick behavior. If the patient is hospitalized, say, "I'll talk with you after we get you into a chair." Or, "It's sure nice seeing you up and about today." Give patients credit for their role in their own improvement: "I know it isn't easy for you. I'm glad to see you forcing yourself to eat everything on the tray."

Dealing with the "organ recital" is a persistent problem in treating patients such as those discussed in this chapter. The patient is likely to have an endless stream of complaints, and we physicians therefore become reluctant to talk with the patient at all for fear that the entire day will be spent dealing with one symptom after another. The best response to this kind of patient behavior is to recognize that the complaints are merely a device for seeking and maintaining a relationship with us and for eliciting our concern and approval. Therefore, whenever possible, avoid dealing directly with the symptoms. Focus on caring rather than curing. Say, "I know you are concerned with your constipation, but I am more concerned with *you*. How are your spirits today?" By doing so, you relieve the patient of the requirement of going through a list of symptoms in order to elicit your concern. It's a rare patient who will be unhappy with this approach, though some will occasionally have to remind you that they do indeed have a problem with constipation that requires your attention.

Bibliography

Adler G: The physician and the hypochondriacal patient. *N Engl J Med* 304:1394–1396, 1981

Aitken C: Psychosocial aspects of disease and their management. *Psychother Psychosom* 42:52–55, 1984

American Psychiatric Association: *Diagnostic and Statistical Manual,* 3rd Ed. Washington, DC, APA, 1980

Barsky AJ, Klerman GL: Overview—hypochondriasis, bodily complaints and somatic styles. *Am J Psychiatry* 140:273–283 1983

Beitman BD, et al.: Steps toward patient acknowledgement of psychosocial factors. *J Fam Pract* 15:1119–1126, 1982

Blackwell P: Munchausen's at Guy's. *Guy's Hosp Rep* 114:257–277, 1965

Chodoff P: The diagnosis of hysteria—an overview. *Am J Psychiatry* 131:1073–1078, 1974

Craig TJ, Vannatta PA: Disability and depressive symptoms in two communities. *Am J Psychiatry* 140:598–600, 1983

Cronkite RC, Moos RF: The role of predisposing and moderating factors in the stress-illness relationship. *J Health Soc Behavior* 25:372–393, 1984

Fairbank JA, McCaffrey RJ, Keane TM: Psychometric detection of fabricated symptoms. *Am J Psychiatry* 142:501–503, 1985

Fleming DM, Elliott-Binns, CP: Disability as identified from general practice records. *Brit Med J* 290:287–290, 1985

Fontaine R, Boisvert D: Psychophysiologic disorders in anxious patients. *Psychother Psychosom* 38:165–172, 1982

Gallon RL (ed.): *The Psychosomatic Approach to Illness.* New York, Elsevier, 1983

Lewis WC: Hysteria—the consultants' dilemma. *Arch Gen Psychiatry* 30:145–151, 1974

Lipp MR, Looney JG, Spitzer RL: Classifying psychophysiologic disorders—a new idea. *Psychosomatic Med* Sept-Oct, 1977

Lipsett DR: Psychodynamic considerations of hypochondriasis. *Psychother Psychosom* 23:132–141, 1974

Little NE: The hysterical and malingering patient. *Emergency Medicine,* Jan 15, 1984, pp 187–201

Looney JG, Lipp MR, Spitzer RL: A new method of classification for psychophysiologic disorders. *Am J Psychiatry* 135:304–308, 1978

Looney JG, Spitzer RL, Lipp MR: Classifying psychophysiologic disorders with DSM III. *Psychosomatics* 22:6–8, 1981

McDougall J: On psychosomatic vulnerability. *Intl J Psychiatry in Med* 14:123–137, 1984

Martin PD: Secondary gain, everybody's rationalization. *J Occup Med* 16:800–801, 1974

Mead BT: Management of hypochondriacal patients. *Postgrad Med* 53:107–110, 1972

Menninger KA: Psychology of a certain type of malingering. *Arch Neurol Psychiatry* 33:507–515, 1935

Nicholas JR: The chains of illness as an old friend. GP 37:112–116, 1968

Parker N: Malingering. *Med J Aust* 2:1308–1311, 1972

Pattison EM, Kahan J: The deliberate self-harm syndrome. *Am J Psychiatry* 140:867–872, 1983

Pugno PA: Screening for hypochondriasis in family practice. *Family Medicine* 16:134–135, 1984

Sarason IG, et al.: Life events, social support and illness. *Psychosomatic Med* 47:156–163, 1985

Sparr L, Pankratz LD: Factitious posttraumatic stress disorder. *Am J Psychiatry* 140:1016–1019, 1983

Thomas EJ: Problems of disability from the perspective of role theory. *J Health Human Behav* 7:2–14, 1966

11

Medical Conditions
in Psychiatric Disguise

Men in general judge more from appearances than from reality. All men have eyes, but few have the gift of penetration.
—Machiavelli

Things are seldom what they seem, Skim milk masquerades as cream.
—Gilbert and Sullivan

This chapter concerns those medical disorders and chemical agents that customarily produce psychiatric symptoms. I have arbitrarily excluded the confusional syndromes, which are discussed elsewhere.

We will talk about various diseases and drugs as "causing" various psychiatric problems. However, there is no clear evidence that these conditions and agents are sufficient causes in themselves. They may simply be contributing factors, only one of many such factors to consider in any given patient. We are discussing them here because statistically they are associated far more than other conditions and agents with what we customarily regard as psychiatric symptoms.

These factors have a dual importance. The importance to the patient of establishing a correct diagnosis for a potentially treatable condition is obvious. Another by no means trivial consideration concerns our professional competence and the vanity associated with it. There is no more embarrassing circumstance for a psychiatrist than to be treating a patient for a year in psychotherapy, only to find that the patient's depression is rapidly cleared by thyroid replacement therapy. Conversely, there are few accomplishments more gleeful for a psychiatrist than to make a correct diagnosis of pernicious anemia on a patient referred by an internist for treatment of family problems. What we are talking about is not so much what is wrong with the patient, as the labels we decide to put on the patient. The labels derive from symptoms or complaints in a given patient, as interpreted by us. Most of us, schooled as we are in the diagnostic rule of parsimony, look for single explanations for multiple findings. The temptation is to say either that the organic disease produced the psychological findings, or that psychological factors produced the appearance of organic disease. It's rarely that simple.

There is no fundamental difference between mind and body. Behavior, thinking, and emotional display are simply the output of one portion of the body, the brain. The brain itself is the most sensitive indicator of body physiology. It has the highest metabolic rate, the greatest complexity, and the most exquisite sensitivity to the juices which nurture it and surround it. As a consequence, subtle symptoms of brain dysfunction occasioned by systemic disease may precede signs of dysfunction in other parts of the body, often by a considerable lead time. What we must struggle to achieve is a sense of the natural history of disease, with psychological function and dysfunction as an integrated part of that evolution. For instance, in pernicious anemia, psychological symptoms may precede hemotologic evidence of disease by many months.

In Table 11.1 I have listed the diseases and agents which most commonly produce psychiatric findings. Lists are a pain, because they seem to invite memorization. On the other hand, they are handy to have for reference. These lists simply include the conditions and agents which are most commonly associated with psychiatric symptoms; literally hundreds of others have been reported as occasionally or rarely being associated with psychiatric symptoms.

In addition to the lists, I am providing a conceptual framework for understanding why certain kinds of physical disease commonly result in the patient's receiving a psychiatric label.

Theory of Similar Consequences

Symptoms feel identical regardless of their cause. How one explains a symptom to oneself depends largely upon family upbringing and the cultural values of one's place and time. Thus, one person who is feeling weak and lethargic may look for an explanation in his or her social life, while another with the same symptoms will look for signs of disease. Physicians are equally prone to biases in this regard.

Any disease which produces lethargy, fatigue, weakness, or other symptoms of sluggishness may be initially labeled as depression, by either patient or doctor. The patient's level of arousal *is* depressed, regardless of the source. The patient *feels* depressed and often ends up thinking unhappy thoughts. As a consequence, calling a patient like

Table 11.1 Physical Diseases and Exogenous Agents Which Commonly Produce Specific Psychiatric Findings

	Anxiety	Depression	Psychosis, behavioral abnormalities
Neurologic disease	Alzheimer's Autonomic epilepsy Multiple sclerosis Delirium and dementia	Parkinson's Myopathies Multiple sclerosis Myasthenia	Psychomotor seizures Wilson's disease (adolescent turmoil) Multiple sclerosis
Nonneurologic disease	Pheochromocytoma Avitaminoses (beriberi, etc.) Uremia Hypoglycemia GI Hyperirritability Thyrotoxicosis Hypoparathyroidism Premenstrual tension Porphyria	Chronic infection (esp. mononucleosis, fungal disease, and tuberculosis) Uremia Diabetes mellitus Neoplasm (esp. lung, pancreas) Anemias (esp. pernicious anemia) Hypopituitarism Hyper- and hypothyroidism Cushing's and Addison's diseases Menopause Pregnancy	Cushing's disease Systemic lupus erythematosis Hypothyroidism (myxedema madness)
Drugs and toxins	Steroids Amphetamines (any sympathomimetic agent as in, e.g., decongestants) Caffeinism L-Dopa Belladonna alkaloids Mushroom poisoning Heavy metal poisoning Dilantin Sedative withdrawal Organophosphates	Steroids Reserpine Bromidism Birth control pills Digoxin L-Dopa Tranquilizers Insecticides Heavy metal poisoning Note: Any drug which has sedative properties	Steroids Hallucinogens Belladonna alkaloids INH (Isoniazide) Mushroom poisoning Bromidism L-Dopa Thyroid supplements Amphetamines Furosemide Heavy metal poisoning

Note: This chart is not intended to serve as an exhaustive resource--it is merely a guide to the most common physical conditions producing psychiatric symptoms this "depressed" is not an error. Unfortunately, however, it is only a partial explanation of what is going on inside the patient.

Conditions which can be understood in this context and are commonly labeled depression in their subclinical or early clinical phases include chronic infections, myasthenia gravis, diverse myopathies, diabetes mellitus, the anemias, and similar diffusely debilitating diseases.

Any condition may be labeled as anxiety if it commonly produces the same symptoms which we ordinarily associate with anxiety: that is, nervousness, palpitations, diaphoresis, agitation, gastrointestinal hyperexcitability, and other symptoms suggesting hyperarousal or hyperirritability. Here again, the description not only sounds like anxiety, the patient *feels* anxious. The patient's thoughts are consistent with anxiety as well, because the way the patient feels helps to determine what the patient thinks about. It is therefore not an error to label this patient anxious, it is simply a partial explanation.

Some conditions which are commonly diagnosed solely as anxiety in their preclinical or early clinical stages include pheochromocytoma, thyrotoxicosis, hypoparathyroidism, caffeinism, and porphyria.

Theory of the Final Straw

People react in strange ways when something is happening to their bodies that they do not understand. People often perceive, in ways which are difficult for them to explain to their physicians, that something just isn't right; and they may respond with varying degrees of malaise and dysphoria. Occult neoplasms, for example, often present in this manner, and even the most articulate of patients is challenged to describe exactly in what way "something isn't right."

Hidden physical disease consequently can result in a patient's decreased adaptability and coping. The practical consequence of this is that the patient then has increasing difficulty in meeting social and professional obligations; he or she experiences increased stress in psychosocial situations and may end up talking a good deal more about the psychosocial stress than the original physical malaise that played an important contributory role.

This will be especially so if the patient was under a good deal of psychosocial stress prior to the development of the physical illness. Recent stress research, in fact, confirms what grandma knew all the time: people who are under a considerable psychosocial stress are more likely to develop physical illnesses of all kinds than people whose daily lives are going smoothly. Stress not only precipitates ulcer disease and heart attacks, it may also be a contributory factor in lowering patients' resistance to carcinoma and autoimmune disorders. Look for sources of psychosocial stress in all your patients, and you will find it in many. But if you focus on the psychosocial factors at the expense of a careful and thorough assessment of the patient's physical health, you will fail to diagnose physical disease which is at a subclinical or early clinical level.

Theory of the Intemperate Labeler

The labels tacked onto any given patient may have as much to do with the person doing the labeling as it does with the person being labeled. A patient's physical illness is likely to be seen as representing a psychiatric problem if a certain combination of circumstances exists:

1. There are zero-to-minimal physical findings;
2. The patient has a history of "psychiatric problems" on the chart;
3. The physician perceives the patient as being unusual or bizarre or difficult;
4. There is an easily elicited history of genuine psychosocial stress;
5. The physical examination is for some reason less than comprehensive; and
6. There is no opportunity to reassess the patient over a period of time.

Sometimes, too, we label patients "psychiatric" as a means of excusing our own ignorance. There is obviously something wrong with the patient; we can't find any explanation for the problem based upon our physical examination and laboratory tests, so therefore the problem must be psychiatric. This kind of thinking puts the problem neatly into the patient's head and relieves us of any further responsibility in the matter.

An alternative approach is to resist the urge to diagnose when the data simply does not justify a diagnosis. For example, "1. anorexia and malaise, unexplained. 2. depression," may accurately describe our knowledge, and relieves us from assuming that the anorexia and malaise are necessarily a consequence of the depression, if the evidence doesn't warrant such a conclusion.

Theory of No Theory

Neither I nor others can explain away the fact that certain diseases, as opposed to others with the same pathology, are associated with psychiatric symptoms with a frequency and/or severity which defies true understanding. Partial explanations are always available, but (at least to me) they do not sufficiently account for this frequency.

Alas, these conditions, such as multiple sclerosis and systemic lupus erythematosis, must be memorized. An alternative is to have ready access to a resource where such information is contained. Table 11.2, I hope, will serve that function.

TABLE 11-2 Physical Conditions Which Commonly Produce Variable or Fluctuating Psychiatric Symptoms

System	Disorders	Comments
Endocrine	Addison's or Cushing's disease	Psychiatric symptoms are the 2nd most important side effect of steroid medication, esp. prednisone, esp. over 40 mg/day
	Hyper- or hypoparathyroidism Hyper- or hypothyroidism Panhypopituitarism	
Metabolic	Pernicious anemia Porphyria Hypoglycemia	From islet cell adenoma, diabetes, or even insulin
	Electrolyte disturbance	Any antihypertensive medication which results in electrolyte abnormalities may be expected to have some psychiatric side effects
Neurologic	Multiple sclerosis Tumors Encephalitis Head trauma	Obviously almost any intracranial disease can produce abnormal behavior or thinking. Most, however, will result in confusional states (see Ch.5) or be associated with physical findings
Immune response	Systemic lupus erythematosis	

Suggestions

Expect psychiatric problems with physical illness, especially with those illnesses and drugs listed in this chapter. Consult the list below for the drugs that are most commonly associated with psychiatric side effects. Do not allow psychiatric signs and symptoms to distract you from potential organic contributing factors.

The following is a list of the most important drugs that produce psychiatric reactions:

Prednisone	Furosemide
Isoniazid	Phenobarbital
Methyldopa	Chlordiazapoxide
NPH Insulin	Aminophylline
Diazapam	

Often you will know from the medical record that a patient has a given disease and that psychiatric symptoms simply indicate either an exacerbation or recurrence of the illness or a side effect from a drug like prednisone. Sometimes patients will give you that information. However, you can't always rely on the patient to make the diagnosis. Just as a patient with a systolic murmur cannot always say that she has aortic stenosis, a patient with increasingly bizarre and manic behavior cannot always diagnose her own myxedema. We, as physicians, have to maintain an index of suspicion.

Frequently, there will be multiple possible explanations for psychiatric findings. For example, consider a woman who develops paranoid delusions over several days. She has systemic lupus, is taking 40 mg of prednisone a day, and has just learned that her husband is filing divorce papers and demanding custody of the children. In such a situation, don't waste time trying to sort out which factor is the crucial one. Instead, regard all factors as contributory, and treat the patient as a whole rather than restricting your focus to any specific contributing factor alone. If there is no laboratory evidence that the patient is having an acute attack of lupus, reduce the prednisone. If the patient *is* having a recurrence of lupus, treat it as you must, but be very wary about raising the dose of steroids beyond the minimum necessary to stem the attack. And by all means, call in a mental health consultant to help you sort out what is going on in the patient's marriage.

Of critical importance to the material presented in this chapter is an understanding of the natural history of any given disease. What appears to be a psychiatric problem now may later become a manifestly organic one. A thorough physical and mental status examination now may pick up subtle signs which a superficial examination would miss. Nonetheless, even the most meticulous of exams cannot pick up findings which will only appear later in time. Follow-up exams are therefore crucial if you are to diagnose correctly many medical conditions which present psychiatrically.

Whenever the clinical picture is unclear or you are tempted to explain the patient's complaints on a psychiatric basis, always make sure that there will be adequate medical follow-up. Be sure that the patient understands your concerns, so that you and the patient are working together rather than at cross purposes.

Bibliography

Craig TJ, Van Natta PA: Medication use and depressive symptoms. *NY State J Med* 82:1439–1443, 1982

Crook WG: Depression associated with candida albicans infection. *JAMA* 251:2928–2929, 1984

Gorman JM, et al.: Hypoglycemia and panic attacks. *Am J Psychiatry* 141:101–102, 1984

Hall RC (ed.): *Psychiatric Presentation of Medical Illness*. New York, SP Medical & Scientific Books, 1982

Heron GB, Johnston DA: Hypothalamic tumor presenting as anorexia nervosa. *Am J Psychiatry* 133:580–582, 1976

Jick H: What to expect from prednisone. *Drug Therapy:* Aug 1975, pp 85–90

Levenson AJ, Hall RCW (eds.): *Neuropsychiatric Manifestations of Physical Disease in the Elderly*. New York, Raven Press, 1981

Lever, EG, Stansfeld SA: Addison's disease, psychosis, and the syndrome of inappropriate secretion of antidiuretic hormone. *Brit J Psychiat* 143:406–410, 1983

Levin HS, Rodnitzky RL, Mick DL: Anxiety associated with exposure to organophosphate compounds. *Arch Gen Psychiatry* 33:225–228, 1976

Lueg MC: Hormones and mental changes. *J La State Med Soc* 134:32–37, 1982

Mackenzie, TB, Popkin MK: Organic anxiety syndrome. *Am J Psychiatry* 140:342–344, 1983

Oppenheim G: Propranolol induced depression. *Aust NZ J Psychiatry* 17:400–402, 1983

Peterson HW, Martin MJ: Organic disease presenting as a psychiatric syndrome. *Postgrad Med* 54:78–82, 1973

Pies R: Change in depression score during mononucleosis. *Psychosomatics* 24:766–767, 1983

Psychiatric Side Effects of Nonpsychiatric Drugs (The Boston Collaborative Drug Surveillance Program). *Semin Psychiatry* 3:406–420, 1971

Rais N, et al.: Thyroxine induced depressive psychosis. *J Postgrad Med* 29:184–185, 1983

Saad MF, et al.: Occult Cushing's disease presenting with acute psychosis. *Am J Medicine* 76:759–765, 1984

Solomon JG, Solomon S: Psychotic depression and bronchogenic carcinoma. *Am J Psychiatry* 135:859–860, 1978

Weizman A, Eldar M, Shoenfeld Y: Hypercalcemia-induced psychopathology in malignant diseases. *Br J Psychiatry* 135:363–366, 1979

Wilson LG: Unmasking the psychiatric imposter. *Emergency Medicine*. May 15, 1983, pp 212–217

12

Consultation and Referral: Calling for Help

Consultant: an expert called in when nobody wants to take the blame for what is going wrong.

—quoted by Sydney J. Harris

An expert is a person who avoids small errors as he sweeps on to the grand fallacy.

—Benjamin Stolberg

We all love to instruct, though we can teach only what is not worth knowing.

—Jane Austen

Anyone who attempts to give patients comprehensive medical care soon learns that no one doctor can do the job alone. Given the complexity of human beings and the diseases which affect them, no individual can master both the material and the art of applying it. Most of us are therefore grateful when we have consultants to give us assistance, or referral avenues along which we can direct our patients for specialized care.

Many complexities intervene in the process of asking for help, or sharing responsibility for patient care. This chapter is designed to give you a greater understanding of these complexities, along with some practical suggestions to assist you in getting the most useful consultations possible. I have focused particularly on psychiatric consultations, but I believe the information will be broadly applicable to other kinds of consultation and referral as well.

General Features of the Consultation Process

Asking for help has always been regarded as good medical practice, and often enough it is a legal requirement too. A physician should know when diagnosis and treatment of a patient's condition with reasonable success is beyond one's skill, and one must advise the patient of this circumstance and bring in other resources. A familiar rule is: If in doubt, bring in a consultant. Another general rule is to bring in a consultant if the patient asks for one. To refuse to do so in the latter circumstance is an affront to the patient's right to self-determination as well as an obvious invitation to a malpractice suit.

Consultations are not without their problems, however, which may stem from features unique to the individuals involved, and sometimes from the nature of the process itself.

The consultation serves a variety of both obvious and subtle functions. Most obvious, it is a request for help in the diagnosis and treatment of a patient and disease. Consultants may be called in to confirm impressions or enhance understanding. They may be requested to participate in formulation of treatment. They may be asked to help assign responsibility for further care, or to advise whether the patient should see another specialist or be sent to another hospital. Less often, they are called in to give advice concerning the doctor-patient relationship itself. Sometimes they may be called in simply to encourage the patient that something is being done. Occasionally, the process of consultation simply serves to avoid or defer action—a written consult request may take a couple of days to get to the consultant, it may be a couple of more days before the consultant sees the patient, and it may be another 24 hours before you are able to read the written report. Finally, a consultation request may disguise the intent to refer, i.e., to bestow (or to dump) responsibility for the patient's further care onto someone else.

Dissatisfaction can stem from discrepancies among the expectations of the patient, the consultant, and yourself. A very common response of the patient, especially if the patient must pay for the consultation out of pocket is, "That doctor came in and asked a few questions but didn't do anything for me. What a rip-off!"

The problems with consultations are not just monetary, however. Most of us learn about the process of consultation when we are in training in busy teaching hospitals, a situation which brings certain difficulties into dramatic relief. In that situation, requesting a consultation from a busy teaching service will mean that the patient will be visited by crowds of white coats, worn by individuals whose faces express varying degrees of interest and disinterest. Such mob scenes rarely do much to foster a good doctor-patient relationship. In addition, the process usually also involves considerable loss of control for the admitting physician, and a diffusion of responsibility for patient care.

The latter deserves special emphasis. The major problem with consultations in a complex medical center, especially with patients who have "interesting" and complicated diseases, is that responsibility becomes maddeningly diffuse—for the patient, as well as for the physicians. Nobody knows what anyone else has told the patient, and no one person has a clear sense of the patient's overall medical and human condition. Often enough, the admitting physician has the least professional clout of any of the doctors involved in the patient's care, and feels not only preempted, but also in a difficult position to do much about it.

For example, consider a male patient with severe myasthenia gravis, numerous respiratory problems (at one point requiring tracheostomy and chest tubes) and an "intriguing" clotting defect. The patient was theoretically the responsibility of the interns and residents on the admitting service (internal medicine); but since he was hospitalized in the respiratory intensive care unit, his case was technically the jurisdiction of the staff physician in charge of the respiratory intensive care unit. However, most of the shots were really called by the consultants: a nationally known myasthenia gravis specialist, an equally famous hematologist, and a chest surgeon with enormous power of personality who was convinced that problems with the chest tubes were the consequence of sloppy nursing care. At least three other consulting services were involved in the patient's treatment—none of whom were around at night when the patient's frustration at his hopeless and powerless condition tended to explode into temper tantrums. The similarly frustrated nursing staff and house officers had to deal with those. I'm sure most readers can think of numerous similar examples.

The point is, simply, that getting assistance from others sometimes turns out to be a mixed blessing and this consideration deserves attention whenever you think about calling for help with a complicated patient. Once the consultants are involved in the act, someone has to take responsibility for coordinating care. The more consultants involved, the more important and difficult is the role of the coordinator.

Collaboration is extremely difficult. It requires professionally mature and confident individuals who are willing to work together as colleagues with a clear eye to the patient's benefit. Collaborators must be keenly aware of their own professional needs and idiosyncracies that tend to shape their relationships with patients. This is particularly difficult when the collaborators are in different stages of their professional careers, and the problem of coordination falls to the individual with the least clinical experience. Almost all consultants tend to see things from a relatively more narrow perspective than does a generalist, and it must be the coordinator's responsibility to see that the disease being treated comes in a human package.

Physicians in general are competitive individuals, whether battling to get through medical school or lunging at the ball on a tennis court. Each is generally committed to a view of illness stemming from personal training experiences and professional identification, which tends to exclude other perspectives. Hematologists look at a patient in terms of blood cells, and psychiatrists look at them in terms of neuroses. Each will take it as an affront if you don't give priority to those views. Each will want to regard the patient as "my patient."

Your expectations of the consultant will vary depending upon you, your own stage of professional development, and your practice setting. Many physicians requesting a consultation expect to continue treating the patient themselves with the collaboration of the consultant's specialized skills, while many consultants' dominant expectation is to have the patient transferred to their own care.

Given that you have called the consultant in for a bona fide reason, the consultant will tend to recommend something. The consultant wishes to demonstrate acumen, and once involved in the case wants to make a contribution. Sometimes the consultant's recommendations have less to do with the merits of the specific case and more to do with that very natural human desire to make a contribution. Neurologists will tend to recommend neurodiagnostic studies, psychiatrists will tend to recommend psychotherapy, and surgeons will tend to recommend surgical procedures. However, if you repeat a consultation by another physician of the same specialty, the initial consultant's recommendations will be confirmed in only a portion of the cases. The percentage varies with the specialty and the individuals involved, but the pattern is consistent. The first consultant makes a contribution by recommending something—anything—and the second consultant can make a consultation not only by recommending something, but by recommending that you not do what the first consultant recommended. Some consultants even believe they can make a contribution by pointing out how stupid you are for having asked for a consultation in the first place, or how inadequate your efforts thus far have been.

The choice of a consultant is an extremely personal one. Occasionally, the choice of the given consultant is inevitable, and your only decision concerns timing. More commonly, you have some leeway concerning which specialty from which to seek consultation, as well as which individuals within that specialty. For instance, I have spent time in a hospital where the orthopedic service liked to confine its attentions to exotic bone diseases. In that setting, the distribution of consults followed a predictable pattern: whenever possible, fractures went to the emergency room, foot disorders went to podiatry, back problems went to neurosurgery, and hand problems went to plastic surgery. The point is that you must trust the judgment and interest of the person whose input you are seeking, and that may have relatively less to do with credentials than one might think. In many complex medical institutions, you will have little choice in the matter: you request a consultation from a department or particular service, and who actually shows up may have nothing to do with your wishes.

In general, your selection of a consultant will tend to favor someone you like (possibly as a friend), whom you respect, who respects you in return, and who is available. You will tend to refer people with specific problems to consultants with specific interests in that problem. You may tend to ask consultants you like to see patients for whom you have affection, and ask consultants about whom you are less enthusiastic to see patients about whom you are less enthusiastic.

Once you have decided on a consultant, you must decide when to ask for the consultant's input. Consultants differ regarding what they consider ideal timing in the transmittal of consultation requests. Some will want a full evaluation, including all conceivably relevant laboratory data already in the medical record, and some will wish to be called at the earliest possible moment. It depends a bit upon the degree to which they regard themselves as diagnosticians as opposed to treatment specialists. For example, having been approached for an obstetrical consult on a patient with a possible ectopic pregnancy, some consultants will ask you if there is "blood in the belly" and some will fly into a fury if you have performed a culdocentesis in their absence.

In general, you will have done best to have performed a good general history and physical and ordered relevant laboratory work, but to have called the consultant as soon as the reason for doing so was clear in your mind. Postponing contacting the consultant until all laboratory results are on the chart makes sense only if the results would significantly alter the need for the consultant. This is especially true in psychiatric consultations. If you have need for a psychiatric opinion, the presence or absence of organic disease should not alter the relevance of the consultation. The presence of organic disease does not exclude psychological contributions to the problem.

The consultation means requesting an opinion. It is not always necessary for the consultant to see the patient in order to be able to give you some suggestions. In that sense, informal consultations can occur in the hallway or over lunch, and nonetheless be quite useful. However, frequently the consultation involves having the consultant see the patient. In these days, when malpractice liability is often such a concern, it is almost always wisest for the consultant to see a patient, do a thorough exam, and write an appropriate note. In this instance, both consultant and patient should be prepared for their meeting.

Always tell the patient that the consultant is coming, and why. Identify the consultant surgeon as a surgeon, and the consultant psychiatrist as a psychiatrist. Explain the reasons for the consultation in as much detail as the patient can absorb. The patient has a right to know. Emphasize that the consultation is for your benefit in your treatment of the patient, and consequently for the patient's benefit as well. Say, "I am asking for an opinion." Dispense with "either/or" thinking. The patient may tend to jump to the conclusion that because a surgeon is being called in, that will inevitably result in an operation, or because a psychiatrist is being called in you think that the problem is all in the patient's head. Say, "The consultant is going to give us an opinion regarding this aspect of the problem; we should know about anything we can do to help." Clarify where control will lie: if you can honestly do so, say, "The consultant is simply giving an opinion; you and I together will decide what to do; how much attention we pay to the views of the consultant will depend upon how valuable those views seem to us to be."

If the patient has had previous unfavorable experiences with consultants, ask the patient to refrain from generalizing on the basis of limited experience. Emphasize your desire to help, rather than any elements of rejection or punishment which the patient may see in your calling in someone else. Help the patient to understand that you will not be abandoning care.

Preparing the consultant is as important as preparing the patient. Give your specific reasons for requesting help. What *is* your question? The more precise you can be at this stage, the more likely you are to get the kind of help you really want. Inevitably, the consultant will want to know the present status of your workup of the patient. Make clear how quickly you would like the patient seen, though both you and the consultant will appreciate some flexibility on the other's part. Air your expectations concerning who will take responsibility for what, including arranging for diagnostic studies, treatment, and writing nursing orders for hospitalized patients. Clarify whether you expect the patient to remain your responsibility or to be transferred to the consultant's care. Tell the consultant that the patient is expecting the visit, and looks forward to (or is anxious about) it. Help the consultant to have a positive view of your patient so that he or she will treat your patient with the respect that you feel is deserved.

Be sure to let the consultant know the patient's understanding of the condition. What does the patient know or not know? How much should the consultant feel free discussing with the patient, how much should be left to you, and how much should the two of you communicate to the patient in a three-way meeting?

After the consultation, make sure the patient is not set adrift. A common error is to send a patient to a specialist for a specific problem (e.g., to an ear, nose, and throat specialist for epistaxis) and forget to arrange appropriate follow-up for basic medical conditions (e.g., the hypertension which may have been an important contribution to the nosebleed in the first place). Many specialists refuse to care for—or to write orders concerning—any matter which is not directly related to their own narrow specialty.

Expectations and Perspectives

Each of the parties involved in the consultation—the consultant, you, and the patient—have your own views and concerns that may affect the consultation process.

Consultants in general like being helpful, appearing skilled, and feeling valuable to someone else. They dislike being taken for granted, doing someone else's scut work, and getting insufficient appreciation.

The consultant who can help you will generally want to, and will appreciate well-intentioned feedback. If a consultant resorts to jargon or obscurities which are incomprehensible to you, it may reflect the consultant's own insecurity. Try to put such a person at ease so you can get maximum value from the contact. Say: "That's really helpful, but I'm not familiar with some of the words you use. I hope you won't think me an idiot, but could you run through that again in simpler terms?"

Some consultants will always feel taken advantage of and will let you know it. If they nonetheless provide useful services, give them more than the usual amount of appreciation. Figure they need it, and things will go more smoothly for all three of you, if you are willing to give an extra measure of gratitude.

Some consultants seem to have learned their lines by watching arrogant professors at wherever they were trained. They assume that their appropriate function is to put you down, point out all your shortcomings, and generally make you feel like a third-year medical student, even though you may have been in practice a number of years. Sometimes you can discuss such behavior directly with the consultant involved, and sometimes nothing seems to do any good at all. Try to avoid becoming defensive or angry in dealing with such prima donnas. Recognize that the behavior is inherent in the consultant and not a reflection of your inadequacies. Simply do the best you can, ask for help when it is in the patient's best interest, and keep your sense of humor.

Most consultants hate *stat* requests, where the crisis nature of the request is largely a consequence of the requesting physician's poor planning or abruptly resolved ambivalence in the requesting of the consult. No busy consultant will be very happy to hear you say: "I'm discharging the patient tomorrow, and I'd just like you to take a look at him before he leaves." Don't hesitate to make the contact when you first think that a consultation may later be indicated. Use the phone freely in advance of emergency situations, and emergency situations will occur much less frequently.

Many consultants have never clarified for themselves exactly what their role involves. If you have had a bad time with a consultant of a given specialty (e.g., a psychiatrist who doesn't treat you or your medical orientation with respect, or a nephrologist who gets sidetracked with petty detail), avoid generalizing from the experience. Keep looking till you find resource people who give you useful services.

Often a consultant may be tempted to treat *you* as a patient. Doctors help patients; in this instance, you have asked for help; therefore, you are to be treated like a patient. Few consultants adopt this attitude in any blatant fashion but the message sneaks out in other ways: they will keep you waiting for what appears to be an unseemly period of time, they will avoid keeping you informed, they will use specialist jargon that you can't understand, or they will simply imply that your time is less valuable than theirs. Rather than responding immediately with rage, you might savor for a moment what it feels like to be a patient. *Then* clarify any possible misunderstanding with the consultant.

Many consultants also like to see themselves as teachers, and get their psychic rewards from feeling that they teach well and are appreciated for this skill. Such individuals will therefore enjoy consulting on patients who provide such an opportunity, and consulting to doctors who are interested in learning. They tend to get a bit testy if they sense that the requesting physician has no interest in what they have to say, instead only wishing them to do something or supply a pro forma note.

Your own expectations may be equally diverse. You may be calling in a consultant to perform a specific procedure or to reassure yourself that you are doing what the consultant would do. You may request a consultation simply because you believe yourself to have a medicolegal obligation to do so, or because you want to demonstrate how smart you are (e.g., when you have made a correct diagnosis on a patient who has vainly sought assistance in the past from physicians in the consultant's specialty). Occasionally, you may call in a specialist to counteract what you believe to be a foolish recommendation by a previous consultant. In that event, you may be asking the consultant to provide you with arms and ammunition, and it would be a courtesy to let that consultant know that he or she may soon be in an adversary role with another specialist. Sometimes some physicians call in a consultant to punish the patient for not getting well or for creating a fuss. For example, the patient may be told, "I think your behavior is inappropriate, and I'm going to call in a psychiatrist to check you out." Sometimes some physicians call in a consultant because they really don't know what else to do, have no specific question in mind, and are simply trying to buy time and give the patient the impression that something is being done.

Mostly, however, physicians call in consultants because they wish to help, in the best sense of that word, and they think the patient will receive better care with another opinion than without it. Physicians who habitually avoid calling consultants usually hold back because they feel demeaned by admitting they need assistance, or are reluctant to share their proprietary role with another physician who might "undermine" their own authority.

None of us, of course, likes to have our ignorance shoved in our face, and we expect the consultant to treat us, our skills, and our patients with respect. We expect consultants to be accessible and to see the patient promptly if that is indicated, unless they have a reasonable explanation for the delay. We assume that the consultant will do a thorough exam and talk to relatives or other individuals whose input will be necessary to develop an informed judgment.

As a practical matter, we expect the consultant to write a legible and practical note, answering our specific questions, adding relevant additional comments, providing useful suggestions concerning further assessment, treatment, and follow-up, including a notation of who is expected to take responsibility for what. Most of us appreciate having the consultant contact us personally to convey all that information verbally, in addition to the written note.

Assuming the patient is aware that a consultation is taking place, or has direct contact with the consultant, most react positively or generally positively with understandable reservations. The latter may be due to concerns about additional cost, if that is a factor, reluctance to having to tell the whole story to yet another physician, fears about additional diagnostic and treatment procedures, or feelings about the particular specialty which the consultant represents.

Some patients—a distinct minority—react adversely to the idea of consultation in general or to specific kinds of consultation ("I don't want any surgery, and I don't want to see any surgeons," or "My sister went to an allergist weekly for three years, and he didn't do anything but steal her money!"). By and large, if you have a decent relationship with a patient and carefully prepare the patient for the consultation, that patient is likely to respond to the idea of a consultation in a manner consistent with whatever feelings you communicate. That is, if you consult reluctantly or with anger ("I'm at my wits' end; call in the damned radiotherapist—or psychiatrist, or surgeon"), the patient is likely to view the consultant with suspicion or even dread. On the other hand, if you give the patient the idea that you eagerly anticipate assistance from the consultant, that consultant is much more likely to find a receptive patient.

Psychiatric Consultations

Psychiatric consults are similar to other consultations in that you are asking a colleague for help concerning a matter relevant to the patient's care. As such, psychiatric consults are subject to all the complexities and subtleties that exist for consults in general.

Psychiatric consults are also distinct in a number of ways. While you would ask a psychiatrist to offer opinions concerning diagnosis and treatment in much the same way you would other consultants, the process often feels different and is different. Sometimes psychiatric consultants can be useful in commenting on the process of treatment itself, and how the psyches of those involved (doctor, patient, family, other health professionals) contribute to potential strengths and weaknesses in the healing situation. In that sense, the psychiatrist may be called upon to give a forthright assessment of you and your particular strengths and weaknesses in a manner which you would never expect from any other kind of consultant. Potential psychiatric consultants vary enormously in their ability to usefully perform this function.

Nonetheless, a major current in recent psychiatric-consultation literature emphasizes liaison psychiatry in which a psychiatrist consults with a ward or medical group or department over time, observing and commenting on the evolving milieu of treatment in a manner that heightens staff awareness of subtleties and facilitates psychologically astute treatment. The psychiatrist may participate in ward rounds, sit in on meetings and conferences, or simply consult directly to you about issues in patient care, without necessarily getting involved in day-to-day patient care.

Another difference about psychiatry consults is that they may not be performed by a psychiatrist. Especially in institutional settings, a "mental health consult request" may elicit a response from a psychologist, psychiatric nurse, or psychiatric social worker, each of whom may provide an excellent service, especially if your request concerns evaluating some psychosocial component of illness or providing ongoing treatment for anxiety or depression or marital or family problems. Though physicians in general are reluctant to accept nonphysician consultations, their availability is not unique to psychiatry. I've met few physicians who couldn't learn something worthwhile from a talented nurse who works in a cardiac care unit, renal care unit, or obstetrical delivery room. Still, the formal inclusion of nonphysicians in respond-

ing to consult requests remains unusual, and is primarily a phenomenon of the "mental health field."

Few individuals are totally dispassionate about psychiatry, and the
idea of a psychiatric consultation is therefore likely to arouse more
feelings than, say, a metabolic consult. Some patients may be concerned about a stigma involved, not only in such areas as job and
security clearance, but also with family. The patient may ask, "What
will people think?" And there is no question that some concern is
understandable. If the issue remains important to the patient despite
reassurance from you, and you nonetheless believe consultation to be
necessary, say, "I need a psychiatric opinion; I will ask the psychiatrist to leave out all personal details from the written report and advise
me orally; the medical record will contain a simple notation that you
were seen in consultation." If the patient accepts, make certain that
the psychiatric consultant understands the terms involved and is willing to proceed on that basis.

The psychiatrist responding to any consultation request within a
general hospital is likely to differ from other physicians in having a
good deal less comfort in a medical-surgical setting. Indeed, many may
have gone into psychiatry in the first place as a means of fleeing from
blood-and-bowels medicine. Psychiatrists also tend to have their days
more highly structured than other physicians. Their schedules are a
series of 50-minute appointments which they are reluctant to interrupt,
and it may be difficult to talk to them on the phone (except 10 minutes
before the hour), and nearly impossible to get them to come to see a
patient on an urgent basis in the middle of a working day. Some have a
near-fetish concerning confidentiality and may be reluctant to confide
in you details of the patient's personal life which they discover and you
yourself do not know. Finally, some psychiatrists may feel that any
opinion they give is premature if given with a superficial understanding
of what makes the patient tick. Definitions of "superficial" vary, but
many would feel uncomfortable commenting on persons whom they
have seen fewer than several times.

Indications for psychiatric consults include any of the issues mentioned in this book when they become relevant to the care of a given
patient. These generally fall into the categories of assessment, treatment, staff-patient relationships—or consultation prior to arranging
patient referral.

It is perfectly justifiable, of course, to initiate a psychiatric consultation request because the patient asks you to do so. However, as a
courtesy to the consultant, you should certainly get some idea of exactly what it is that the patient wishes and some idea of the dimension
of the problem. How detailed an inquiry you make into the patient's
thinking depends on you and your relationship with the patient, and

your knowledge of available resources. Once you get an idea of the general nature of the problem, you are in a much better situation to request appropriate consultation: a patient who is hearing voices should probably be seen by a psychiatrist, whereas the options may be much wider for a patient who would like some marital counseling.

Referral

Referral is subject to many of the same kinds of considerations as consultation, but often means that you are far more likely to wash your hands of the patient once the process is accomplished. After you have referred a patient, you may never see that person again. Referral means giving the responsibility for care—or at least some aspect of it—to someone else. The referring physician may retain some interest in collaborating with the physician referred to, but an element of control is always sacrificed.

Referral is often usefully preceded by a consultation, especially if you know you will be having no further contact with the patient. Consultation in advance helps to ensure that the patient won't get lost through the many cracks in the health care system. If you are referring the patient to a psychiatrist, the same considerations apply as for psychiatric consults discussed earlier. You will particularly want to discuss referral to the psychiatrist if you are thinking of psychiatric hospitalization. Psychiatric hospitalization per se is not necessarily curative or even helpful; there are numerous advantages and disadvantages. A strong case can be made for alternatives to psychiatric hospitalization when these are available (including outpatient care, day hospital, visiting nurses); and you should know what options are available to this specific patient. It is also useless to discuss brief hospitalization with the patient if the only psychiatric facility available tends to keep patients for months rather than days.

If you are referring a patient for outpatient psychotherapy, it's useful to keep in mind the patient's monetary resources and location of residence. Eligibility for psychiatric care is far more restricted than eligibility for medical and surgical services. If you are sending a patient to an agency or an institution which provides psychotherapy, the patient's eligibility may well be determined by the catchment area in which he or she lives.

Don't send the patient to a psychiatrist who is not prepared to treat the patient. Some psychiatrists don't wish to work with patients who are physically ill; others may lack skill or inclination; some may simply be too busy. The primary consideration is finding a skilled clinician with whom the patient will feel comfortable, and who is available.

Remember not only with psychiatrists but also with most specialists who take a particularly focused view of patients (e.g., ophthalmologists, oral surgeons, and the like), that very few will do thorough and competent physical examinations of the patient, or really take responsibility for general health care. It is up to you and the patient to see that ongoing general health problems are not neglected.

In general, the fewer credentials a therapist has, the less expensive the services will be. Psychiatrists will charge more than Ph.D. psychologists, who will charge more than nurse clinicians and social workers. Individual therapy will cost more than group therapy. Any psychotherapy which leaves a family financially depleted is unlikely to be beneficial to that family's mental health. You will want to adjust your referral accordingly whenever this is an important consideration.

When preparing your patient for a psychiatric referral, it is useful to have a spiel that will cover the essentials. I usually tell patients that psychotherapy is an intensely personal experience and it's important to find a psychotherapist one can be comfortable with. I recommend comparison shopping. Interview potential therapists, and pick the one that's right for you. Check out a potential therapist at least as well as you would anyone else from whom you are seeking a service. Ask for an estimate of the cost and length of treatment. If the therapist says that this will require a more detailed evaluation, ask for the usual cost and length of the evaluation. Keep clear your priorities and what you want. If you aren't sure of your priorities, ask the therapist what he or she thinks is a reasonable length of time to devote to clarifying such issues. Then choose the therapist who seems to provide the most reasonable answers.

Bibliography

Abram HS: Interpersonal aspects of psychiatric consultations in a general hospital. *Psychiatry Med* 2:321–326, 1971

Brantley JT, Jr., et al.: Consultation-liaison fellowships—effects on internists' attitudes toward psychiatric consultation. *Psychosomatics* 26:18–28, 1985

Carson NE: The referral process. *Med J Aust* 1(Feb 20):180–182, 1982

Cummins RO, Jarman B, White PM: Do general practitioners have different 'referral thresholds?' *Br Med J* 282:1037–1039, 1981

Fauman MA: Psychiatric components of medical and surgical practice—referral and treatment of psychiatric disorders. *Am J Psychiatry* 140:760–763, 1983

Hodge JR: *Practical Psychiatry for the Primary Physician.* Chicago, Nelson–Hall, 1975

Linn LS, Daniels M: Social and structural factors affecting psychiatric consultation. *Intl J Psychiatry in Med* 14:77–86, 1984

Ludke RL: An examination of the factors that influence patient referral decisions. *Med Care* 20:782–796, 1982

McCarthy EG, Widmer GW: Effects of screening by consultants on recommended elective surgical procedures. *N Engl J Med* 291:1331–1335, 1974

Patterson CW: Psychiatrists and physical examinations—A survey. *Am J Psychiatry* 135:967–968, 1978

Phillips S, Sarles RM, Friedman SB: Consultation and referral—when, why and how. *Pediatric Ann* 9:269–275, 1980

Pullen IM, Yellowlees AJ: Is communication improving between general practitioners and psychiatrists? *Brit Med J* 290:31–33, 1985

Schwab JJ, Brown J: Uses and abuses of psychiatric consultation. *JAMA* 205:65–68, 1968

Weissberg MR: Emergency room medical clearance. *Am J Psychiatry* 136:787–790, 1979

13

The Family: Whose Patient Is This?

A family is a unit composed not only of children, but of men, women, an occasional animal, and the common cold.

—Ogden Nash

The opinions which we hold of one another, our relations with friends and kinfolk, are in no sense permanent, save in appearance, but as eternally fluid as the sea itself.

—Marcel Proust

It's no fun to be a martyr if the martyr knows that the family knows that the martyr likes it.

—Zona Gale

Illness is a family affair. Disease occurs in vivo, not in vitro, and people live in vivo, not in vitro—though the latter is easy enough for us to forget when we see a patient alone in our office or, worse, as a glorified biologic preparation in the hospital. My views on this subject are admittedly personal, having beeen substantially influenced by my experience with considerable illness in my own family.

I remember sitting in the waiting room of an intensive care unit, waiting for my five-minute allowed visiting time out of every two hours—which, as it turned out, was quite enough for both my patient-relative and myself. I busied myself with reading and curious side-glances at the other families who had been encamped in the waiting room, frightened and depressed for days. An earnest physician came in to explain to one family what was happening to their father/brother/husband, who was a postcardiotomy patient. The physician did his damnedest. He recited the electrolyte levels, the enzyme levels, and the renal function studies. He went into enormous detail, and the family sat there listening numbly. Finally, he told them that he would talk to them again tomorrow, and then left. The family anxiously conferred. What had the doctor said? No one knew. He had, in good faith, spent his precious minutes to reassure and inform, and totally misread his audience. What they wanted to know was: Will he be okay? Will we be okay? Is there anything we can do that we aren't doing? What I think they really wanted was to be told: "All of you except one, go home and sleep; there's nothing to be done here except for your ritual visits five minutes every two hours."

Treating patients and their families effectively remains the most complicated level of clinical care. Every family is different, and both specialty and hospital-based medicine usually screen out subtleties of family interaction from the clinical situations. Therefore, in dealing with patients' families, you will often be proceeding in ignorance with regard to the family in question, basing much of your approach on preconceived assumptions concerning families in general. Frequently, these assumptions will reflect experiences within your own family and with families of similar cultural and socioeconomic background.

Though the family remains the single most important social unit for most of us, its role in both health and illness has changed considerably over the lives of our parents, grandparents, and our selves. Historically, disease was treated within the family unit, among close relationships, and treatment was interwoven with the fabric of life. The family is now far more vulnerable than it has been, and illness has become a major stress for many, in ways we will discuss shortly. The vulnerabilities of the family stem from the increasingly small size of the nuclear unit, the isolation of that unit from other family units that might provide potential support, and the decreased sense of neighborhood that has occurred in so many cities and which heretofore had provided an extra measure of protection to families under stress. Internal pressures upon the family arise in the changing role of the woman/wife/mother and the concomitantly changing expectations of the man/husband/father.

In this time of changing values, family stability is far more fragile than at other times, and we as physicians have to be cautious about making assumptions concerning any patient's family and how it will function with the added stress of illness. Nonetheless, assuming the patient does have a family, there are certain issues that almost inevitably arise and to which the astute clinician will be alert.

One important function of the family is to decide if the patient is really sick, and what degree of dependence is allowable given the patient's condition. Does the family answer these questions in the same way I do? Another function is to help provide home treatment and to determine the appropriateness and frequency of seeking professional help. Do I have the family's confidence as well as the patient's? Do they have mine? Will we be working together or at cross purposes?

There is no question that families and the ambiguities of family life can have profound effects on not only illness behavior, but also on basic disease processes themselves. The role of parental deprivation in producing illness in infants is indisputable, and it's tempting to extrapolate to adults. Certainly there is now good evidence that morbidity across many categories is greater among those who are not involved in stable marriages. Family problems not only complicate illness, in some diffuse manner they seem to predispose an individual to illness. If you buy the notion that illness is, among other things, one potential response of the organism to stress, then the presenting illness may well be only our point of entry into a complicated and troubled family situation.

Reaction of Family to Illness

The impact of illness on any family is related to that family's customary pattern of dealing with stress, attitudes toward sickness in general, the prognosis of the particular illness involved, feelings about the patient, the patient's role in the family, and how that role will be altered by the illness. Though sometimes illness can serve positive functions, such as drawing a family closer together, illness almost always results in some turmoil even in smoothly functioning families. Illness of one member results in some disruption of daily life for all. There is usually considerable inconvenience of time, effort, and mobility, with increased demands and responsibilities on the healthy members. Illness, like any other crisis, brings emotions to the surface; common themes include depression, loneliness (if the ill person can no longer function as a companion), fear for the future, frustration of goals, anger at the patient (usually expressed indirectly) for "causing" so many inconveniences, and guilt because of these feelings of anger.

The family must have some equilibrium to continue to function as a unit. If the illness is to be a prolonged one, the family has to decide how much dependency they will allow or encourage on the part of the sick person, as opposed to how much self-sufficiency can reasonably be expected. If the family feels very stressed, the illness itself becomes not only a source of strain, but also a potential weapon in struggles for control. The condition of illness—and the patient's implied lack of responsibility for the condition—can become a frequent justification for decision making. Under such pressures, feelings of guilt abound, and patient and family may tend to withdraw from one another, emotionally if not physically.

Obviously, the impact of illness depends heavily on which member of the family is affected. It's difficult to generalize about the functions served by various members of the family, because the nature of the family itself and sex roles in our culture generally are currently in such flux. While everything I say must be qualified by this awareness, the prevalence of such uncertainty itself suggests certain kinds of pressures.

A typical family now (increasingly) is a unit isolated from other relatives, composed of only two adults, each with only partially defined roles, held together only by emotional attraction and generally elusive traditions of family stability. The welfare of the children per se is less a stabilizing force toward marital stability than it has been in the past. If one adult becomes seriously ill, the other may have relatively few resources available to shoulder the responsibilities heretofore carried by two able adults—plus the additional strain and financial obligations incurred in the course of caring for the sick individual. In such circumstances, many families become heavily dependent on institutional resources and the sometimes impersonal and seemingly insensitive individuals who staff them.

While sexual stereotypes are changing, the traditional stereotypes are easiest to talk about. I ask that you make whatever extrapolations are necessary when the family you are caring for has a woman as principal breadwinner, or a house-husband, or a single parent struggling to carry the roles of both mother and father.

The stereotypic male/husband/father sees himself as being an active person, the family's primary financial provider, and a source of personal strength to his family. In the face of impaired ability and increased passivity that illness so often involves, he feels anxiety and even shame. He sees illness not only as an unpleasant experience, but also as an emasculating one. His illness impairs his ability to provide financially and the family may lose prestige in their community as well. The typical young family is plagued by debt, and cutting down current spending may barely diminish monthly cash outlays over the near future. When the husband comes home from the hospital, he must be cared for by the wife, who can no longer fully care for the children, who in turn often have difficulty understanding their mother's limitations. In addition, their father's presence in the home during the daytime may seem disruptive to all concerned: he isn't used to being there, he feels uncomfortable being there, and he intrudes upon interactions which previously belonged solely to mother and children.

The traditional woman/wife/mother sees herself and is seen by her family as being the house organizer, the glue that holds the family together, the primary nurturing agent for all the others. Her illness typically results in considerable domestic disorganization. There is no one to look after the others, and no one else to look after her. Home

care during illness of most family members is usually the family responsibility of the mother; when she is sick, everyone else has to pick
up the burden, but generally without her skills.

Illness in children, however heartbreaking or painful, is usually the
least disruptive of all, so long as the two adults are healthy. However,
anyone who knows a family in which one child has had a serious or
prolonged illness knows that this "least disruptive" circumstance can
still be very disruptive indeed. The sick child can consume enormous
parental time and emotional energy. The parents consequently have
less of these qualities to devote to one another or to the children.
Sibling rivalries with the sick child, tinged with envy and guilt, are the
rule; and the ostensibly healthy children often tend to develop somatic
complaints with which the parents may have relatively little patience.

The Family and the Hospital

It used to be that illness was handled within the family and within the
home. The physician, to be sure, might often make house calls to
continually assess progress and make technical suggestions, but it was
the family who provided nursing care, and the home was the arena in
which care was delivered. People went to hospitals only to die. Hospitals became a locus for delivering care to nonterminal patients not only
as a consequence of technical medical knowledge and the centraliza-
tion of sophisticated equipment and personnel, but also because the
modern, intensely busy, nonextended family tends to be poorly organized to provide sick care in a home setting. The hospital therefore
often provides a functional alternative to the family itself, and many of
the stresses and virtues inherent in its function can be laid to this fact.
Hospitalizing a patient takes enormous pressure off a family in most
instances, but it also serves as a stimulus for envy and hostility. Like a
mistress who serves a recognizable need, the hospital is nonetheless
often resented for providing a service many guiltily feel should be
taken care of at home.

It's a problem not only for the family, but for the staff as well. The
staff keenly feels its role as surrogate family, though most members of
the staff don't articulate these feelings quite so blatantly. Nonetheless,
staff commonly act in a manner which says: "I know what's best for
the patient, and the family doesn't. I am acting in the patient's best
interests, and the family isn't. If the family cared as much for the
patient as they should, they would act in thus-and-so manner." The
end result, sometimes, is to pit staff and family against one another in
mock combat for the distinction of having the patient's best interests at
heart. This is particularly likely to happen with long-stay patients, with
whom staff develop personally important relationships.

When family members enter the hospital, in the course of their concern for the patient, they tend to become dominated by the hospital atmosphere. Yet they often feel peripheral to what is going on. The doctor and staff tend to concentrate on the patient. In general, the more complex the hospital setting, the less time and interest staff have for family. Family members are tolerated usually within narrowly prescribed visiting hours, but their attendance is often not encouraged.

In fact, family members usually feel—and are often regarded by staff as being—in the way. Whenever anything important is to happen with the patient—a lumbar puncture, a catheter change, a trip to radiotherapy—they are asked to leave and wait elsewhere. As a consequence, many family members feel a sense of alienation from their patient-relative, and they feel isolated from and ignorant of the evolution of events which play an important role in their own lives. They may in such circumstances view doctors and other hospital staff not as allies, but as barriers between themselves and their relative. They may see *you* as a divisive factor in their own family, and they may be jealous of your intimacy with their relative at the same time they are being estranged.

Members of the family, waiting among faceless strangers in a frightening and morbid environment, have a lot of time to brood over such matters. They are likely to become emotionally and physically fatigued, and tempers get frayed. Meetings in hospitals in the event of family sickness may represent a significant occasion for family members to get together who haven't seen one another for months or years. If relationships were strained before, the hospital gatherings may be marked by guilt, resentment, and blaming. It's not surprising that hospital staff sometimes get some of the spin-off.

Under the circumstances, physician and staff may be reluctant to get involved with the family, even if their usually hectic schedules allow them an opportunity to do so. If you don't know what family members think or want, you don't have to respond. If you suspect that family interactions are like a tag-team wrestling match, it feels safer to avoid contacts completely. This "avoidance" line of thinking is certainly understandable, but it represents a narrower approach to human health care than most of us are capable of.

Besides, in moments when we aren't under stress or facing multiple demands on our time and energy, it's easy to empathize with our patient's families. They are in a lousy situation. Many of us have faced illness in our own families and have struggled with the human problems involved. However, for us it's always easier than for the average family member of a hospitalized patient. We know the language and the territory—we can sort out the competent physician, technician, and nurse from the incompetent. We know how to use the system to the benefit of those we love, and we know how to make our voices heard. The average family is less likely to have such advantages.

Assessing Families

While finding out the bare outlines of what is going on in a family can sometimes be difficult, usually it is not. If you make yourself available, show your interest, ask a few questions and then be quiet and listen, you can usually expect a gush of information. The areas to be concerned about are the following:

1. In what way is the family at risk? How was the family system functioning before the illness, and how has the fact of illness altered the balance? Who is carrying the patient's responsibilities, and is anyone overburdened? In what ways are the patient and family able to help one another, and in what ways do they add to one another's burdens? Do family members have access to whatever resources they need to cope effectively? What are the epidemiologic risks, and how are these perceived by the family? Is anyone concerned about infectious or genetic or indirect effects on other family members, and does the family need counseling or further discussion in this regard?

2. What is the family's role in this patient's care and treatment? What are the strengths of its members? What are the family's views of illness in general? Do members regard the illness as a stigma or punishment for previous sins, or as a ticket to avoiding responsibility? Are their views consonant with those of the patient, yourself, and other medical personnel involved? What are their views on medical care? Do they view you and the medical profession generally positively or negatively? Will you be working together on the patient's treatment or at cross purposes?

3. With the hospitalized patient, are members of the family able to spend quality time with the patient? Do they have reasonably private moments together, free of staff and activity? What can be done to help them find some moments together?

4. How do the hospital staff and you view this family? Do you think of the family in respectful terms? Are you beginning to think of members of the family as nuisances, idiots, turkeys, or adversaries? How much are staff attitudes contributing to interactional problems? In what ways can attitudes be altered to facilitate more empathetic and effective treatment?

Guidelines in Dealing with Families

It's possible to treat the disease and not the patient, and it's possible to treat the patient but not the family. The more broadly you conceptualize your role, the more the potential rewards and hassles. Treating families is complicated business, and the process becomes particularly difficult if you work in a setting where you provide episodic care without any long-term understanding of the family as an evolving unit. In order to avoid enormous frustration in your attempts to be helpful to the family, you have to recognize your personal limitations; you can seldom do everything that you or the family might wish you could do.

I offer the following suggestions as a foundation for developing a useful philosophy of family-oriented patient care. If you don't like my suggestions, come up with your own, but try to make explicit the values upon which you base your actions.

Treat the patient in context. Try to get some sense of how what you say or do, or what you ask the patient to do, will affect the patient's life. Telling a mother of three small children to go home and elevate her feet all day may make great medical sense but little common sense. Ask the patient for feedback about your therapeutic recommendations, and search for realistic compromises.

Treat family members as allies in a common cause. Keep open lines of communication. Show respect for them by asking their opinions and treating their suggestions thoughtfully. Even when you disagree with their perspective, say, "I can understand how you feel as you do; I feel somewhat differently; let's see what we can work out." Avoid criticizing or scapegoating members of the family in the event of disagreements or when things don't go as you might have planned. Avoid setting yourself up as a more accurate judge than they of what is good for the patient. Tell them you value their role as quality-control monitors of the patient's care and will appreciate their feedback. Encourage them to express their gripes to you and, if appropriate, to others.

Focus on the family's welfare. From time to time, ask relatives, "How are you doing in all this?" Observe, "Illness is hard on a family, isn't it?" or "You look really worn out by what you've been going through." See that the family gets to spend some good time with the hospitalized patient, ideally without the constant distraction of machines and monitors and procedures by staff. Help the family to feel involved in the treatment process, rather than extraneous to it, by asking for their help. Allowing someone to feel useful is sometimes one of the finest things you can do. Ask them to help with feeding, use of bedpans, or bathing and turning the patient when appropriate. Help the nursing staff not to feel threatened by the family's "intrusion" into providing good, routine nursing care. Help family members to accept their own limitations in the same way that you seem to be accepting of yours.

Urge the family not to fight with the patient over such issues as compliance with medical regimens; e.g., when a patient "cheats" on a low-salt diet: "The patient is old enough to take responsibility for her own body. It's frustrating, but we have to recognize our limitations. I won't fight with the patient, and I urge you not to also." Help them to see the complexity of such situations: "In not arguing, we lose some ground on the water and salt retention, but we help the patient retain some sense of control over her own treatment and allow her some forbidden pleasure with appetizing food. Let's be patient and see if her behavior doesn't gradually improve over time."

Give the family information in a manner in which they can *hear* it. That may take patience, repetition, and privacy to allow for asking questions. The family may be unable to incorporate all the information you give them when they first hear it. Start by explaining the acute condition and work in more information with time. Remember, family members are seldom as interested in data as we are; test results are usually of more interest as an indicator of improvement or deterioration, or of evidence that "something is being done," than for their numerical value per se. If the family requests detailed laboratory data, you can give it to them, but say, "I don't want to get bogged down in detail with you. What you want to know are the implications of my findings, and I will share those with you willingly. Where conclusions are a matter of medical judgment, where my judgment might differ from that of other conscientious qualified physicians, I will tell you. Where conclusions are a matter of human values and where professional qualifications take a second seat, I will tell you that also." Of course, we ourselves have to be aware of such distinctions, and focus attention on making them, before we can convey them to the patient's family.

Anticipate common family problems associated with serious illness and hospitalization, and counsel the family accordingly. A little anticipatory guidance will help prevent staff-family conflict and will reveal you to the family as someone who is empathetic, concerned, and knowledgeable. If you anticipate a postoperative confusional episode, warn the family so they won't be terrified to see the patient "losing his mind." Warn them about the apathy, depression, regression, and anger that are a natural consequence of prolonged hospitalization. Prepare them for the expected evolution of their own feelings if, for example, the patient is terminal. Emphasize that a sequence of emotional responses is the rule, and they needn't be ashamed of their feelings.

Set up communication patterns in a manner that will be comfortable for those concerned, including yourself. Say, "I don't have time to meet with each of you separately, but I would be glad to meet with all of you at once or speak with one person who will act as a representative." Be careful about privileged information; in general, don't divulge any of the patient's confidences without the patient's permission. If the family asks you about such a matter, say, "You'll have to ask the patient about that." If that results in some awkwardness for you, say so: "Frankly, I would prefer to be able to discuss everything openly with you; if you and the patient can reach an agreement, I'll be happy to abide by your mutual decision." In general, refer questions from friends of the family to the family itself, unless you are explicitly advised otherwise by the patient.

Treat the angry or accusative family member with patience and understanding. Avoid a defensive posture. Remember that frustration, irritation, and anger are normal responses in the illness situation. With your demeanor as well as your words say, "Given your experiences and perception, it's certainly understandable that you feel as you do." After a family member has had a chance to ventilate his or her feelings, say, "Given that you feel as you do, I'm certainly glad you expressed yourself rather than keeping everything bottled up inside. Now, let's see if we can deal with some of your concerns."

Preparing for Discharge and Home Care

Medical training for physicians has tended to focus on hospital care of the seriously ill, and most of us have a tendency to neglect posthospital care. If we get our satisfaction from care of the acutely ill patient, the rehabilitative aspects of the patient's treatment is likely to get inadequate attention unless we make sure that someone else picks up where we leave off. Ideal discharge planning involves developing a program that won't disrupt family life, treats the family unit with respect, utilizes the patient's and the family's retained skills, and allows the family to have input and to make choices when acceptable alternatives are available.

The higher the criteria for patient well-being prior to discharge, the fewer detailed plans are necessary for postdischarge care. However, if you are under considerable pressure from a hospital utilization review committee to discharge patients as soon as they are able to go, you may need to devote more attention to planning for home care. In addition, the patient who adapts best to being in the hospital may in fact be the least prepared to leave. Anyone who is totally passive, compliant, and happy in the hospitalized patient role may not only be reluctant to leave the hospital, but may not put a lot of energy into self-care after discharge.

The transition from hospital to home is often a difficult one for both patient and family. The patient tends to be weak and relatively more helpless than normal, ability to cope with stresses is reduced, and there is consequently the likelihood of increased susceptibility to stress. The family, too, may be fearful of what new responsibilities may be required of them, as well as their lack of knowledge in dealing with medical signs and symptoms. It's helpful if they can get good instruction in such matters from nursing staff prior to discharge, and even more helpful if they have an opportunity to practice routine nursing care.

After a prolonged hospitalization, it is not uncommon for a patient to develop a recurrence of presenting symptoms prior to discharge; e.g., MI patients may develop some angina. Patients become concerned about their ability to perform adequately without supervision. It's easy to empathize with patients in this regard when we reflect about the kinds of anxieties which perfectly competent interns and residents are likely to have at the conclusion of their training; the idea of being out on one's own without supervision, again a novice struggling with the unknown, creates understandable concerns. Some debilitated patients, especially the elderly, fear leaving the hospital because they are reluctant to become dependent upon individuals who are not paid to take care of them. They feel keenly their lack of ability to be of assistance in return. Whatever the specifics, the transition from hospital to home often results in some emotional ups and downs, with some irritability on the part of all involved.

For some, recuperation involves a loss. A patient leaves a hospital, in which he or she was surrounded by caring people, to go home to a situation where daytimes may be quite lonely, with everyone else at work or school and no one available to provide support and nurturance. The patient will miss the hospital staff's understanding, concern, and assistance with daily tasks.

If the family is to experience a major dilemma once the patient is home, the difficulty commonly centers on issues of dependence and independence, promoting invalidism at one extreme versus premature activity and unrealistically high expectations on the other. The physician wonders, Will detailed discharge planning foster prolonged social dependency, or does sending the patient out of the hospital on his or her own constitute a form of abandonment? The best course usually is to bring the issue out in the open, and help patient and family make informed decisions which rightly belong to them.

Community Resources

The primary problem with community resources concerns helping patient and family know about what is specifically available to them among a seeming abundance of potential aids. Stumbling blocks commonly are accessibility and eligibility. Some skilled social workers, psychiatrists, or clergymen are extremely knowledgeable about such resources, while others are not. Often patients with similar health problems can provide useful consultation. Persistent individuals can gain assistance from reference librarians in the public library or even by combing through the yellow pages of the phone book and calling likely looking numbers under such headings as associations (fraternal, religious, et cetera), charitable organizations, social service and welfare organizations, health agencies, and the like. However, mobilizing all potentially available resources will often require aggressive prodding by family and patient.

Potential resources may depend on the patient's race, religion, place of residence, ethnicity, previous military service, age, and membership in fraternal or other organizations. Resources for particular patients with particular problems may be available free, subsidized, on a volunteer basis, or on a sliding scale. Many disabled individuals qualify for state or federal monthly stipends or are eligible for low-cost loans or for payments for special purposes. The availability of special services covers a broad range which most patients wouldn't even think to ask about: license plates for the disabled that allow special access parking, free bus tickets for companions traveling with handicapped persons, transcribers and readers for the visually impaired, and so forth. Attendant care is sometimes available to help with errands, chores, and housework. Other potential resources include employment counseling, legal aid, housing assistance, educational guidance, and personal counseling. The point is that there is often a great deal of help available which patient and family may never know about unless someone takes the responsibility for nudging them in the appropriate direction.

All available community resources are potentially useful; actual usefulness must be decided by recipients of services. If you know a particular service to be especially helpful, tell the family, but avoid cramming it down their collective throat. If you think a given service is unlikely to be helpful, say, "I don't believe you will find that useful, but you might." Since you can never know for sure, don't say, "You don't need that."

Few families are set up for home care of the seriously ill individual, but lately there has been a resurgence of interest in what traditionally had been regarded as a common family responsibility. The task is often emotionally wearing, with many procedural difficulties, but it offers the interested family a challenge with enormous potential pleasure and satisfaction too.

If a family decides to take on the responsibility for home care of a seriously ill person, help them to anticipate potential difficulties and give them some idea of how to arrange phone consultations when they need them. A doctor who gives a damn will be an enormous comfort. Equally important, the family should have a network of friends, neighbors, or relatives to make a successful go of it.

If the patient is to have significant problems with pain, nausea, and vomiting, or open wounds and bedsores, you can expect to hear about them and guide the family at that time. You are somewhat less likely to hear about bowel or bladder incontinence unless you ask specifically, and almost no family complains about patient-generated odors—sometimes a major source of frustration at home. Families are least likely to complain about low-level confusional episodes, though you will want to be alert to their potential diagnostic importance and will want to know when they occur. Confusion is also something the family can often do something about, with your help, and which will make home care much more pleasant for all concerned.

Some circumstances are filled with so much pathos that they will break your heart, and you will wonder how the family manages to survive, let alone in good spirits. The loneliness and frustration of the dysphasic hemiplegic patient and the family are terrible to observe.

Where possible, suggest that the family find simple chores for the patient, both so the patient can contribute to household work, and as a way of preserving self-respect. Remember, any family who undertakes home care of a seriously ill patient deserves your respect and understanding. They also need a break from time to time, too. "Social admissions" have traditionally provided this kind of relief, but are becoming much more difficult to sneak past utilization-review committees and third-party payers, but they remain a humane and sometimes necessary tool for a stressed family doing its best under difficult circumstances.

If a family declines to attempt home care, or members find themselves unable to continue once begun, avoid becoming judgmental. The difficulty is at least as attributable to changing social patterns as to any basic abdication of responsibilities by the specific family involved. The latter will have to struggle with their own guilt and fears and inadequacies; don't make it any worse for them.

Bereavement, Grief, and Mourning

Notifying the family of the death of a loved one is something no doctor enjoys doing. I always hate the task, even when I know that the family will be relieved to hear that the patient's suffering is over. Even when I, too, am relieved that the patient is dead, I feel a vague sense of guilt and failure at my inability to forestall the inevitable. My feelings must show a bit too, because even though I do my best to comfort and console the family, it's disconcerting to find how often they try to console me in return: "It's okay, Doctor, I know you did what you could." Actually, that usually makes both of us feel better, a helpful recognition that we're all human and caring can be reciprocal.

Bereavement refers to the state of being deprived of a loved one by death. Grief and mourning are common experiences for the bereaved person. Indeed, some writers believe they are a necessary part of a long-term adjustment to significant personal loss.

The initial reaction depends upon the person's relationship to the deceased, the nature of the death, whether it was expected or unexpected, and whether the person feels in any way responsible for the occurrence. Responses may cover a broad range of emotions including shock, disbelief, grief, emotional dullness, feeling "numbed," despair, resentment, guilt, anger, emptiness, and loneliness. The duration of the initial response may be a few hours to a few weeks. Commonly, the intensity of the response is at its peak a day or two *after* first notification of death.

The long-term response to bereavement may last months or years. After the death of a significant loved one, persons often go through a persistent depression, getting little pleasure out of their normal activities, often withdrawing from social contacts, performing poorly on the job or at school, and becoming vulnerable to a variety of physical problems. There is a tendency to be neglectful of oneself, to lose one's customary regard for personal safety, to become bored with life, and to become overly dependent upon alcohol. Many individuals become obsessed with thoughts of death; questioning the meaning of life, blaming and punishing themselves for things they did that they wish they hadn't, and things they did not do that they wish they had done.

Your approach to the bereaved family or bereaved individual depends upon when you see them. If long-term contact is possible, that will provide you with an extra tool to work with, and you needn't feel that you have to accomplish everything in one sitting. Regardless of what you say and how you say it, your interchange with the family will probably go better if it takes place in reasonable privacy. Get the family out of a busy waiting room or noisy corridor and into a place in which you can talk with at least a semblance of intimacy. Your goals are to help the survivors live with decreased stress, increased comfort and productivity, and decreased morbidity and mortality.

In dealing with acute grief, the most common urgent need is for catharsis. Encourage bereaved persons to let their feelings out. They should not be left alone at this time; someone needs to be with them, but it needn't be you. If you need to leave to see another patient, tell them, "Take as much time as you need; I'm going to step out and see another patient, but I'll be back shortly." After a suitable period of ventilating feelings, the bereaved person is ready to leave, but again should be encouraged to have someone with whom to stay. Many individuals appreciate some sedation for the first night or two after the death of a loved one. Before the bereaved person leaves, encourage them to be patient with themselves. Help them to understand that their feelings are natural and serve an important function. Say, "What you will feel in the days and weeks ahead is the cost of loving someone." Encourage the bereaved to find someone with whom they can discuss their feelings on a continuing basis in the months ahead. If you will be filling this function, you will want to keep the following considerations in mind:

Bereaved persons need stability. Caution them against making major changes until they make a reasonable accomodation to the recent dramatic loss in their life.

Caution bereaved persons to pay special attention to their physical health over the months ahead, and to see their own physician for a physical examination and continuing health maintenance. The loss of a loved one is the single most serious threat to one's own resistance to disease, and therefore a bereaved person can expect to be at risk for illness across a broad spectrum. Warn family members to look after one another in this regard.

Encourage the bereaved to share their distress in order to help moderate it. Potential counselors include funeral directors, church members, various self-help groups, friends and family, and of course their physician. Warn them that others in the family will be bereaved too, often feeling a broad range of emotions, often with little patience for one another. Under the circumstances, it may be hard for one family member to provide much nurturance for another. Warn them: "People will feel awkward with you, and many won't know what to say. Though you want people to be patient and understanding with you, the people around you will be most helpful to you if you are flexible in receiving the kind of help that they can give."

Warn them that the process of mourning is something which takes time. For some people it goes on months and even years. You needn't tell them this all right away, but you should understand it yourself and be able to give insight and perspective as called for. The bereaved person can expect listlessness, feelings of emptiness, and emotions to evolve through a natural dynamic process. In the meantime, they will do well to be patient with themselves, taking one day at a time. Over the long haul, they may have difficulty associating the manifestations of the grieving process with the loss itself. Grief comes out in strange ways: in dreams and nightmares many months hence, in "strange" reactions to events and places associated with the deceased loved one, and in "anniversary reactions" for landmark events over the years ahead.

Often bereaved persons go through a period in which there is a tendency to idealize the deceased person. That, too, is natural enough; but some persons need to ventilate negative feelings regarding the deceased in order to see the dead person as the human being, good and bad, that he or she really was.

Over the long haul, the life and death of the deceased person is a part of the personal history of the survivor. Putting one's own personal history in perspective is an opportunity for personal growth available to all of us. Dealing effectively with the mortality of those we love can be a useful step in helping us to come to terms with our own mortality. But don't ever tell anyone that it will be painless.

Bibliography

Anstett RE, Poole SR, Morrison J: The single parent family. *J Fam Pract* 14:581–586, 1982

Beam IM: Helping families survive. *Am J Nursing* February 1984, pp 228–232

Bergquist B: The remarried family—an annotated bibliography, 1979–1982. *Family Process* 23:107–119, 1984

Boyle JF: The diminishing family and its impact on health. *Del Med J* 55:515–525, 1983

Burns CE: The hospitalization experience and single parent families. *Nurs Clin No Amer* 19:285–293, 1984

Frey J: A family systems approach to illness maintaining behaviors in chronically ill adolescents. *Family Process* 23:251–260, 1984

Gilliss CL: Reducing family stress during and after coronary artery bypass surgery. *Nurs Clin No Amer* 19:103–112, 1984

Hagen DQ: The relationship between job loss and physical and mental illness. *Hosp Comm Psychiatry* 34:438–441, 1983

Haggerty JJ: The psychosomatic family. *Psychosomatics* 24:615–623, 1983

Howard J: *Families.* New York, Simon & Schuster, 1978

Jaffe DT: The role of family therapy in treating physical illness. *Hosp Community Psychiatry* 29:169–174, 1978

Keith PM, Schafer RB: Role behavior and psychological well-being—a comparison of men in one-job and two-job families. *Amer J Orthopsychiat* 54:137–145, 1984

Leavitt MB: *Families at Risk.* Boston, Little, Brown, 1982

Litman TJ: The family as a basic unit in health and medical care—a socio behavioral overview. *Soc Sci Med* 8:495–519, 1974

Northouse L: The impact of cancer on the family. *Intl J Psychiatry in Medicine* 14:215–228, 1984

Racy JC: The family and chronic disease. *Ariz Med* 40:854–857, 1983

Richtsmeier AJ, Waters DB: Somatic symptoms as family myth. *Am J Dis Child* 138:855–857, 1984

Sabbeth B: Understanding the impact of chronic childhood illnesses on families. *Ped Clinics No America* 31:47–57, 1984

Spanier GB: The changing profile of the American family. *J Fam Pract* 13:61–69, 1981

Stubbs DE, Yates A: Stress and the role of the family in psychosomatic illness. *Ariz Med* 41:324–327, 1984

Taylor RB: The extended family encounter. *Am Fam Physician* 22:119–121, 1980

Walker LG, Thomson N, Lindsay WR: Assessing family relationships. *Brit J Psychiat* 144:387–394, 1984

Wessel MA: A death in the family. *Medical Opinion,* April 1976, pp 32–35

14

Psychotherapeutic Medications in the Physically Ill

The desire to take medicine is perhaps the greatest feature which distinguishes man from animals.
—Sir William Osler

I firmly believe that if the whole materia medica, as now used, could be sunk to the bottom of the sea, it would be all the better for mankind—and all the worse for the fishes.
—Oliver Wendell Holmes

One should bear in mind that to take anti-psychotic drugs, one must be crazy, either literally or figuratively.
—Leo Hollister

Though in general I encourage you to use human rather than chemical treatment, psychochemotherapeutic agents can be useful; and, when they are needed, they are a godsend.

Before discussing specific agents and situations, I would like to emphasize several basic principles.

1. Use only a few medications and know them well. It is difficult for most of us to remember all the details concerning all the drugs mentioned in this chapter, especially if we use them infrequently. We needn't apologize for the limitations of our knowledge so long as we know what they are and know where to look up additional information when the necessity arises.

2. With any given patient, use the least possible number of drugs. Medication errors, in and out of the hospital, are extremely common, with the likelihood rising in direct proportion to the number of drugs used. Error can take the form of the wrong drug being given, the right drug being given to the wrong patient, mistake in dosage, and mistake in timing. In addition, the more drugs used, the greater the chance of

side effects, idiosyncratic reaction, and drug reaction. While some drug interactions are well known and have been included in this chapter for your reference, almost nothing is known about interactions which develop when *more* than two drugs are being used simultaneously. Proceed with caution.

3. Whenever you use a psychotherapeutic medication, have a specific target symptom in mind by which you can judge the effectiveness of your treatment. Global or vague indications, such as "bizarre," "psychotic," "nuts," are seldom enough. Be as precise as you can. If your target symptoms consist of auditory hallucinations, attempt to understand exactly what the voices are saying to the patient so that you can continually assess the patient's intellectual functioning for their presence. you can't know if your treatment is successful when you don't know what you're trying to treat.

4. If you are attempting to modify the patient's behavior, ask To whom is this behavior troublesome? Is the behavior in fact adaptive for the patient? For example, restless pacing is one adaptive way to deal with anxiety. The pacing may bother other people around the patient, but not the patient. You may end up dealing with the patient more effectively by trying to direct the pacing, rather than by subduing it with medication. For instance, you might suggest that the hospitalized patient walk in the lobby rather than in the ward corridor at night when the other patients are trying to sleep.

5. Initially, give medications in divided daily doses until you learn how much medication the patient needs on a daily basis. If the patient requires maintenance medication, try switching to a single h.s. dose. Virtually all phenothiazines, butyrophenones, thioxanthenes, and tricyclic antidepressants can be prescribed on a once-a-day schedule. Advantages include reducing the need for nighttime sedation, increased dispensing convenience, focusing mild bothersome side effects (such as dry mouth) at night when the patient is asleep, and establishing a regimen which is easier for the patient to continue as directed.

6. Adjust the dosage to your specific patient. Most psychotherapeutic agents can be used across a wide dosage range. Don't be afraid of high doses in carefully monitored situations, especially in the hospital in an acute situation, but avoid high doses for maintenance.

7. Tell the patient what medication you are giving him, for what indications, and on what schedule. It is, after all, the patient's body that is being medicated, and he or she has a right to know what is going into it. In addition, the knowledgeable patient, whether having hallucinations or not, is always a potential asset in his or her own treatment. The frequency of medication errors can be minimized if you keep the patient informed. Remember that in our increasingly complex health care system, more and more patients are under the care of multiple

physicians and therefore may be getting prescription drugs you will only know about if you remember to ask.

8. Do whatever you can to keep total drug dosage down in patients who are on maintenance medications. Consider "drug holidays" in which some or all medications are discontinued for brief periods at regular intervals (e.g., each Sunday or each weekend). This helps to minimize total drug dosage, minimizes side effects, reduces cost, and gives the sensitive physician an opportunity to assess the patient's functioning during drug-free intervals of various lengths.

9. Continually assess whether the medication is doing the job you have in mind for it. If patients don't show the expected response to any given psychotherapeutic agent, first determine if they are taking the medication as you prescribed it. In the hospital, tablets and capsules are particularly likely to be sequestered in the mouth and then spit out when the nurse has gone elsewhere. Elixirs are much less likely to avoid ingestion (though more complicated if your pharmacy operates on a unit-dose system), and parenterally administered agents are by far the most reliably incorporated into the body. If the patient has not been taking a medication as prescribed, it is time to sit down with him or her and ask why. Maybe there's good reason.

With any psychotropic medication, you must consider the possible deleterious effect of overdose. If a given patient uses a prescribed medication in an overdose, how serious will the consequences be? This question should be asked with any patient who is depressed, or whom you don't know very well. Never supply the patient with a potentially lethal dose of medication unless you are confident that there is absolutely no risk of overdose. If in doubt, discuss the matter frankly with the patient, including your own reluctance to be the instrument of some else's death.

The following represents the ratio between the potentially lethal dose and the average daily dose for a given patient. For example, a ratio of 12:1 means that a 12 day supply is potentially lethal. Consequently, the figure after each agent represents the maximum supply of drug which can be given to a patient with reasonable comfort by the clinician. Each figure represents an approximation, designed to give a workable order of magnitude only:

Monoamine oxidase inhibitors: 10 to 12 days

Tricyclic antidepressants: 5 to 7 days

Benzodiazapines: 30 to 60 days

Phenothiazines: 30 to 60 days

Suppose a patient has been maintained on a psychoactive medication for appropriate indications and, during the course of maintenance therapy, develops an infrequent but known and serious complication: e.g., a patient taking thioridazine develops bone-marrow depression. You discontinue the drug, treat concomitant problems (e.g., infection), the complication remits after a week or two, and then the original psychiatric symptoms return. Assuming that either the patient or those in the environment find those symptoms intolerable, your treatment options are several: gingerly reinstitute the same medication, switch to another drug in the same pharmacologic group (i.e., a congener), change to a drug in another group entirely, or institute nondrug somatic therapies, (for example, electroconvulsive therapy). You will probably want to have a psychiatric consultation in such matters (especially, of course with ECT) not only for the decision itself, but because the person who will have ongoing responsibility for the patient's care deserves an opportunity to voice an opinion in major therapeutic decisions.

In the pages that follow, I will focus on patterns of drug usage and side effects in the physically ill. The specifics are included primarily to emphasize areas of concern. You know that styles change in drug treatment as they do in everything else and that new indications, contraindications, and side effects will be discovered, while others are discarded, as time goes along. My expectation is that you know of all the drugs mentioned here, at least by name, and I won't discuss their structure, general uses, or metabolism. Before you use any of these agents, you will obviously want to have a fuller understanding of the pharmacology than can be gathered from this one brief chapter.

Though the evidence is sometimes flimsy for linking a specific drug with a specific idiosyncratic reaction, I have included it anyway. Simple prudence dictates that we avoid prescribing a specific agent whenever suspicion exists that doing so will cause more harm than good.

Drug Interactions

The list of drug interactions (Table 14.1) serves primarily to place patterns of drug behavior in a readily accessible place. You are unlikely to remember many such details unless you prescribe a given drug frequently, but as long as you remember that tricyclic antidepressants have many drug interactions, you can return to this chapter to remind yourself of the specifics.

Most interactions simply create difficulties in juggling dosages and titrating the medications against troublesome, but not very dangerous, side effects. The relatively few interactions that pose potentially grave dangers are 1) monoamine oxidase inhibitors narcotics, sympathomimetics, or tyramine, 2) antipsychotics and lithium*, and 3) anticoagulants with phenobarbitol and other enzyme-inducing drugs.

Table 14.1. Catalogue of Major Drug Interactions

Primary psychoactive agent	Interacts with
Monoamine oxidase inhibitors	Amphetamines, anticholinergics, barbiturates, carbamazepine (TEGRETOL), dextromethorphan, doxopram, ephedrine, L-dopa, methyldopa (ALDOMET), methylphenidate (RITALIN), guanadrel, metaraminol (ARAMINE), methotrimeprazine (LEVOPROME), meperidine (DEMEROL), phenylephrine, phenylpropanolamine, propranolol (INDERAL) succinyl choline, sympathomimetics, tricyclic antidepressants, tyramine-containing foods or drinks (e.g., Chianti, cheese, yogurt)
Tricyclic antidepressants	Monoamine oxidase inhibitors, ethchlorvinol (PLACIDYL), meperidine (DEMEROL) and narcotic analgesics, coumarin compounds, barbiturates, levodopa, sympathomimetic amines (e.g., epinephrine, ephedrine, phenylephrine, norepinephrine, amphetamines), in elderly patients any drug with anticholinergic effects (e.g., antihistamines, antiparkinsonians, glutethimide, phenothiazines), and many antihypertensives
Haloperidol	Lithium, indomethacin, barbiturates, phenytoin
Lithium	Haloperidol, methyldopa, amphetamines, indomethacin, phenothiazines, and most diuretics
Meprobamate	Coumarin compounds
Disulfiram (ANTABUSE)	Ethanol (topical, oral, parental), benzodiazepines, isomiazid paraldehyde, coumarin compounds, phenytoin
Benzodiazepines	Cimetidine, disulfiram
Phenothiazines	Levodopa, propranolol, guanadrel, barbiturates, guanethidine, phenytoin, lithium

Concurrent use of one agent while the other is physiologically active in any given patient may result in significant potentiation of, or deleterious side-effects by, one or both agents, making combined use ill-advised or contraindicated. Do not use together without careful study of reference material.

---

* The combination of lithium and various high-potency antipsychotic drugs has been implicated in a variety of neurologic syndromes, some quite severe and irreversible. Though the final word is not in, cautious non-psychiatrists should get consultation before administering these drugs in combination.

Increased or decreased responses are not always harmful, and may even be helpful. Usually they simply constitute more details to be kept track of.

There are several kinds of drug interactions which I have not bothered to list. All readers will be familiar with the fact that central nervous system depressants in general tend to have a synergistic effect when prescribed with one another. For example, benzodiazapines and narcotics both may produce central nervous system depression, the combined effect of which will be greater than with either agent used alone, but their combined usage is still acceptable on an empirical basis. However, prudence is the rule, and both you and the patient must be aware of potential problems. Neither have I made any attempt to list drug interactions which don't require special precautions beyond the kind of observation that one would expect from physicians when they are treating a medical condition which warrants the use of a specific drug; e.g., any patient whose hypertension is sufficiently severe to warrant treatment with guanethidine will presumably be monitored more closely than a hypertensive patient who is being treated with hydrochlorothiazide.

Drug Side Effects

The list of drug side effects (Table 14.2) is largely for reference and to jog your memory: I assume you are already familiar with important side effects of drugs you prescribe. If in doubt, consult the standard references on clinical pharmacology, the appropriate resources cited at the end of this chapter, or a knowledgeable pharmacologist or pharmacist.

The list of drugs in each class and the brand names for each listed drug are not intended to be comprehensive. Psychochemotherapeutic agents are among the most numerous medications, and brand name preparations are proportionately plentiful.

My categorization of the frequency of side effects is based upon those reported in the literature and my own experience. The intent is to give a general sense of how often you are likely to encounter certain problems, but the lists are by no means exhaustive. Other writers would maintain that some of the findings I list under "Other adverse and toxic effects" should really be listed under "common side effects," or, in other cases, under "idiosyncratic and hypersensitivity reactions." You can safely assume, however, that none of what I labeled idiosyncratic reactions would be called a common side effect by someone else or vice versa.

The term *anticholinergic side effects,* which appears often in Table 14.2, refers to a set of phenomena with which most physicians are quite familiar. Mostly, these include bothersome but not very dangerous occurrences such as blurred vision, dry mouth, minor constipation, et cetera. However, in elderly and debilitated patients, the same pharmacologic effects can assume far greater importance. In such patients, watch for paralytic ileus, closed-angle glaucome, urinary retention, and the like.

Minor Tranquilizers

The so-called minor tranquilizers are used primarily for the symptomatic treatment of anxiety. The benzodiazapines are the mainstay of this group, though the propanediols and various antihistaminic and sedative hypnotics are sometimes substituted. Drug tolerance develops with virtually all of these agents, so whereas it makes sense to prescribe them for a few days or on an occasional as-needed basis there are few indications for prescribing these medications on a recurrent daily basis. Chronic medication-taking by the patient depends largely upon chronic medication-prescribing by the physician, and neither doctor nor patient are at their best with chronic use of minor tranquilizers.

The benzodiazapines themselves are remarkably safe. It is usually possible to find a dose which is therapeutic without being toxic. The danger of serious interactions with other medication is small, though of course there is some danger of synergism with other central nervous system depressants at high doses.

Hydroxyzine (ATARAX, VISTARIL) is regarded by many as a safe alternative to the benzodiazapines. So far as we know, there is no hepatotoxicity and no bone-marrow depression associated with this medication. Though experience with this medication is more limited, side effects appear to be of the minor, bothersome variety.

There are many additional nonbarbiturate hypnotics that are sometimes used for their antianxiety properties, particularly for insomnia. These mostly share the side effects of the barbiturates. However, these agents come from a variety of chemical classes, and keeping track of idiosyncratic reactions for them is very difficult, unless you use them frequently or have a particular affinity for such detail. Examples of such agents include ethchlorvynol (PLACIDYL) and methyprylon(NOLUDAR).

Major Tranquilizers

The major tranquilizers are variously also called neuroleptics and antipsychotic agents. The phenothiazines are by far the most commonly used and best studied of these drugs. The thioxanthenes closely approximate the phenothiazines in structure and function, but the bu-

276

Table 14.2 Side Effects of Psychotherapeutic Drugs

Class and Drug	Common side effects	Other adverse and toxic effects	Idiosyncratic and hypersensitivity reactions
Propanediols Meprobamate (MILTOWN, EQUANIL) Tybamate (SOLACEN, TYBATRAN)	Drowsiness; ataxia; incoordination; dizziness; hypotension; tolerance and physical dependence	Alcohol intolerance; rashes; vomiting; paresthesias; blurred vision	Blood dyscrasias; stomatitis; mastitis with lactation; ? teratogenicity (first 6 weeks); bullous dermatitis; precipitation of seizures; erythema multiforme
Benzodiazepines Chlordiazepoxide (LIBRIUM) Diazepam (VALIUM) Oxazepam (SERAX) Flurazepam (DALMANE)	Drowsiness; ataxia; tolerance and physical dependence; mental obtundation	Hypotension; confusion; agitation; excitement; hallucinations; nightmares; depression	Rash, photosensitivity, purpura; leukocytosis; cosinophilia; ? cardiac arrest (VALIUM IV): ? teratogenicity (first 6 weeks); ? hepatotoxicity (rare)
Antihistaminics Diphenhydramine (BENADRYL) Hydroxyzine (ATARAX, VISTARIL) Promethazine (PHENERGAN)	Drowsiness; blurred vision; local discomfort (Parenteral)	Diplopia; nausea; vomiting; hypotension; CNS depression	Seizures in epilepsy; rash; urticaria; granulocytopena; teratogenesis ?
Chloral hydrate	Gastric irritation; hangover effect	CNS depression; ataxia; tolerance, physical dependence	Effect potentiated; liver and kidney disease; rash, urticaria
Barbiturates	Drowsiness; hangover effect; tolerance, physical dependence, ataxia	CNS depression; coma; rash	excitement; trigger acute porphyria; rash, urticaria; fever; megaloblastic anemia

Phenothiazines A. *Aliphatic subgroup* Chlorpromazine (THORAZINE)	Sedation; postural hypotension anticholinergic effects; reduced gag reflex	Parkinsonism, akathisia, dystonic reactions; tardive dyskinesia; impaired ejaculation; proteinuria; photosensitivity; rashes; pigmentation of skin and eye	Cholestatic jaundice: blood dyscrasias
B. *Piperadine sub group* Thioridazine (MELLARIL)	Ejaculatory problems; male impotence; anticholinergic effects; sedation; postural hypotension; reduced gag reflex	Pigmentary retinopathy; EKG abnormalities; arrhythmias; parkinsonism, akathisia; dystonias, tardive dyskinesia	Blood dyscrasias; cholestatic jaundice
C. *Piperazine subgroup* Fluphenazine (PROLIXIN, PERMITIL) Perphenazine (TRILAFON) Trifluoperazine (STELAZINE)	Prakinsonism; akathisia, dystonias; anticholinergic effects; reduced gag reflex	Postural hypotension; photosensitivity; ejaculatory problems; tardive dyskinesia; ocular pigmentation; sleep disturbances	Cholestatic jaundice; blood dyscrasias
Thioxanthenes Thiothixene (NAVANE) Chlorprothixene (TARACTAN)	Drowsiness; anticholinergic effects, including hyperpyrexia	Parkinsonism; akathisia, dystonic reactions; postural hypotension	Blood dyscrasias; photosensitivity; rashes; cholestatic jaundice
Butyrophenones Haloperidol (HALDOL)	Akathisia, dystonic reactions, parkinsonism; anticholinergic effects, including hyperpyrexia	Blood dyscrasias; tardive dyskinesias; postural hypotension; tachycardia, laryngeal-pharyngeal dystenia	Cholestatic jaundice; rashes; photosensitivity

(continued)

Table 14.2 (*Continued*)

Class and Drug	Common side effects	Other adverse and toxic effects	Idiosyncratic and hypersensitivity reactions
Tricyclic Antidepressants Amitryptiline (ELAVIL) Desipramine (NORPRAMIN) Doxepin (SINEQUAN) Imipramine (TOFRANIL) Nortyptiline (AVENTYL)	Anticholinergic effects; blurred vision; dry mouth; hypotension	Cholestatic jaundice; tremor; rashes; first-degree heart block	Bone-marrow depression; epileptiform seizures; sudden death (cardiac patients); peripheral neuropathy; jaundice; myoclonus; tinnitus; severe hyponatremia
Monoamine Oxidase Inhibitors Isocarboxazid (MARPLAN) Phenelzine (NARDIL)	Restlessness; insomnia; nausea, dizziness; dry mouth	Tachycardia; palpitations; blurred vision	Hepatitis; rashes; tinnitus; muscle spasm, tremors; paresthesias; urinary retention; blood dyscrasias
Lithium carbonate (LITHANE) (ESKALITH)	Fine rapid tremor; polyuria; pruritis; slurred speech; sluggishness	Cogwheel rigidity; reversible goiter; hypokalemia; cardiac arrhythmias; renal damage (prolonged treatment); vomiting; diarrhea; blurred vision; tinnitus; rashes; proteinuria; diabetes insipidus	hypothyroidism and hyperthyroidism

CNS–Central nervous system

tyrophenones—while resembling the piperazine phenothiazines in function—represent a distinct chemical group. We have accumulated less extensive clinical experience with some of the newer major tranquilizers (e.g., the dihydroindolones and diabenzoxazepines), and so I have not included them here.

In general medical-surgical hospitals, contrary to popular expectations, the primary diagnosis of those receiving phenothiazines is not psychosis but rather neoplasia. This perhaps reflects the use of phenothiazines in the treatment of anxiety associated with physical disease, and also for nausea and insomnia. The most frequent significant reported side effects involve the central nervous system (drowsiness, disorientation in the elderly, respiratory depression, extrapyramidal symptoms, etc.) with hypotension following close behind.

The major tranquilizers are among the safest categories of drugs in medical practice. We now have an enormous accumulation of experience with use of these agents in high dosages in literally millions of patients. The common side effects tend to occur early in treatment, and are more annoying than dangerous: sedation, weakness, fatigue, mild anticholinergic effects, etc. Side effects tend to be lowest when the dosages are lowest and the agent is used for a short duration, as in for acute anxiety or nausea. Using chlorpromazine as a standard, low dosage is anything less than 100 mg per day.

SIDE EFFECTS OF MAJOR TRANQUILIZERS

Central nervous system side effects of the major tranquilizers take a variety of forms. Of major importance, particularly with the sedating phenothiazines, is the toxic confusional syndrome which can present significant problems in elderly patients. With this single exception, all central nervous system side effects of the major tranquilizers affect neuromotor behavior. Be wary of depressed gag reflexes in patients who are supine, especially if they vomit and are restrained: aspiration may be the primary source of mortality among medical-surgical patients treated with major tranquilizers.

Acute dystonic reaction

This event almost always occurs early in treatment, often following the initial dose within a matter of hours. It is most common with piperazine phenothiazines and can often make its appearance with dramatic intensity. Typically, the patient first complains of "muscles tightening up" and the sensation of an enlarged tongue. Muscle spasms are usually particularly prominent in the head and neck, but may go on to affect the entire body, in extremus producing opisthotonos, carpopedal spasm, and oculogyric crisis. Acute dystonia responds rapidly

to antiparkinsonian agents or diphenhydramine (BENADRYL), prefera-
bly given parenterally if the condition is severe.

Akathisia

This term represents an emotional state which is characterized by a
subjective desire to move and be active. Most patients have a great
deal of difficulty in describing this sensation, though observers may say
that the patient acts as though he "has ants in his pants." The condition usually is mild and requires not treatment. However, if it is sufficiently bothersome, most but no all cases respond to either a decrease
in dosage or the use of antiparkinsonian agents for several days.

Pseudoparkinsonism

This side effect usually occurs early in treatment, and its manifestations are similar to those of parkinsonism itself: poverty of movement
and expression, arms and body held in a flexion posture, a shuffling
gait, a pill-rolling movement of the hands, and excess salivation. Sometimes the condition is only mildly bothersome and requires no special
treatment. Some cases respond to a decrease in dosage and/or antiparkinsonian agents for a few days, while other cases can be more
persistent.

Tardive dyskinesia

This is a phenomenon which, as the word "tardive" suggests, occurs well along in the course of treatment. The dyskinesia consists of
rhythmic involuntary movements, usually concentrated in the tongue,
lips, and cheeks, so that the patient appears to be repeatedly puckering
and smacking the lips. The condition may occur after treatment is
discontinued or while the patient is taking the drug. In the former event
the condition will sometimes be masked if the medication is reinstitu-
ted. With this exception, the condition is usually not reversible and
there is no known treatment.

Other effects

Other long-term effects of phenothiazines, when the total lifetime
dosage is measured in pounds rather than in milligrams, include a
bluish-grayish discoloration of the skin in areas exposed to sun and
pigmentation and/or opacification of various parts of the eye, including
the anterior lens, the anterior cornea, the posterior cornea, the con-
junctiva, and the retina.

Jaundice was a common side effect in the early years of chlorpromazine, but it is now uncommon. When it occurs it is of the cholestatic
variety, and customarily reversible.

To prevent postural hypotension from becoming a problem in an
ambulatory patient taking, e.g., chlorpromazine, warn the patient to

rise slowly. If the patient is not responsive to your instructions, make sure someone else is present when the patient arises. Postural hypotension is rarely a problem in the bedridden patient, since hypotension does not become manifest until the patient leaves the supine position.

Because of the adrenolytic properties (i.e., α blocker) exhibited by phenothiazines, treating profound hypotension—especially that associated with anaphylaxis—is complicated by the "paradoxical effect" of increased hypotension (from β stimulation) when epinephrine (an α and β stimulator) is given. Therefore, epinephrine is to be avoided in patients taking phenothiazines, and it is contraindicated in patients who are hypotensive and on phenothiazines.

Bone-marrow depression, while listed as a potential side effect, is rare in all the phenothiazines. However, since it is potentially lethal when it occurs, it is a problem of which the physician must continuously be aware. It is more common in the elderly, especially women, and tends to occur only with prolonged use; i.e., more than a couple of weeks. However, if a person hasn't had problems with bone-marrow depression in the first three months of taking phenothiazines, the problem is unlikely to develop subsequently.

Because of induction of prolactin secretion, some clinicians believe that phenothiazines should not be used in patients with breast carcinoma. Therefore, probably some nonphenothiazine should be used for the nausea associated with, e.g., radiation sickness. In the case of hallucinations and/or delusions associated with brain metasteses from breast cancer, haloperidol is probably the drug of choice.

Of the various antipsychotic agents, the piperadine phenothiazines are those most likely to interfere with normal sexual function. Male patients taking thioridazine (MELLARIL) report major problems in achieving and maintaining erections, as well as ejaculatory difficulties including retrograde ejaculation. Some patients regard this as only a minor, bothersome problem, while others find it very upsetting and depressing. Consider the patient as well as the drug in prescribing.

Another potential problem with the piperadines concerns their electrocardiographic effects. T-wave effects are most common with this group, and tend to be worse in the presence of hypokalemia. The problem usually responds positively to the administration of potassium and is customarily reversible by discontinuing the drug, which is usually a prudent course to follow.

ANTIDEPRESSANT AND ANTIMANIC DRUGS

Of all psychotherapeutic agents, those used in so-called affective disorders are the most complicated to administer and the most toxic. The therapeutic effect of each develops only with extended treatment, so that the decision to undertake therapy should be based at least in part upon the risk of side effects with extended treatment, and the patient's ability to responsibly self-medicate if he or she is to be an outpatient.

The monoamine oxidase inhibitors are so dangerous, it seems to me, that they should only be administered to young, physically healthy individuals in a supervised setting such as a psychiatric hospital. Many clinicians, however, would believe that I have overstated the case.

Fatal hypertensive crises can occur in patients taking monoamine oxidase inhibitors concurrently with tricyclic antidepressants, sympathomimetic amines (e.g., in a decongestant preparation or nose-drops), or foods containing tyramine (e.g., ripe cheeses, Chianti).

The tricyclic antidepressants are far safer than the monoamine oxidase inhibitors, but do have some important cautions: because they have been implicated in sudden deaths of individuals with cardiac histories, they are contraindicated in such people. Because of anticholinergic effects, they should be used with great caution in the elderly. Before elective surgery, as with most agents that affect the cardiovascular or respiratory system, the drug should be discontinued for as long as the clinical situation will permit, because activity of anaesthetics including side effects may be potentiated.

The newer "second-generation" antidepressants have not to date been demonstrated to offer significant clinical advantages over their better-known forebearers, and therefore will not be discussed further here.

Lithium is used primarily in individuals with manic-depressive illness, largely for prophylactic purposes. The therapeutic levels of lithium are perilously close to the toxic levels and—because of possible tissue retention—serum levels do not always accurately reflect total body lithium. Lithium is contraindicated in patients with significant cardiovascular or renal disease or evidence of brain damage. Toxicity is related to the effect of lithium on sodium metabolism, including decreased reabsorption in renal tubules.

Safe Drugs in Unsafe Patients

There is precious little information about the safe use of psychotherapeutic agents in the medically ill. In general, the more sick the patient, the less precise our information. Most data have been accumulated from extrapolation from side effects, anecdotal information, and reports of catastrophes. Only a fool would do controlled experiments in the presence of serious illness, challenging individuals with drugs of known toxicity. For example, I shudder to think of a controlled experiment measuring the relative respiratory depressive effect of various drugs in patients designated respiratory cripples. The information that follows reflects my own prescribing practices, and in general, I hope, errs in the direction of the patient's safety. The clear bias of this book is to avoid psychochemotherapeutic agents whenever possible, so I'm proceeding with the assumption that a given patient, in your considered judgment, needs medication and the decision now is to decide which medication to use.

CARDIAC PATIENTS

Virtually all of the minor tranquilizers, the piperazine phenothiazines, the thioxanthenes, and the butyrophenones can be safely used with cardiac patients, assuming the clinician proceeds with reasonable prudence.

Because the aliphatic phenothiazines so often cause postural hypotension, they are best either avoided, or used with special care. None of the major tranquilizers has a predictable direct effect on myocardial function, with the exception of the piperadine phenothiazines, which may produce T-wave changes at therapeutic doses and whose use is therefore not advised. Some authors would stress that phenothiazines are safe only so long as the patient is *not* hypokalemic.

Antidepressants and antimanic drugs of all categories are to be avoided in patients with cardiac disease, especially those with preexisting conduction defects. The monoamine oxidase inhibitors have significant interactions with many drugs used in the treatment of cardiac disease. The curious phenomenon of occasional sudden death in cardiac patients taking tricyclic antidepressants remains rare, but is so devastating when it does occur that tricyclics should not be used in cardiac patients. Lithium likewise should not be used because of its multiple effects on the myocardium, which may result in T-wave abnormalities, ventricular irritability, various conduction defects, and even myocarditis. That leaves us with few pharmacologic arrows in our therapeutic quiver, instead requiring us to substitute verbal forms of psychotherapy, therapeutic reserve, or electroconvulsive therapy in severe cases. Tricyclics have, however, been used safely in pacemaker patients, though investigators urge great caution.

RESPIRATORY CRIPPLES

Proceed gingerly with all psychotherapeutic drugs in such patients. Start with low doses, and raise dosages gradually and by small increments.

Virtually all sedatives and tranquilizers produce respiratory depression with resultant decreased arterial pO_2 and increased pCO_2, and most articles and texts warn that the potential for ill effects can't be overemphasized. However, psychotherapeutic agents can produce decreased anxiety with subsequent decreased metabolic requirements, often producing less air hunger and greater patient comfort, so clearly the pros must be carefully weighed with the cons in each case.

Most psychotherapeutic agents, in combination, produce a synergistic respiratory depression effect such that two drugs together produce an effect greater than either one alone. The piperazine phenothiazines and haloperidol are probably safer than most other major and minor tranquilizers, given that they tend to be less sedating in general.

THE RENAL PATIENT

Watch for excess sedation in all renal patients taking psychotherapeutic agents. With this caution, you may prescribe any psychotherapeutic agent other than lithium to patients with renal disease, and you can prescribe virtually all psychotherapeutic agents including lithium to a patient on dialysis.

Short-acting barbiturates are excreted by the liver, and long-acting barbiturates are excreted partly by the liver and partly by the kidney. Virtually all are dialyzable. Like all the other drugs discussed for kidney patients, dosages may need to be reduced or given less frequently.

Both the benzodiazapines and meprobamate are metabolized primarily by the liver. Though the former is not dialyzable and the latter is, either one may be prescribed so long as you observe the patient closely and adjust dosages accordingly.

Both the penothiazines and the tricyclic antidepressants are excreted primarily by the liver and are not dialyzable. Both may be used in renal patients, though often at reduced dosage levels, with a particular watchfulness for such anticholinergic effects as urinary retention in elderly patients. Renal patients tend to have more unstable blood pressure than normals, and may therefore be more susceptible to hypotensive effects of aliphatic phenothiazines. In the case of the tricyclics, watch particularly for drug–drug interactions with other therapeutic agents.

Lithium is excreted by the kidney, and may be directly toxic to the kidney, particularly in the presence of hyponatremia. Therefore, the drug is not to be used in patients with renal disease, though you may use it in anephric patients because the agent is so readily dialyzed.

HEPATIC DISEASE PATIENTS

Patients with liver disease are very sensitive to sedation. Prolonged administration of sedatives of any variety are an important precipitant of coma in patients with hepatic disease. Clinicians who prescribe psychotherapeutic agents to hepatic patients often worry about 1) direct hepatocellular toxicity or cholestatic jaundice, 2) increasing the functional burden for drug metabolism on an already overburdened liver, and 3) potential drug overdosage at therapeutic levels because of impaired metabolism. However, though these concerns are justified, most psychotherapeutic agents (with the exception of monoamine oxidase inhibitors) may be used, but with cautious attention to size and frequency of dosage.

The barbiturates, despite the fact that they rely upon the liver for partial excretion, are often quite well tolerated by patients with chronic liver disease. In fact, some hepatic functions (e.g., bromosulfophthalein excretion, reduction of serum bilirubin) may actually improve with phenobarbitol administration.

Distinctions among members of the benzodiazapine group have been subject to considerable discussion. Oxazepam is reportedly eliminated normally in patients with parenchymal liver disease, and therefore represents a good choice antianxiety agent. Diazepam seems to be well tolerated clinically, but pharmacokinetic studies suggest impaired clearance in chronic liver-disease patients. It seems reasonable to me to use any of the benzodiazapines, but watch the patient carefully and adjust the dosage downward at any evidence of obtundation.

Though phenothiazines can produce hepatic side effects, they are uncommon and reversible. In particular, cholestatic jaundice is a recognized but infrequent complication which usually appears after one to four weeks of continuous administration. Phenothiazines may be prescribed for hepatic patients, but usually at decreased dosages, with reduced frequency, and increased careful observation of the patient. Phenothiazines tend to remain in the system for 24 to 36 hours in healthy patients, and longer in hepatic patients, so—if you develop problems with a particular agent in a particular patient—they are unlikely to disappear abruptly after the drug is discontinued.

Monoamine oxidase inhibitors have been reported to have specific hepatocellular toxicity, and therefore are contraindicated in patients with hepatic disease.

In the case of tricyclic antidepressants, some hepatitis has been reported, mostly as presumed hypersensitivity reactions, and are in any event uncommon. I think it is reasonable to use tricyclic antidepressants where indicated, but to do so with caution and only when the patient can be carefully observed.

HEMATOLOGIC PATIENTS

At this writing, benzodiazapines appear to be the only psychotherapeutic drugs you can give without fear to patients with bone-marrow depression. Almost all of the major tranquilizers, meprobamate, and possibly some tricyclic antidepressants have been named in drug-induced blood dyscrasias, though rarely so and even more rarely so with short-term use. If dyscrasias are to occur, they usually do so after at least one week's treatment and usually before three months. If it is necessary to treat a blood-dyscrasia patient with a major tranquilizer, do so warily and limit the duration of treatment wherever possible.

Do not give barbiturates or glutethimide to patients receiving coumarin drugs because of their anticoagulant inhibition effect and the dangerous anticoagulant rebound effect if the sedatives are discontinued.

The benzodiazapines and any of the major tranquilizers may be given to patients on coumarin drugs.

SEIZURE PATIENTS

Many psychotropic drugs have been regarded to be epileptogenic, meaning that even if they don't cause seizures, they are likely to produce electroencephalogram changes consistent with a seizure disorder. This is rarely a problem in patients lacking a predisposition, but in brain-damaged patients or those with known seizure histories, one must proceed with caution, choosing psychotropics carefully, raising doses gingerly, and perhaps juggling anti-seizure medicines as well. Some authors recommend serial electroencephalograms in high-risk patients. The most dangerous epileptogenic drugs are the sedating phenothiazines (especially chloropromazine) and lithium, and these should be avoided. The other antipsychotics and antidepressants are of intermediate risk and may be used with care. The minor tranquilizers, especially the benzodiazepines, have antiseizure activity and may be used freely—though one must, as a consequence, use care in discontinuing them.

THE PREGNANT PATIENT

As with the rest of the pharmacopoeia, a good general rule is to avoid the use of any psychotherapeutic agent in the first trimester. Absolutely safe use of any drug during pregnancy (and lactation) has not been established and is unlikely to be established, because such experiments simply will not be performed.

However, in view of the millions of women treated with phenothiazines, the absence of any clear evidence implicating them in fetal malformations speaks for itself. If any risk exists at all, it is small. The phenothiazines given in the last trimester, however, may produce a transient syndrome in newborns marked by hypertonicity, agitation, and irritability. This is rarely serious, but often bothersome and sometimes frightening to those in attendance, and is of course to be avoided whenever possible.

There have been isolated reports of limb deformities in babies born to women taking haloperidol in the first trimester. This is particularly worrisome in a drug of such recent vintage, and therefore haloperidol is probably the major tranquilizer of last choice in first-trimester patients.

Clinicians must use caution in prescribing all of the minor tranquilizers in pregnant patients. Very cautious clinicians would avoid them completely. At least two studies suggest that diazepam may be teratogenic in the first trimester, producing cleft lip and/or cleft palate. Meprobamate and chlordiazepoxide may likewise be teratogenic, but the major studies are conflicting.

All addicting psychotherapeutic agents, including most particularly the barbiturates, when given to the mother may affect the newborn infant by direct pharmacologic effects after delivery, including hypotonia and respiratory depression as well as subsequent symptoms related to withdrawal syndrome.

The tricyclic antidepressants have been implicated in multiple fetal abnormalities and are clearly to be avoided, even though the final verdict is not yet available.

Lithium has now been established as a teratogenic agent, and may produce lethargy, respiratory depression, and cyanosis in the newborn infant for a matter of several days.

Remember that any drug that can produce sedation or anticholinergic properties or extra pyramidal symptoms in the mother can likewise do so in the newborn.

With regard to the breast-feeding mother, the safest course is not to prescribe any medications. With that said, it is useful to know for perspective that most drugs excreted in the milk appear there in very small concentration relative to the mother's blood levels. Our concerns relate primarily to cumulative effects secondary to chronic maternal ingestion or to specific metabolic deficiencies in the infant. The literature suggests that any of the major tranquilizers or the tricyclic antidepressants are usually compatible with breast feeding. Some authors would say the same about the benzodiazepines, while others are concerned about possible infant sedation. Of all the psychotropics, lithium causes the most concern, with reports of electroencephalogram and symptomatic changes, though other authors believe these worries to be overstated.

THE ELDERLY PATIENT

Psychotherapeutic agents must be used cautiously in virtually all elderly patients, and for a variety of reasons. The elderly are uniformly more susceptible to side effects, especially confusion, which is most likely to occur at the beginning of treatment and at night. Because so many are on other medications, there is also a greater probability of drug–drug interaction. When confusion does occur as a side effect, those in attendance are likely to attribute the confusion to old age, senility, and disease; and a common response is to increase drug dosage until the patient becomes almost comatose.

A good general rule therefore is to discontinue whatever drugs can be discontinued in elderly patients and evaluate the patients in a drug-free state. Continue medications only if such discontinuance results in relapse of significance symptoms.

In particular, remember that tricyclic antidepressants, phenothiazines, and antiparkinsonian agents all have major and potentially additive anticholinergic effects including paralytic ileus, closed-angle glaucoma, urinary retention, and an atropinelike psychosis which usually resolves in a day or two if the drugs are discontinued.

Medications in general tend to go a long way in elderly people, who consequently need smaller dosages and need them less frequently. A good general rule is to start your dosages low, at perhaps from 40% to 50% of the level you would use for a middle-aged person, and increase dosages more slowly than you would in a younger person. If the patient's spirit is younger than the chronological age, you can proceed with greater therapeutic vigor.

Bibliography

Abbott R: Hyponatremia Due to antidepressant medications. *Ann Emerg Med* 12:708–710, 1983

Adverse interactions of drugs. *Med Letter Drugs Ther* 23(578):17–28, 1981

Alexopoulos GS, Shamoian CA: Tricyclic antidepressants and cardiac patients with pacemakers. *Am J Psychiatry* 139:519–520, 1982

Ananth J: Side effects in the neonate from psychotropic agents excreted through breast feeding. *Am J Psychiatry* 135:801–805, 1978

Applebaum M: Drug toxicity and visual fields. *J Am Optom Assoc* 51:859–62, 1980

Bader TE, Newman K: Amitryptiline in human breast milk and the nursing infant's serum. *Am J Psychiatry* 137:855–856, 1980

Beeley L: Adverse effects of drugs in later pregnancy. *Clin Obstet Gynecol* 8:275–290, 1981

————: Adverse effects of drugs in the first trimester of pregnancy. *Clin Obstet Gynecol* 8:261–274, 1981

Bennett WM, Singer I, Coggins CJ: A guide to drug therapy in renal failure. *JAMA* 230:1544–1553, 1974

Bloomer JR, Boyer JL: Phenobarbital effects in cholestatic liver disease. *Ann Intern Med* 82:310–317, 1975

Bowes WA: The effect of medications on the lactating mother and her infant. *Clin Obstet Gynecol* 23:1073–1080, 1980

Brophy JJ: Suicide attempts with psychotherapeutic drugs. *Arch Gen Psychiatry* 17:652–657, 1967

Campbell, HD, Moffic HS: Guidelines for combination of lithium and neuroleptics. *Tex Med* 79(9):60–62, 1983

Cohen WJ, Cohen NH: Lithium carbonate, haloperidol and irreversible brain damage. *JAMA* 230:1283–1287, 1974

Coull DC, et al.: Amitriptyline and cardiac disease. *Lancet* 2:590–591, 1970

Decina, P, et al.: Effect of lithium therapy on glomerular filtration rate. *Am J Psychiatry* 140:1065–1067, 1983

Drug interactions update. *Med Letter Drugs Ther* 26(654):11–14, 1984

Evans DL, Martin W: Lithium carbonate and psoriasis. *Am J Psychiatry* 136:1326–1327, 1979

Flaherty JA, Lahmeyer HW: Laryngeal-pharyngeal dystonia as a possible cause of asphyxia with haloperidol treatment. *Am J Psychiatry* 135:1414–1415, 1978

Fleckenstein L: Adverse effects of drugs on the liver—update. *Alta Bates Hosp Drug Info Newsletter* 7:24–38, 1975

Glassman AH, Johnson LL, Giardina EV, et al.: The use of imipramine in depressed patients with congestive heart failure. *JAMA* 250:1997–2001, 1983

Grogono AW: Anesthetics—drugs: problem combinations. *Drug Therapy,* January 1976, pp 58–68

Hall MRP: Drug interactions in the elderly. *Gerontology* 28 (Suppl 1): 18–24, 1982

Hollister, LE: Second-generation antidepressants. *Ration Drug Ther* 16(12):1–5, Dec 1982

————: *Clinical Pharmacology of Psychotherapeutic Drugs* (2nd ed). New York, Churchill Livingstone, 1983

Jaffe CM: First-degree atrio-ventricular block during lithium carbonate treatment. *Am J Psychiatry* 134:88–89, 1977

Janke W (ed.): *Response Variability to Psychotropic Drugs*. Elmsford, NJ, Pergamon Press, 1983

Jeste DV and Wyatt RJ: Therapeutic strategies against tardive dyskinesia. *Arch Gen Psychiatry* 39:803–816, 1982.

Kantor SJ, Glassman AH, Bigger JT, et al: The cardiac effects of therapeutic plasma concentrations of imipramine. *Am J Psychiatry* 135:534–538, 1978

Klotz U, Reimann L: Delayed clearance of diazepam due to cimetidine. *N Engl J Med* 302:1012–1014, 1980

Kotin J, Wilbert DE, Verberg D, et al: Thioridazine and sexual dysfunction. *Am J Psychiatry* 133:82–84, 1976

Lippman S, Moscovitz R, Otuama L: Tricyclic-induced myoclonus. *Am J Psychiatry* 134:90–91, 1977

Matthes KJ: Drug-induced proteinuria. *Contrib Nephrol* 24:109–114, 1981

Miller FA, Rampling D: Adverse effects of combined propranolol and chlorpromazine therapy. *Am J Psychiatry* 139:1198–1199, 1982

Moir DC: Tricyclic antidepressants and cardiac disease. *Am Heart J* 86:841–842, 1973

Nasrallah HA: Factors influencing phenothiazine-induced ECG changes. *Am J Psychiatry* 135:118–119, 1978

Norton JC, Ludwig AM: Medical treatment of psychiatric patients–possible polypharmacy problems. *Hosp Comm Psychiatry* 33:305–307, 1982

O'Brien JP: A study of low-dose amitriptyline overdoses. *Am J Psychiatry* 134:66–68, 1977

Penovich P: Drug-induced hyperpyrexia and heat stroke. *Drug Ther* Aug 1976 pp 6–7.

Pope HG, et al.: Toxic reactions to the combination of monoamine oxidase inhibitors and tryptophan. *Am J Psychiatry* 142:491–492, 1985

Racy J, Ward-Racy EA: Tinnitus in imipramine therapy. *Am J Psychiatry* 137:854–855, 1980

Rao JM, Arulappu R: Drug use in pregnancy. *Drugs* 22:409–414, 1981

Reus VI, Gold P, Post R: Lithium-induced thyrotoxicosis. *Am J Psychiatry* 136:724–725, 1979

Roos JC: Cardiac effects of antidepressant drugs. *Br J Clin Pharmacol* 15:439S–445S, 1983

Roxe DM: Toxic nephropathy from diagnostic and therapeutic agents. *Am J Medicine* 69:759–766, 1980

Sack RL, Shore JH: Psychopharmacology in medical practice. *West J Med* 134:223–233, 1981

Safra MJ, Oakley GP: Association between cleft lip with and without cleft palate and prenatal exposure to diazepam. *Lancet* 2:478–480, 1975

Shull JH, Wilkinson GR, Johnson R, et al.: Normal disposition of oxazepam in acute viral hepatitis and cirrhosis. *Ann Intern Med* 84:420–425, 1976

Siris SG: Comparative side effects of impramine, benztropine, or their combination in patients receiving fluphenazine decanoate. *Am J Psychiatry* 140:1069–1071, 1983

Szefler SJ: Drug excretion in human breast milk. *J Ped Gastroent Nutr* 2 (Suppl 1):S120–126, 1983

The transfer of drugs and other chemicals into human breast milk. *Pediatrics* 72:375–383, 1983

Turan MI, Soldatus C: Epileptogenic side effects of psychotropic drugs. *JAMA* 244:1460–1463, 1980

Weiner MF: Haloperidol hyperthyroidism, and sudden-death. *Am J Psychiatry* 136:717–718, 1979

15

Coping and Occupational Hazards of Physicianhood

We are confronted with insurmountable opportunities.

—Pogo

In times like these, it is helpful to remember that there have always been times like these.

—Paul Harvey

The recurring theme of this book is that origins of problems between doctor and patient are as likely to reside in the doctor or in the treatment milieu as in the patient. Yet most of our therapeutic efforts are directed at the patient, though occasionally we make a conscious effort to try to change in some way the hospital, clinic, or office setting in which we practice.

This chapter is directed at us, at you and me and our colleagues, as we struggle to do our best to provide quality health care to our patients. The foundation of good medical care is giving a damn; most of us already know how to practice far better medicine than we do. Usually, when I don't do as well by a particular patient as I might have, the primary obstacle is *me;* my lack of interest or enthusiasm or energy. Clinical work then becomes drudgery, which not only results in poorer treatment, but my satisfaction from the process tends to diminish proportionately, and something unsavory happens to my self-respect as well.

In order to respect ourselves, we have to respect what we do. In order to respect the process of caring for patients, I believe we have to respect the patients themselves.

Certain kinds of vulnerabilities represent a phenomenon widely shared by medical colleagues. Suicide is the second most common cause of death among medical students, and is more frequent among physicians than the *combined* deaths from automobile accidents, plane crashes, homicides, and drownings. Vaillant's 20-year-long prospective study of physicians *preselected* for mental health revealed that dependency on drugs and alcohol represented a substantial problem, and was responsible for one-third of the time spent in the hospital by members of that group. Anyone who sits on department executive committees or medical society good and welfare committees knows that alcoholism is routinely associated with impaired performance, even (and perhaps especially) among those with the most impressive credentials and the highest medical school grades. Most of us have read reports that physicians are prone to certain kinds of marital and family problems, and while the facts are by no means clear, juggling the competing priorities of profession and personal life presents a continuing challenge to many.

These facts have been so widely disseminated that they now often seem boring with their dreary familiarity, yet their implications for the pedestrian aspects of patient care often remain elusive. "So what?" ask many physicians, practical creatures that we are. "What the hell should *I* do about it?"

Physicians' Expectations of Their Work

The test of a vocation is the love of the drudgery it involves.
—G. K. Chesterton

Actually, there is quite a bit that most of us can do to lessen the grief we experience in our professional lives, because much of it is self-inflicted—albeit aided and abetted by others—a natural consequence of the jarring clash we experience between the highly romanticized expectations we bring to our work and the realities, which in contrast, often seem grim and disillusioning.

Our expectations from our clinical activities relate to both what we wish from work generally, and what we wish specifically from our contact with patients. Doctoring may be a profession or a calling, but it is also a job; to find satisfaction in patient care, you must also find satisfaction with the specific job that is your vehicle for taking care of patients.

The irony is that many students and young professionals approach their vocation without much appreciation that it, like all others, will be work—meaning that it entails its full measure of drudgery, tedium, routine, paper shuffling, office politics, and mundane hassles. Medicine, many suppose, is not supposed to be work. One does not "work" medicine as one works construction or works selling or does secretarial work. Instead, we "practice" medicine, with the implication that it's an ongoing learning experience, a gradually refined form of sport or art analogous to practicing a golf stroke or practicing the piano.

It may be instructive therefore to look at the most common motivators which keep people going to their jobs day in and day out. People work to involve themselves in one or more processes: (1) earn money, (2) make social contacts, (3) structure time, (4) gain a sense of identity, and (5) give meaning and purpose to activities in life itself.

Money is the easiest to talk about of the various reasons for working. It's the most concrete, and successful attainment of the goal is presumably the easiest to measure. While physicians do very well financially compared to the population at large, they are more likely to compare themselves to persons of similar social class, age group, and social aspirations.

In particular, physicians in people-oriented specialties are prone to compare themselves to medical classmates who have gone into procedure-intensive specialties: the occasional, but highly visible, colleagues who shell out cataracts or prostates on lucrative production lines, or the cardiac surgeon who specializes in coronary artery bypasses at tens of thousands per chest cracked. It's no secret to the public at large that the medical profession has been entirely too concerned with its own financial enrichment. It's all well and good to earn a comfortable income in medicine, but if you put those dollars ahead of the profession's function—providing quality health care to our citizens—then you are in trouble and so is everyone else. Unless you run a procedure-mill or some sort of medical extravaganza, you will make a middle-class income—one on which you can be comfortable to be sure, but hardly one to support all the care-free perquisites many believe all rich doctors can afford. The days are gone when a young physician could expect to hang out a shingle and join the country club in the same day, but for perspective you have to keep in mind that more than 80% of all *households* in the United States live on less than $37,000 a year. How greedy we have become when we physicians grouse about incomes of $60,000, $80,000 and $100,000!

I'm spending so much time on this subject because so many physicians are obsessed with the topic and contemplate their financial circumstances with such unhappiness. Financial counselors of my acquaintance confirm that, as income increases, so too does the income of the reference group. The ideal income tends to remain elusively at 10% to 20% above current income, even at the very highest socioeconomic strata. Depending on income as the primary source of job satisfaction, therefore, tends to lead consistently to frustration: it's never enough. Paradoxically, one's income becomes increasingly satisfying in inverse proportion to the importance attached to it. If you get pleasure from other aspects of your work, you are far more likely to be content with your income, no matter how high or low it may be.

The importance of work in providing social contacts varies across the course of one's life. Variables include marital status, accessibility of family and relatives, the presence of a non-work-related network of friends, and the fluctuation of one's interpersonal neediness. Even where work-related social contacts seem unimportant, their effect remains pervasive. Try working with a bunch of people you can't stand or who bore you and you'll see what I mean. Conversely, you may sometimes stay in a particular clinical setting with onerous technical requirements, simply because you like the people and they like you.

Many of us have difficulty appreciating the importance of structuring time until we are faced with a period of time lacking in structure. The retired executive provides a readily recognizable example: post-retirement anxiety and depression are common afflictions until retirees find something to keep them busy. Physicians of my acquantance seldom are very comfortable with amorphous days. If they don't have work to keep them occupied, they impose an avocational structure to their hours which marshals one activity after another: hobbies, games, sports, projects, adventures, travels, reading, writing, or socializing.

One's work also provides a sense of identity separate from the work one does. With the possible exception of being a member of a super-rich family, occupation is the principal determinant of status. Our occupations label us in ways that have connotations for many people we meet. Each of the following labels conjures up different stereotypes, though each may have little accuracy in describing a particular person who carries the label: police officer, ballet dancer, day laborer, medieval historian. Some labels are high in identity value (e.g., Supreme Court justice), while many are not. Depending on the job market, some carry high employment and geographic options, and some do not. Whereas historically being a physician identified one as being among the most highly educated members of a community, that may now be less so in a sophisticated urban community where PhDs drive taxicabs and work as carpenters. Whereas being a physician historically meant that everyone else who worked with patients would automatically defer to our judgment, that is no longer necessarily so. The "identity value" of being a physician is changing in important ways, which in turn will result in potentially significant changes in the way we see ourselves.

Separate from everything else, work has the potential for providing a sense of meaning and purpose to life—but often it does not. We are all familiar with statements such as: "it's just a job," or "I just put in my eight hours a day," or "don't ask me; I just work here." The emphasis in each of these statements is on the "just." Whatever else people get from such employment, they don't get a sense of meaning. In contrast, for those physicians who really enjoy their work, achievement of a sense of meaning assumes an important role in their reward systems, however they define it.

Whichever goal(s) of work you emphasize obviously reflects personal values, and patterns vary among physicians. I've been struck, however, by the sense that physicians—ambitious creatures that we are—have uniformly high expectations of our work. The average physician wants the profession to supply substantial monetary rewards, fascinating and admiring social contacts, an aesthetic structure to daily living, a prestigious and gratifying identity, and a satisfying sense of meaning. Total success on all counts not surprisingly remains the exception rather than the rule.

For balance, we should recognize that diminished job satisfaction results from aversive factors as well as the lack of rewards. In Studs Terkel's book, *Working,* two factors emerge again and again as being a hateful part of far too many occupational settings: being oversupervised, and feeling a lack of identification with the quality of the endproduct or service.

Changing Social Values

> In the medical corporation we know about, the general practitioner's role is usually somewhere near the front door of the corporation, triaging the patients and in some cases regulating the use of services. These are low-level tasks and are rewarded accordingly.
> —G. Gayle Stephens

> [I]n the 1970s in this country, medicine went up for sale. The age of the supermarket mentality in medicine was born. . . . Increasing corporate involvement in health care means, in human terms, that the grey flannel suit is replacing the white coat. . . . Certainly physicians still see the patients and prescribe pills, but their influence in shaping the important decisions in the health field is now greatly diminished.
> —Stanley Wohl

The mystique that heretofore surrounded medicine has become tarnished. We live in a culture that places increasing priority on health education for the average citizen, who in turn feels an increasing right to decide not only about personal health care, but about the social policy that will determine the structure in which health care is given and received. Physicians and other health professionals are still seen as valuable resources by most persons; but, as war is too important to be left to generals, health policy increasingly is seen as too important to be left to physicians. We are seen not only as fallible, but as subject to making decisions biased by self-interest.

H. L. Mencken defined self-respect as "the secure feeling that no one, as yet, is suspicious." Even if you don't accept Mencken's cynical definition, this is a difficult time for physicians whose self-respect depends on the secure sense of the public's trust. Many patients who trust us at their sickbed are uncertain whether they can trust the medical profession in general if left to its own devices. The rise of health consumerism as well as state and federal monitoring agencies as representatives of the patients' interests, bears continuing witness to the suspiciousness of our clientele.

The changes in health care in the past quarter-century have been numerous and dramatic. The most obvious and most discussed change, the one which most easily can be seen as the parent of the others, is the incredible rise in health-care costs. Health care is now the single largest industry in this country, overshadowing defense by two or three times, depending on who tallies the figures. In the wake of that dominant reality, the second most dramatic change is the controlling role of institutions in almost every aspect of patient care—from the regulating and bankrolling federal government on the one hand to the various interconnected Wall Street firms on the other: the giant hospital chains, the insurance firms, the various suppliers and organizers whose very products and marketing practices determine what the phrase "standard of care" will mean. And the third change, more subtle but no less pervasive than the others, is the growing estrangement of doctor and patient by the removal of decision making from the clinical interface to regulatory and administrative bodies with no knowledge of—and not much interest in—the human beings involved. For example, physicians now rarely decide whom to resuscitate (ACLS* standards dictate: everyone), or can use discretion in electing to report a parental temper tantrum (child-abuse statutes require: everyone), or exercise judgment in how much sensitive psychiatric information to put in a chart (malpractice liability decisions dictate: be complete, write down everything). Who can be hospitalized, for how long, with what treatment, all are increasingly subject to public policy decisions.

Medicine is no longer a cottage industry, with a physician in charge of each little cottage. In 1966, when I graduated from medical school, almost all of my classmates elected to go into private fee-for-service practice—I was somewhat of a weirdo in looking forward to some variant of salaried and/or group practice. My goals were heavily influ-

---

*Advanced Cardiac Life Support

enced by my parents' politics, and by some financially devastating illnesses among family and friends. Students graduating now, however, whatever their politics and expectations, are very likely to end up as corporate employees at some stage of their medical careers.

Money makes a difference to people, including our potential patients. Our services, however much or however little training preceded them, are worth only what people are willing to pay for them. Because the vast majority of health-care visits require little in the way of technical skill or sophistication on the part of health-care providers, our would-be clientele are developing decreasing interest in paying physicians' high fees. Instead, they turn to health-care discounters and "Doc's-in-a-box," where economies of scale keep the rates down. Practice opportunities will follow patient dollars, and physicians will increasingly be working in such locations, needing to adjust their patient management skills accordingly.

Our nonphysician co-workers also regard us differently from how they have in the past, and want to be regarded differently in return. Many feel that they have received a disproportionately small share of the health-care dollar compared with physicians, and they want that situation changed. Many feel capable of more responsibility than the laws allow them, and they feel resentful when their competent work must be rubber-stamped by a physician in order to be validated. Many experienced nonphysician clinicians (nurses, health technicians, psychologists, for instance) rebel at always having to be subservient to physicians who may be less competent and less experienced than they in performing some specific task. The public, as represented by legislators, is increasingly sensitive to the plight of such individuals, and the role of the physician vis–à–vis co-workers will be changing by legislation in the years ahead, as well as by the informal arrangements which are already familiar to many of us.

Central to our adaptation to the evolving realities is an understanding that the professions are being bureaucratized and the bureaucracies are becoming professionalized, so that it is harder and harder to tell the two apart.

Historically, professions were said to have special characteristics. These included a generally recognized, intellectually based competence, extensive autonomy for each professional, and a capacity for, and dedication to, self-regulation. Authority within the professions presupposed competence and accomplishment, with the tacit understanding that one mature professional *advised* another—one did not *order* a professional to do anything.

In contrast, a bureaucracy is characterized by the hierarchial specialization of roles and tasks, with task-completion dependent upon appropriate orders emanating from an appropriate level in the hierarchy. In a bureaucracy, authority is granted by fiat, and a supervisor need not necessarily have technical expertise comparable to that of the people supervised. The sole job is to organize the technicians effectively, each to do one portion of a given task, so that the task as a whole is done efficiently.

Persons who regard themselves as professionals tend to perform poorly and with considerable discomfort in a bureaucracy. They are reluctant to sacrifice autonomy and accept conformity. They don't like having tasks assigned indiscriminately to them nor do they like having to accept a goal which is chosen for them. They are particularly uncomfortable in being evaluated on the basis of their adherence to bureaucratic performance standards rather than on the basis of professional accomplishment. Typically, the professional is reluctant to punch a time clock or to do paperwork.

The difficulty for most of us is that while we think of ourselves as professionals, the clinical work of medicine is increasingly subject to bureaucratic overtones. As a consequence, we have dual membership in two fundamentally different organizational systems. We must not only master professional knowledge and skills, but if we wish to get anything done we must also learn to function effectively in that bureaucracy. Getting essential tasks done, either for ourselves or for our patients, often requires an intimate knowledge of, and a willingness to play by, the bureaucratic rules.

The evolution of health policy has recently been, and will continue to be, dominated by the growing awareness that health care is a limited national resource. The notion of "maximum therapeutic effort for everyone," which was such a fundamental assumption inherent in my own medical education, is now being seriously questioned. Many feel that the severely and critically ill, on whom complicated medical teaching centers concentrate, have been getting a disproportionate share of health-care resources, with discouragingly small impact on mortality, and sometimes even an adverse effect on quality of life. Medicine no longer can write a blank check on the public till. Our resources are finite, and cost-effectiveness studies, one hopes balanced by humane clinical judgment, will be the basis for allocating resources.

All of these considerations place an unsettling stress on our self-image as physicians. Physicians are learning of the personal and social costs of total dedication to work, but deciding to devote more time to our nonprofessional lives is seldom totally free from guilt: can a doctor who is partially committed to patient care render the same quality of service as one who is totally committed? Do we derogate patient care by devoting so much time to finding satisfaction elsewhere, in leisure activities and in nonprofessional settings?

Values Inherent in Medical Education

Life was something you dominated, if you were any good.
                                                   —F. Scott Fitzgerald

We simply can't get around the fact that we are overpaid and overtrained for most of our practice.
                                                   —David W. Crippen

Medical schools in my experience have had a discouragingly similar character. The students begin the first year with laudable amounts of intellectual curiosity, optimism, and empathy for patients; and, for far too many, leave at the end of the fourth year feeling cynical, regarding many patients with blatant hostility, and viewing the process of patient care as perhaps interesting but not a whole lot of fun. It's not a universal pattern, but I believe it to be distressingly common. I also believe it to be a product of our medical-education system itself.

While students may be the relatively more innocent victims, the faculty often becomes victimized too. Even the best potential clinicians among junior faculty members because of institutional pressures tend to become insensitive and impatient with both individual patients and individual students, withdrawing from continuing empathetic care of the one in favor of the processing of the many. Time for clinical work is likely to be regarded as a duty rather than as an opportunity, and heavily weighted toward episodic care with unfamiliar patients, using a disease-oriented focus. Conflicting administrative and research obligations account for too many demands on time and are too important for progress up the department ladder. Human and family-oriented care inevitably is slighted, and the young faculty member's development of potential humanistic traits tends to be neglected. How, then, can the young faculty member teach these qualities to students?

Students learn values by example, and examples tend to be consistent from one department to the next. Clinical care is relegated to the least-experienced persons around—students and house officers—with faculty members darting in and out to provide episodic supervision. The result is a subtle downgrading of the value of patient contact; anyone with seniority and clout soon flees from continuing daily contact with patients to other and presumably more attractive and important activities.

Faculty members seldom can get to know their students as human beings or watch them evolve over four years. Instead, they measure the students by the amount of data the students can master and divulge on request, and by the technical procedures they can perform. Faculty members, because of their other obligations, seldom have the time to assess more subtle skills derived from patience, empathy, understanding, and integrity. By implication, the student finds these qualities less of an asset in getting through medical school than mastery of cognitive detail; and, even if the former qualities don't wither, they are unlikely to flower in a medical school setting.

Intensive involvement with patients who are sick and in pain and needy is often itself painful, even for an experienced clinician, and certainly for a novice. Where is the student to learn to experience such involvement with an acceptable degree of comfort? Who among the professors or junior faculty have both the time and skill to demonstrate the process? Students who suffer noisily, like patients who suffer noisily, are commonly either ignored, regarded as a pain in the neck, or referred to a psychiatrist. Suffering is seldom viewed as a potentially enriching experience for a clinician, which calls for patient and empathetic listening by colleagues. The unspoken message is, "If you're having troubles, keep them to yourself. Suffering shows weakness, and a real professional has to be tough." I believe that message provides a lousy standard for an evolving physician, and I think the values on which the message is based serve our profession poorly.

Medical school usually teaches you that you can never be bright enough, never know enough, never work hard enough to be worthy to practice medicine. The explicit message is that every missed fact, any oversight on your part, can be the death of someone—literally! You are told that perfection is not merely the elusive ideal, but rather, the daily standard by which you must measure your performance. You neither expect nor receive plaudits for a job "just" well done when perfection alone is the standard. Only deviation from perfection stands out, and that constitutes disaster. You are not permitted to see yourself as what you are: bright, capable, hard-working, but nonetheless a human being and therefore fallible, vulnerable and subject to making judgments distorted by fatigue, personal values, and considerations other than merely "objective" measures of health.

In many respects, you are not only too smart for much of what you need to do in the practice of medicine, your intelligence is too restless. By virtue of getting into medical school, you are a straight A undergraduate student or nearly so, and capable of a stunning performance in your Medical College Admissions Test. By virtue of getting through medical school, you demonstrate your mastery of the Krebs cycle and an unending flow of exotica. As you go through one class, one rotation after another, your mind becomes accustomed to constant stimulation, the recurrent exposure to new and obscure conditions and diseases. Yet these qualities will not help you in the *practice* of 90% of what you will do. Whether you are a family practitioner or a thoracic surgeon, after your apprenticeship is complete, the measure of your happiness will lie in the mastery of what after a while becomes routine. The stuff you see day in and day out, the things that you do almost as a matter of habit, make it seem easy because you know it so well and can do it so well without being bored by the repetition.

But medical school's biggest failing, in my view, is its emphasis on pathology. Not only the focus on disease per se, but on patients as bearers of disease, as persons who are themselves diseased. In the process, we neglect to see our patients as colorful human beings, living lives of quiet and personal drama and comedy, each with their own very human stories to tell. Someplace in the curriculum, students should be helped to focus on the wonder of it all—not just the wonder of the electrons spinning in their orbits and electrolyte transport at the cellular membrane, but the extraordinary ability of people to cope in the face of illness and the mundane stresses of life. Most of us find it difficult to see heroism in the low-back-pain sufferer, but that doesn't mean it isn't often there. We only begin to understand the phenomenon when we ourselves develop some sciatic pains and somehow manage to discharge our responsibilities despite the aggravating burden of day-in-and-day-out discomfort. If we look for valor of spirit in our patients, expecting to find it, we will often be successful; if we look for psychopathology in our patients, expecting to find it, we will be successful in that search too. But we will seldom find the discovery ennobling to ourselves or our patients.

Models of the Doctor-Patient Relationship

> *It is an occupational hazard, I thought. Everyone gets contemptuous after a while of his clients. Teachers get scornful of students, doctors of patients, bartenders of drinkers, salesmen of buyers, clerks of customers.*
>
> —Robert B. Parker

So what does all this have to do with the kinds of relationships we have with our patients? The one truth which surely must be apparent from what has been discussed so far is that our relationships with our patients can be extraordinarily complex and necessarily evolve not only with our own personal development, but also with the changing realities of contemporary medical care.

The central issue in these relationships is how responsibility and authority for decision making are allocated. Each physician will approach the issue in a personal fashion, but one hopes with flexibility enough to adjust personal style to the needs and wishes of individual patients and families.

The pleasure a physician gets from contact with a patient reflects not only the kind of individual each may be, but what each wants from the other. The manifest requests are important, but so are unspoken and perhaps more amorphous interests and needs. Every patient comes to us with a set of expectations, conscious or not, about what the experience will be like. The patient may approach us expecting a tender healer, a stern authority figure, an accepting parent, or a blundering fool. We, in turn, may expect the patient to act in a dependent, stoic, sneaky, seductive, or some other manner. These expectations may have little to do with any specific patient, or they may be brought out primarily by certain categories of patients.

A classic example is a case of a physician who places great emphasis on the healer role and a patient who is on the road to becoming a career disability-compensation patient. The doctor in essence says, "I'm going to cure you if it kills you," and the patient responds, "I will do everything in my power to frustrate your desire to heal me." Another common but somewhat more subtle example involves the patient who, in addition to organic disease, would also like to feel taken care of and "special" to doctors. When a patient like this is looked after by a researcher-scientist who values objectivity, personal distance, and data, there is bound to be a clash.

Such physician and patient expectations and attitudes in themselves are neither good nor bad. We can ignore them, fight them, or find some way of using them to enhance patient care and the satisfaction we get from our clinical work. In this broadened sense, these phenomena are inappropriate only when they constitute barriers to optimal health care and a sense of satisfaction in the participants.

Various models of physicianhood and patienthood are summarized in Table 15.1. The models clearly are not mutually exclusive. Most of us will see ourselves as fitting into more than one category, and the same is true for many patients that we see. As a consequence most of us are simultaneously seeking rewards from diverse roles that call for (often) conflicting behaviors. Often it's difficult to know what we really wish for ourselves, and we end up seeking rewards that don't give us the pleasure we anticipated.

In many respects, our training years teach us to be students rather than physicians. As a consequence, our personal reward systems, as molded early in our careers, often emphasize the role of patient as "learning material" rather than human being. Some physicians can find no pleasure in contact with patients unless they have "interesting" or unusual diseases. This circumstance is truly unfortunate, because as Table 15.1 demonstrates, there are many potential rewards to be gotten from patient contact in addition to those sought by the pure student.

Specific kinds of illnesses often have the capacity for bringing out or frustrating different kinds of role functions in patients and physicians.

Depending upon the kinds of contribution each of us enjoys most, we may prefer patients with conditions which are acute or chronic, straightforward or complicated, which either do or don't foster patient neediness, or which lend themselves to clinical study or reporting in scientific journals.

One contemporary reality deserves special attention, in part because the discrepancy between physician and patient perspectives can be so profound, and in part because my personal experience with this discrepancy was so dramatic.

Several years ago, I was a member of the audience at a conference on traumatic injuries, where the following problem was presented to experts on a panel: You are an emergency physician at a small community hospital. An eight-year-old boy is brought in after a bicycle accident, from which he sustained a 15-minute loss of consciousness. The exam is entirely normal (except for minor contusions and abrasions), as are all x-rays and lab work. According to protocol, such patients are admitted for observation to the pediatric service, which in this case means old Doc Jones, who phones in orders without ever seeing the patient. To make a long story short, over the next 6 hours the patient becomes marginally more obtunded, not alert and bright as usual, and somewhat lethargic. Because you are interested and concerned, you repeat your neurologic exam, finding no "hard" signs of neurologic damage. You call Dr. Jones, describe the situation and your concern about a slowly evolving intracranial bleed, and suggest transferring the patient to the nearest hospital with a CT scanner. Dr. Jones politely but adamantly refuses, saying he is confident the patient can be safely observed in this hospital. Now, what do you do, given your concern? The expert panelists suggested a variety of options: demand that Dr. Jones come in to examine the patient himself; call Dr. Jones' department chief; call in a surgeon for a second opinion; call the hospital chief-of-staff; or as a last resort, transfer the patient to another hospital on your own authority, however flimsy. Then yours-truly piped up from the audience with the following suggestion: how about talking with the parents, explaining that you and Dr. Jones have a difference of opinion (as can happen between any two competent professionals), but that since it was their son who was involved, you thought they deserved to be informed, so they could influence what happened next, if they so chose.

Well, you would think I had advocated that chiropractors be allowed to perform neurosurgery. Every one of the panelists thought that my suggestion was the worst thing that could be done in the circumstances—and, if a single physician in the audience of 300 or so thought my suggestion had any merit, no one mentioned it to me. If that's all there was to the matter, there would be no point in mentioning it. I

Table 15.1 Models of Physicianhood and Patienthood

Model	Physician's role	Patient's role	"Payoff" for physician	"Payoff" for patient
Anthropologic	Healer. Shaman	Sufferer. Supplicant	Cure rates. Individual cures. Power in the tribe or community	Renewed health. Personal cure. Religious experience
Professional	Expert	Client. Patient. Lay person	Esteem of colleagues. Professional achievement	Prestigious care. Care conforming to professional standards
Bureaucratic	Bureaucrat. Purveyor of health services	"Visit" statistic.* Recipient of services	Volume processed. Efficiency (no problems for the system). Task completion. Bureaucratic advancement	Getting entitlement. Efficiency (minimum of red tape)
Market economy	Entrepreneur. Merchant. Competitor	Customer. Consumer. Doctor-shopper	Maximize money, profit. Minimize losses. Security. Number of customers (size of practice)	Value for money spent
Psychologic	Parent-figure (friend)	Child-figure (friend)	Being a "good parent." Feeling loved. Feeling responsible, adult, in control	Being a "good patient", (childlike). Feeling loved, special. Gratification of dependency
Scientific	Investigator. Researcher	Experimental subject. Repository of data	Data, hypotheses. Papers. Scientific acclaim	Contributing to scientific progress. Other compensation. Sense of altruism, contribution to posterity

Religious	Priest. Guru. Spiritual leader	Pilgrim. Spiritual seeker	Followers. Giving guidance. Moral rectitude	Enlightenment. Understanding. Receiving guidance. Religious experience
Educational (medical training variety)	Student	Learning material	Knowledge. Approval of teachers. "Graduating" to next level	Altruism (?). Vicarious satisfaction in Doctor's education
Educational (patient-teaching variety)	Teacher	Student	Knowledgeable patients. Self-sufficient patients	Knowledge. Approval of teachers. "Graduating" to self-sufficiency
Career patient	Credentialing agent	Worker. Achiever. Recipient of funds ("salary"?)	Helping patient advance up disability ladder†	Being certified "ill." Achieving successive disability levels. Adequate "salary," job security, stimulation on the job

* In most bureaucracies each patient contact (no matter how complex) is counted as one patient "visit." In general, visits per unit of time are regarded as an important measure of physician efficiency; and are therefore a criterion for promotion and salary increases.
† Physicians characteristically find few rewards in helping patients become more disabled, and this is a source of significant tension between physicians and patients bent on a career of disability.

have been wrong many times in the past, and certainly could be in the present example.

The interesting thing is that as I have re-told the story to various lay people, not a single person agreed with the panelists— and many parents were vehement in asserting their "right" to know in such circumstances.

The point here simply is that there is an enormous backlash against medical paternalism, wherein a physician makes a decision for a patient, presumably with the best of intentions and for the latter's good, without the patient and the patient's family being aware of it.

As you find models of the doctor-patient relationship, which comfortably fit your own style and values, you will want to keep these ongoing developments in mind. To ignore the patient's wishes in such circumstances is to invite his or her wrath—and to burden yourself with responsibilities which can reasonably be shared with those most intimately involved: the patient and the patient's family.

Values for an Evolving Clinician

> *Idealism increases in direct proportion to one's distance from the problem.*
>
> —John Galsworthy

> *The most utterly lost of all days is that in which we have not once laughed.*
>
> —Sebastien Roch Nicolas Chamfort

> *Many of our prayers were not answered, and for this we are now grateful.*
>
> —William Feather

Writers seldom come to their subjects by accident. My own interest in writing this book arose from a very early and definitely naive biopsychosocial idealism, which I found extremely difficult to implement in practice. At one stage, my natural but occasionally superficial optimism was seriously threatened by a brooding pessimism about the doctor-patient relationship as it seemed likely to unfold in the years ahead. During that period, I wrote a book about my flirtation with disillusionment called, *The Bitter Pill: Doctors, Patients, and Failed Expectations,* which was widely perceived to be about physician burnout and even impairment. As is the norm with such things these days, I was sent on the talk-show circuit by my publisher. On one such program, I was introduced by the talk-show host, who said: "And here, to talk about the important subject, is Dr. Martin Lipp, himself a burned-out and impaired physician."

The introduction caught me by surprise, and I categorically denied it, but it forced me into a careful self-assessment. I will admit to being singed about the edges even as I have avoided burnout at the core, and I certainly acknowledge that the process of relinquishing illusions has been a painful one. My point in mentioning all this here is simply to emphasize that the values I advocate below are not simply derived from scholarly study, but rather are an outgrowth of my own painful experiences and those of colleagues and friends. While others with parallel experiences inevitably would come up with a different list, the following are a representative sample of ideas worth pondering, and perhaps adopting as guidelines in our continuing pursuit of satisfaction in patient care.

Respect for the patient as an individual. If you can't respect the patient, you won't respect what you do with, or for, or to the patient. If you don't respect the process of giving care, how can you respect yourself? The irony of all this is that disrespect for the patient may ultimately be more harmful to ourselves than to the patient. I need to value what I do, even if the patients don't think they need it for themselves. I need to keep alert to the person who is my patient, that amalgam of feelings and thoughts, experiences and hopes, strengths and limitations, which makes each of us unique. I need to keep open my own soul's eye for the soul who is my patient.

Acceptance of self as person. We need to accept that the demands of being a human being supersede those of physicianhood. How we practice medicine will be heavily influenced by the events in our personal lives: birth of children, death of parents and friends, disruption of important relationships, illness, joys and sorrows. Being a physician does not insulate us from the need for sympathy, tenderness, support and occasional guidance from those around us, including co-workers and patients. Learn not only how to give, counsel, and succor, but how to receive in return.

Recognition of personal vulnerability. One of the paradoxes of the good clinician is that the professionally useful quality of sensitivity to the patient as a person in turn makes the clinician potentially vulnerable as a human being who may suffer along with the patient. While recognizing that many ventures worth pursuing nonetheless involve some potential for discomfort, the pain itself never feels good and can sometimes become a major burden. Such stresses affect each of us differently, but once a certain variable threshold is passed, the stress takes its toll of physicians no less than patients. The consequences may include impaired health, depression, excessive use of alcohol or substances, and impaired clinical performance. Be alert to such difficulties in yourself and in your physician colleagues; shared concern and support can lighten many burdens.

Self-respect independent of human limitations. At various stages in my training, I was told implicitly or explicitly: "If you don't know everything, you will kill someone. If you don't know everything, you will be a lousy doctor, and you don't belong in clinical medicine." That, of course, is the Big Lie—and probably the source of more unhappiness and guilt and personal suffering in physicians than all other misbeliefs put together. Each of us has our limitations. No one knows it all, and no one can do it all. The complete physician doesn't exist. These limitations don't make us bad clinicians; they are the basis for our empathy with patients whose illnesses give them such a keen awareness of their own limitations. The only truly terrible things that happen in association with limitations come as a consequence of refusing to recognize their existence and substituting arrogance for humility.

A safe doctor is one who knows his or her limitations, and calls for help when the demands of a situation exceed ability. None of us need feel diminished in requesting assistance from others. All care must be collaborative, and we deserve to respect ourselves even as we respect the nurses, social workers, patients, and others with whom we collaborate.

Effective limit setting. Setting reasonable limits involves two steps: first, knowing what they are; and second, acting on them in a way that demeans neither ourselves nor our patient. You can't meet all of your patient's expectations or all of your own expectations, let alone do so every day. There are differences among "there is nothing I can do," "there is nothing that can be done," and "there is nothing you can do." The irony is that patients are often better able to accept our limitations than we can ourselves, as long as we don't communicate these limits in a way that implies that the patient is somehow responsible for them. Acknowledge the patient's needs and feelings, take responsibility for what you can't or don't wish to do, and then try to find some reasonable alternative. Understand that clashes between expectations and reality are inevitable. While ambition is useful and often praiseworthy, try to avoid the trap that captures so many physicians: substituting rapacious financial ambition for success in the less tangible and sometimes more elusive interpersonal arena.

Setting priorities and cultivating resources. The limits you set will depend upon what you value and what you specifically dislike. We will sometimes choose to emphasize one function of work over another, or one model of the doctor-patient relationship over another. The kinds of choices we make will depend not only upon the rewards we perceive, but also upon the resources we have to draw upon. A recurring question will be, How much can I give at the office and still be able to give at home? We must be able to give our family, friends, and colleagues enough time so that they will be able to replenish us when we need replenishment. Clinical work is hard work, often emotionally draining.

We must be able to share time of high quality with those we care about, in order to get back valuable support in return. We need to honor the need for selfishness in its purest form: attention to self. When we are confident of our own resources, we will feel more comfortable "giving at the office." Take your positive strokes where you can find them. Learn to take satisfaction from small successes, even when—and perhaps especially when—larger successes seem less frequent.

Acknowledging the natural course of events. Some fights are worth fighting even though we are bound to lose by objective standards. In a clinical setting, we must acknowledge that the inexorability of some disease processes and the inevitability of death will overcome any efforts on our part. The physician who regards such an eventuality as a failure has set standards which no human being can hope to meet. We have to believe that providing palliation and comfort constitute worthy contributions, separate from the predictable conclusion of the disease process. Each of us inevitably will have our failures as a part of our professional life. The coping styles we urge upon patients faced with burdensome stresses are no less relevant for ourselves. We need to acknowledge events as they occur, acknowledge our feelings and their appropriateness, and allow them time to evolve. Time soothes wounds for us as well as for our patients.

Limitations of physician authority. In recognizing that physicians are not omniscient, not gods or even godlike, we must also understand that our patients and our nonphysician co-workers will seldom take our requests as divine instruction. Many of us entered the medical profession thinking that, by virtue of being a physician, we would be "in charge," and relinquishing control has not always been easy. The public is increasingly skeptical of our technology and wary of iatrogenesis. Fortunately, we are much less likely to harm wary patients than those who try to abdicate all responsibility to us. However, in respecting the patient's fundamental right to make decisions concerning matters of personal health, we must still live within the legal constraints that put so much of the responsibility for patient care on the physician's lap. Malpractice law must be altered to reflect the acknowledged virtue of the patients' rights movement and its claim that each patient is ultimately responsible for his or her own body.

Personal and professional evolution. A century ago, saddle sores constituted an occupational hazard for the physician on the American frontier. Today, the physician faces a new hazard: "triplicate-form amblyopia." Different times, different frustrations, different rewards. Your life will be more interesting and complicated than you ever imagined it could be, with plenty of unanticipated and unpredictable turns.

Nonetheless, the crucial importance of sustaining high morale while practicing good clinical medicine remains the same. Clinical skill evolves, and inherent in that evolution is an understanding of the universality of human suffering and an alertness to the often subtle manifestations of human nobility in its various guises. The essence is respect for ourselves, respect for our patients, and respect for the process of treatment itself.

Sense of humor. Finally, few qualities will serve you as well in the practice of medicine—and in life—as your sense of humor. You will be confronted again and again by life's absurdities, and they must be recognized for what they are. Often, laughter, if not the only response, is clearly among the best. Believe in human folly; wisdom often creeps into our foolishness if we have the wit to see it. And sometimes the reverse also is true: we who aspire to be so wise can often seem foolish and amusing to others. The practice of medicine can be, in addition to everything else, a great deal of fun, but, like so much in life, what you get out of it is largely a reflection of what you bring to it.

Bibliography

Bittker TE: The industrialization of american psychiatry. *Am J Psychiatry* 142:149–154, 1985

Bosk CL: Occupational rituals in patient management. *N Engl J Med* 303:71–76, 1980

Burnham JC: American medicine's golden age—what happened to it? *Science,* 215:1474–1479, 1982

Cassell EJ: The nature of suffering and the goals of medicine. *N Engl J Med* 306:639–645, 1982

Charles SC, Wilbert JR, Francke KJ: Sued and non-sued physicians' self-reported reactions to malpractice litigation. *Am J Psychiatry* 142:437–440, 1985

Crippen DW: Emergency medicine redux—the rise and fall of a community medicine specialty. *Ann Emerg Med* 13:539–542, 1984

Ehrenreich J (ed.): *The Cultural Crisis of Modern Medicine.* New York, Monthly Review Press, 1978

Ginzberg E: The monetarization of medical care. *N Engl J Med* 310:1162–1165, 1984

Illich I: *Medical Nemesis—The Expropriation of Health.* New York, Pantheon Books, 1976

Jonsen AR: Watching the doctor. *N Engl J Med* 308:1531–1535, 1983

Knowles J (ed.): *Doing Better and Feeling Worse.* New York, Norton, 1977

Kramer M: *Reality Shock—Why Nurses Leave Nursing.* St. Louis, CV Mosby Co., 1974

Kubie LS: The retreat from patients—an unanticipated penalty of the full-time system. *Arch Gen Psychiatry* 24:98–106, 1971

Lipp MR, Weingarten R: Hazards in the practice of medicine. *Am Fam Physician* 12(4):92–96, 1975

Lipp MR: *The Bitter Pill—Doctors, Patients and Failed Expectations.* New York, Harper & Row, 1980

Machie RE: Family problems in medical and nursing families. *Br J Med Psychol* 40:333–340, 1967

May HJ, Revicki DA: Professional stress among family physicians. *J Fam Pract* 20:165–171, 1985

Needleman J: *The Way of the Physician.* San Francisco, Harper & Row, 1985

Reidbord SP: Psychological perspectives on iatrogenic physician impairment. *Pharos,* Summer 1983, pp 2–8

Relman A: The new medical-industrial complex. *New Engl J Med* 303:963–970, 1980

Starr P: *The Social Transformation of American Medicine.* New York, Basic Books, 1982

Stephens GG: Family practice—The renaissance is over. *J R Coll Gen Pract* 31:460–466, 1981

Terkel S: *Working—People Talk About What They Do All Day and How They Feel About What They Do.* New York, Pantheon Books, 1972

Thomasma DC: Beyond medical paternalism and patient autonomy. *Ann Intern Med* 98:243–248, 1983

Vaillant GE: Physicians' use of mood-altering drugs—A 20-year follow-up report. *N Engl J Med* 282:365–370, 1970

Appendix:
Putting the Patient's
Mind at Rest

The various techniques discussed in this section currently belong to the margins of science, or beyond: prayer, concentrated routinization of behavior, systematic relaxation, meditation, and hypnosis. Some critics would maintain that their use by a medical practitioner constitutes nonprofessional conduct or even quackery. This is why I have placed them in the appendix rather than in the body of the text: I didn't want their inclusion to detract from other ideas in this book.

Someone once defined a quack as "a person who continues through time to please his clients but not his colleagues." This apt observation reminds us that there is much we can do for the patient's benefit which nonetheless varies from orthodox medical teaching. If the risk of adverse consequences remains small, why not give some of the techniques a try?

Each approach *works,* at least with some physicians with some patients in some situations. No one technique has universal application.

True believers in any of these techniques will feel that my coverage is superficial and simplistic; the validity of their criticism is acknowledged. I wish simply to provide a precís account of various useful techniques many physicians don't commonly consider. If what you read here makes sense, you will want to look for more information elsewhere. If, on the other hand, you approach each technique seeking to find shortcomings, you will certainly find them, but you will deprive yourself of some interesting and useful skills at the same time.

I have specifically excluded any techniques that require special equipment (e.g., biofeedback, acupuncture, electrosleep), even though they may be particularly useful for any given patient. The only equipment you need for any approach mentioned here is yourself.

Each technique will be most useful if the patient comes to you with a predisposition in favor of it, and you yourself are optimistic. However, neither factor is absolutely necessary. You should try to conceive of each not simply as a device for enhancing peace of mind separate from the rest of the patient's life, but rather as part of a multilevel therapeutic relationship with you. Helping patients put their minds at rest will promote positive feelings about you and augment your therapeutic potency.

Each approach has many subtle gradations, and variations are as numerous as those who utilize them. You should feel free to experiment as you wish. As you read through each, you will find certain themes that are common to all, both in the implementation of the technique and in the response elicited—Dr. Herbert Benson calls this the "Relaxation Response." To the variable degree that each technique has been measured, changes in physiologic function, when they occur, are in the direction of decreased oxygen consumption, decreased respiratory rate, decreased blood pressure, and decreased muscle tension. Therefore, in circumstances these changes are desirable, any technique that is acceptable to both you and the patient should be worth trying.

Dr. Benson believes that all techniques that elicit the relaxation response contain four basic elements: (1) a quiet environment, or the patient's ability to selectively exclude environmental distractions; (2) an object to dwell upon, usually a word, a phrase, or a visual object; (3) a passive attitude, in which the patient ceases to be concerned about how well the technique is being performed; and (4) a comfortable position. You may wish to keep these in mind as we discuss each in turn.

Prayer

How ironic that prayer should be tucked into the Appendix. Prayer was one of the chief therapeutic tools of the nineteenth-century physician, but more recently prayer has been squeezed out of the therapeutic setting by chemicals, machines, and heroic surgical procedures. In including it here, I don't mean to confine religion to the limited role of an anxiolytic technique; I am simply saying that prayerful contemplation, especially when used regularly, can have a remarkable calming effect in receptive individuals.

The physician need not be religious in order to help religious patients draw strength from their beliefs. I am not religious, and I am not a prayerful person, yet I have often asked patients in great stress, "Have you ever found comfort in prayer?" While many haven't been inside a house of worship for years, some will acknowledge that prayer has been helpful in the past. If so, I will ask, "Do you think prayer might be helpful now?" Sometimes I even ask the patient to pray for all of us who are looking after him or her. If the patient agrees, I sit quietly while the patient says the prayer, whether aloud or silently. When the patient is through, I thank the patient for including me in the prayer (if that seems appropriate). Given a willing patient, this technique has without exception resulted in greater calmness for the patient and a closer therapeutic relationship between the patient and myself.

If the patient is not interested in prayer, I never push the matter. Persons who are nonreligious, or even antireligious, want their preferences respected too.

Concentrated Routinization of Behavior

This technique becomes particularly useful when a patient is incapacitated by anxiety, perhaps sobbing uncontrollably or desperately hyperventilating, and when personal loss of control is at issue. The approach depends upon you, the physician, taking control of the situation, getting the patient passively to perform simple behaviors repetitively, pointing out the patient's obvious ability to perform these behaviors, clarifying that the patient retains more control than may have been expected, and gradually transferring control back to the patient. The end result is often remarkably reassuring, not only to the patient, but to family members who can easily be taught to fill in for you as the occasion requires.

The specific tactics include establishing physical contact, distracting the patient from the source of anxiety by focusing attention on rote behavior, reinforcing the process with a soothing patter, and gradually slowing the rate at which the behavior is performed to both reflect and foster gradual lessening of anxiety.

One example will give you the idea: a woman in her late thirties is sobbing hysterically, grief-stricken by the death of her teenage son in an accident on a motorcycle purchased for him by his parents only the previous month. The patient's hysterics are now beginning to undermine the coping efforts of her husband and other relatives. You have already given her ample opportunity to ventilate, but she remains inconsolable, and you are concerned that she might talk herself into a psychotic decompensation if she can't recapture some sense of self-control. Filling her with sedatives doesn't seem a totally comfortable alternative. The following interaction represents one approach to such a situation. Say to the patient: "Take my hand. I want you to get up. You need to get control of yourself, and I'm going to help you. Take hold of my hand with one hand, and your husband's (or other relative or friend) with the other." If the woman needs more physical support than merely holding onto two hands, have her put one arm over your shoulder and one arm over the other person's, and start walking with her between you. Tell the patient, "Every time you step on your left foot, I want you to say, 'Left.' Call it out with me: 'Left, left, left, left.''' The patient's attention may tend to stray; keep bringing attention back to the act of walking itself. Alternatively, you can have the patient count out each step: "One, two, three, four, one, two, three, four." Almost always, if you can get the patient to keep moving and focus on the rote behavior itself, the anxiety will gradually decrease and the patient's sense of control will increase. Gradually slow down the pace. Say: "I want you to be very aware of your feet and legs. You are moving your own body. We are simply providing you with some support. You have more control of yourself than you realize. Keep counting out each step, and try to gain strength from the act of walking itself." When you feel the process is well along, you can step aside and ask another family member to take your place. That will give them a sense of participation, and help decrease any fear they may have about coping with similar behavior at home.

The same general procedures can be applied to persons confined to bedrest, by asking them to do sit-ups or leg-raises, or by counting breathing.

Systematic Relaxation

Telling a person to relax is one thing; teaching someone how to achieve that goal is quite another. The amazing thing is that many people don't know how to relax. Systematic relaxation (sometimes called "Jacobsonian relaxation," after the man who originated the technique) supplies one method for individuals to try.

The advantages of this method include its relative simplicity, and its freedom from mystic or philosophic implications. The technique usually appeals to those who like nitty-gritty formal instruction and who tend to be organized and physically, as opposed to spiritually, oriented. The role of the physician is simply to introduce the patient to the method; persistent benefit for the patient depends on regular practice over time. The method is valuable for the physician as well as the patient because it tends to be relaxing for both parties. I therefore tend to look forward to teaching a patient systematic relaxation on a day when I'm feeling particularly tense too.

Ideally, you and the patient should be in a quiet, somewhat darkened room. The patient should be supine on a comfortable bed or couch, and, if you wish to gain some relaxation too, you should be seated in a comfortable chair.

Do not tell the patient to try to relax the mind; that will usually follow as a matter of course as he or she learns to relax muscles. Encourage the patient to think of a previous experience of comfort and relaxation, such as a visit to the beach or woods, a vacation, whatever. Tell the patient: "Choose a single moment and try to think of details—

sensations of taste, hearing, seeing, feeling. Vividly picture the event. Allow yourself to savor the moment and let your eyes gradually close by themselves." Then proceed to help the patient perceive tension in muscular groups within his or her own body by drawing contrasts between strong muscular contraction and subsequent relaxation. No gross movements need occur; most muscle contractions ideally will be isometric. For your own benefit, try doing the exercises at the same time, though optimal benefit always occurs when the instruction comes from a source external to the person trying to relax.

Jacobson's original method proceeds slowly, beginning with the right upper extremity (which requires six days of practice), then to the left upper extremity, the right lower extremity, the left lower extremity, trunk, neck, forehead, brow. Each session involves simultaneous performance of previously learned exercises along with those new ones scheduled each day. Jacobson's entire course takes from 10 to 12 weeks of daily practice.

The following set of instructions is too much for one 20- to 30-minute session, but it needn't be stretched out over three months, either. Allow yourself to experiment. Many patients appreciate a great deal of detail (e.g., focusing separately on the index, middle, and other fingers), whereas others find detail distracting.

Tell the patient: "In order to relax, you must know when you are tense. We will gradually go through your body, first tensing, then relaxing each group of muscles. Now, clench your right fist as tight as you can. Hold the fist tight, tighter, tighter, for as long as you can. Feel the tension in your fist and your forearm. Keep your fist as tight as you can as long as you can. Now quickly relax; let your hand go limp. Feel the difference. Savor the relaxation." You can repeat this several times, each time drawing the patient's attention to the tension, and then the relaxation. When the patient appears to be able to fully relax with the hand lying limply at the side, you can begin to progress to other parts of the body, to the forearm, upper arm, other upper extremity, and so on. This technique has its most dramatic impact when patients begin to perceive tension in muscles that are habitual targets of stress. Muscles that commonly carry such a burden include the temporalis, masseter, and trapezius and the rhomboid. When you have practiced with enough muscles for one session, encourage the patient to let go of all tension. Say, "Feel the deep relaxation everywhere you find it in your body. Lie comfortably and enjoy the relaxation. When you are ready, feel free to get up slowly, and arise refreshed." As corny as all this sounds on paper, patients who are willing to give it a try seldom regret the experience.

Once you have introduced patients to systematic relaxation over one or more sessions, and assuming they have found the experience useful, you may have them practice on their own. Since the subject's passivity usually adds to the experience, the exercises are best done when someone else is available to give instructions (e.g., a friend or relative observing the procedure) or by listening to a "relaxation tape." The latter is available from many suppliers. Look for advertisements in behavioral psychology journals; one such source: *Psychology Today Cassettes,* Department A0530, P.O. Box 278, Pratt Station, Brooklyn, New York 11205.

Meditation

Different styles of meditation abound, many of them going back thousands of years. In general, persons who practice meditation regularly regard their activity as a part of a system of beliefs, intimately connected with a personal pursuit of understanding or enlightenment. A patient's receptivity to meditation as a relaxation technique therefore often depends in part on receptivity to mysticism and philosophic perspectives that are not a part of mainstream Western culture. Anyone who seriously investigates meditation will rapidly encounter variations stemming from Zen, Buddhism, yoga, or other forms of Hinduism, and other philosophic traditions.

The variations are endless, but by no means of trivial importance to adherents. The most pervasive approach, taught by followers of the Maharishi Mahesh Yoga, is called Transcendental Meditation (TM). The basic technique is to assume a comfortable position, with eyes closed, think or recite a mantra (usually a Sanskrit word or phrase especially chosen for the meditator by a teacher), and repeat the exercise for 20 minutes twice a day. Other schools of meditation tend to regard TM as simplistic. I don't presume to do justice to either sets of views.

If you have a patient who has practiced meditation in the past, the technique represents a resource for the two of you in the present. The only way you can know if the patient has tried meditation is to ask— once you know that a patient has previously tried meditation and is agreeable to doing so again, encourage its use daily, regardless of your own particular views on the subject. If you wish, record the patient's vital signs both before and after meditation periods, to convince both of you of its usefulness.

Meditation becomes a greater resource if you personally can teach receptive patients how to meditate. Physicians who meditate and have the time and energy to teach others to meditate offer a useful technique to receptive patients.

Hypnotism

Hypnotism has long been endowed with overtones of magic, mysticism, and the supernatural. Although there has been a tendency to associate its use with unorthodox practitioners and unseemly show-manship, the development of the technique largely derived from the efforts of turn-of-the-century general practitioners working with "psychosomatic" patients.

My focus here is on the relaxation functions of hypnosis; I do not dispute that it has a valid role as well in diagnostics and specific therapeutic situations.

The key to induction of hypnosis is understanding that which will happen anyhow and then offering the subject "strong suggestion" to help him or her along an inevitable pathway. The specific techniques of induction are far less important than the subject's willingness to believe that the technique will work and the lack of any obvious discordance between the hypnotist's manner and the subject's expectations.

Always tell the patient that ultimate control lies with the patient; no one can be forced to do anything he or she does not wish to do. Your function is simply to help the patient relax, and that will occur more easily if he or she lies still and silent unless specifically directed otherwise.

Usually the hypnotist starts by fixing the subject's attention, often with something bright, often requiring the subject to look upward at the object. Upward gaze is difficult for most persons to sustain, and the hypnotist rarely loses in predicting that "your eyes are getting very, very tired." Let the subject know what is expected (e.g., feelings of lassitude), and set up circumstances so that the result becomes nearly inevitable. Speak in a soothing manner, using language that is comfortable for the patient. Tell the subject that he or she will experience refreshing relaxation and will awaken on command feeling much better. If the subject actually falls asleep, you can awaken him or not as circumstances dictate. Some hypnotists feel the subject should always be explicitly awakened, even when you don't believe you have succeeded in hypnotizing the patient at all. There are numerous methods for deepening a hypnotic spell or trance—e.g., "Now, allow your relaxation to deepen. Feel the relaxation getting deeper and deeper. Imagine yourself going down on an escalator, down, down, down."

Variations are endless, with usefulness depending on the specific patient and your comfort with the process. Depending upon your interest, basic hypnotic skills are all potentially within the competence of the general physician.

Bibliography

Benson H: *The Relaxation Response.* New York, Wm. Morrow, 1975

Chaves JF, Barber TX: Hypnotic procedures and surgery—A critical analysis with applications to acupuncture analgesia. *Am J Clin Hypn* 18:217–236, 1976

Erickson MH: The interspersal hypnotic technique for symptom correction and pain control. *Am J Clin Hypn* 3:198–209, 1966

Frank JD: The medical power of faith. *Human Nature,* August 1978, pp 40–47

Goldberg RG: Anxiety reduction by self-regulation—theory, practice, and evaluation. *Ann Int Med* 96:483–487, 1982

Herbert CP: Teaching hypnosis within a family practice residency program. *Family Medicine* 17:77–78, 1985

Hiebert B, et al.: Self-instructed relaxation—a therapeutic alternative. *Biofeedback Self Regul* 8:601–617, 1983

Jacobson E: *You Must Relax,* 4th ed. New York, McGraw-Hill, 1962

Le Cron LM, Bordeaux J: *Hypnotism Today.* North Hollywood, CA, Wilshire Book Company, 1976

McIntosh IB, Hawney M: Patients' attitudes to medical hypnotherapy. *Practitioner* 228:345–348, 1984

Martin IC: Relaxation on record. *Lancet* 2:1340, 1969

Shorokey JJ, Price WA, Chiasson SW: Hypnosis in medicine—a brief overview. *Ohio State Med J* (December) 1983, pp 935–947

Smith A: *Powers of Mind.* New York, Ballantine Books, 1975

Spiegel D: Hypnosis with medical-surgical patients. *Gen Hosp Psychiatry* 5:265–277, 1983

Stone P: Relaxation techniques in general practice. *Aust Fam Physician* 12:729–730, 1983

Warwick HMC, Salkovskis PM: Reassurance. *Brit Med J* 290:1028, 1985

Index

Resources
  assessment of, in psychiatric emer-
    gency, 55
  community, 263–264
  cultivating of, 308–309
  health care, 298
  related to emergency, 51–52
  for suicidal patient, 65
Respiratory care unit (RCU), 41
  human problems in, 44t
Respiratory cripples, psychotherapeutic
    medication for, 283–284
Responses, overinterpreting of, 58
Reward system, 302
Rigidity, 4
  paratonic, 107–108

S

Satisfactions, finding of, 33
Scale, economics of, 30
Scare techniques, related to invalidism,
    217
Schizophrenia, relationship to psychosis,
    59
Schizophrenic, chronic, 24
  managing medical problems, 25–26
  problems in caring for, 24–25
  reasons for seeking care, 25
Secobarbital, 203, 204
Seductive behavior, dealing with, 20–24
Seizure patient, psychotherapeutic medi-
    cations for, 286
Self
  dangerousness to, commitment for,
    86–87
  use of, in crisis situation, 53
Self-acceptance, 307
"Self-actualization," 170
Self-determination, patient's right to, 71–
    72, 172
  competence and incompetence issues,
    77–80
  discharge against medical advice, 81–
    83
  informed consent, 74–77
  legal criteria, 73
  limiting of, 72–73
  refusal of treatment, 80–81
  related to commitment, 84–89
Self-help groups, for psychological prob-
    lems, 186
Self-image, 28
  physician, 298
Self-respect, 296, 307–308
Sense of humor, 310
Sensitivity, 32
Sensorium, evaluation, for confusional
    state assessment, 105–106

Sensory deprivation, confusional state
    and, 100, 111–112
Services, utilizing of, 29
Sexual activity
  for cardiac patient, 143
  of renal dialysis patient, 45–46
Sexual function, psychotherapeutic
    medication affecting, 281
Similar consequences, theory of, 231,
    233
SLANT technique, for anxiety and
    depression, 165
Sleep deprivation, confusional state and,
    100
Social contacts, through work, 294
Social values, changing, 295–298
Speech, evaluation, for confusional state
    assessment, 105
Special care units, 41–42
  doctor's role, 42–43
  human problems, 43–44
  nurse's role, 43
  types, 41
"Spiritual integration," 170
Spouse, response to disfigurement, 125
Staff
  constancy, for confused patient, 111
  -family relationships, 256
  -patient relationships
    in dialysis unit, 47
    surgery and, 39
STELAZINE. See Trifluoperazine
"Street addict," 201–202
Stress
  confusion and, 91–92, 97–98
  coping with, 175–178
    See also Coping
  in crisis situation, 51
  in doctor-patient relationship, 1–2
  heart attack and, 139
  physical disease resulting from, 206,
    233–234
  in suicidal patient, 65
  surgery and, 38
Suck-and-snout reflexes. See Oral root-
    ing reflexes
Sudden death, 126
Suffering
  physician's, 300
  usefulness of, 173
Suicidal patient, 62–63
  assessment, 63–64
  characteristics, 63
  commitment, 86
  handling of, 65–66
  protection of, 64–65
  response to, 64
  stresses, 65